Reggie Zhan, M.D.
Kaiser Permanente
Dept. of Pathology
6111 Executive Blvd.
Rockville, MD 20852

12/10/2010

Rockville, MD

Atlas of Bullous Disease

Atlas of Bullous Disease

Robert E. Jordon, MD

Jack S. Josey Professor and Chairman
Department of Dermatology
University of Texas Medical School
Houston, Texas

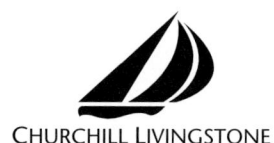

CHURCHILL LIVINGSTONE

A Division of Harcourt Brace & Company
New York, Edinburgh, London, Philadelphia, San Francisco

CHURCHILL LIVINGSTONE
A Division of Harcourt Brace & Company

The Curtis Center
Independence Square West
Philadelphia, Pennsylvania 19106

Editor: Liz Fathman
Project Manager: Carol Sullivan Weis
Designer: Mark A. Oberkrom

NOTICE

Medicine is an ever-changing field. Standard safety precautions must be followed, but as new research and clinical experience broaden our knowledge, changes in treatment and drug therapy may become necessary or appropriate. Readers are advised to check the most current product information provided by the manufacturer of each drug to be administered to verify the recommended dose, the method and duration of administration, and contraindications. It is the responsibility of the treating physician, relying on experience and knowledge of the patient, to determine dosages and the best treatment for each individual patient. Neither the publisher nor the editor assumes any liability for any injury and/or damage to persons or property arising from this publication.

ATLAS OF BULLOUS DISEASE   ISBN 0-443-05863-6

Copyright © 2000 by Churchill Livingstone

All rights reserved. No part of this publication may be reproduced or transmitted in any form or by any means, electronic or mechanical, including photocopy, recording, or any information storage and retrieval system, without permission in writing from the publisher.

Churchill Livingstone® is a registered trademark of Harcourt Brace & Company.
™🜋 is a trademark of Harcourt Brace & Company.

Printed in the United States of America.

Last digit is the print number: 9   8   7   6   5   4   3   2   1

Contributors

Javier Alonso-Llamazares, MD
Dermatologist
Department of Dermatology
Hospital Severo Ochoa
Leganés, Spain

Grant J. Anhalt, MD
Professor
Departments of Dermatology and Pathology
Johns Hopkins Medical Institutions
Baltimore, Maryland

Bita Bagheri, MD
Resident
Department of Dermatology
Columbia-Presbyterian Medical Center
New York, New York

Samuel F. Bean, MD
Clinical Professor
Department of Dermatology
University of Texas Medical School
Houston, Texas

Martin M. Black, MD, FRCP, FRCPath
Chairman
Department of Dermatopathology,
Guy's Kings and St. Thomas School of Medicine;
Consultant Dermatologist
St. John's Institute of Dermatology
St. Thomas Hospital
London, England

Philip R. Cohen, MD
Private Practice
The Woodlands, Texas;
Associate Professor
Department of Dermatology
University of Texas Medical School
Houston, Texas

Kevin D. Cooper, MD
Professor and Chair
Department of Dermatology
Case Western Reserve University;
Director
Department of Dermatology
University Hospitals of Cleveland
Cleveland, Ohio

Luis A. Diaz, MD
Professor and Chairman
Department of Dermatology
University of North Carolina at Chapel Hill
Chapel Hill, North Carolina

Conleth A. Egan, MB, MRCPI
Dermatology Resident
Department of Dermatology
University of Utah School of Medicine
Salt Lake City, Utah

Manish J. Gharia, MD
Department of Dermatology
Medical College of Wisconsin;
Attending Physician
Froedtert Memorial Lutheran Hospital
Milwaukee, Wisconsin

Russell P. Hall III, MD
Professor and Chief
Division of Dermatology
Department of Medicine
Duke University Medical Center
Durham, North Carolina

Rachel E. Jenkins, BSc, MD, MRCP
Dermatology Senior Registrar
St. John's Institute of Dermatology
St. Thomas Hospital
London, England

Robert E. Jordon, MD
Jack S. Josey Professor and Chairman
Department of Dermatology
University of Texas Medical School
Houston, Texas

Neil J. Korman, MD, PhD
Associate Professor
Department of Dermatology
Case Western Reserve University;
Attending Physician
Department of Dermatology
University Hospitals of Cleveland
Cleveland, Ohio

Kristin M. Leiferman, MD
Professor of Dermatology
Mayo Medical School;
Consultant in Dermatology
Director
Immunodermatology Laboratory
Department of Dermatology
Mayo Clinic and Mayo Foundation
Rochester, Minnesota

Mong-Shang Lin, PhD
Assistant Professor
Department of Dermatology
University of North Carolina at Chapel Hill
Chapel Hill, North Carolina

Zhi Liu, PhD
Associate Professor
Department of Dermatology
Medical College of Wisconsin
Milwaukee, Wisconsin

Jose M. Mascaro Jr, MD
Research Fellow
Department of Dermatology
Medical College of Wisconsin
Milwaukee, Wisconsin

Pamela G. Nemzer, MD
Department of Dermatology
University of Utah School of Medicine
Salt Lake City, Utah

Hossein C. Nousari, MD
Senior Clinical Fellow
Department of Dermatology
Johns Hopkins Medical Institutions
Baltimore, Maryland

Edel A. O'Toole, MB, MRCP(1)
Specialist Registrar in Dermatology
Department of Dermatology
Royal London Hospital
London, England

Margot S. Peters, MD
Private Practice
Rochester, Minnesota

Thomas T. Provost, MD
Professor
Department of Dermatology
Johns Hopkins Medical Institutions;
Attending Physician
Department of Dermatology
Johns Hopkins Hospital
Baltimore, Maryland

David T. Woodley, MD
Professor and Co-Chief
Division of Dermatology
The Keck School of Medicine at the
    University of Southern California;
Department of Dermatology
USC University Hospital
Los Angeles, California

John J. Zone, MD
Professor and Chairman
Department of Dermatology
University of Utah School of Medicine;
Chief
Dermatology Section
Veterans Administration Medical Center
Salt Lake City, Utah

This book is dedicated to my family

*Mary Ann, Jim, Kathy, Marie, and Nita
And Jim and Kathy's spouses,
Kirsten and Mike*

*They have supported my pursuits in
academic dermatology and our various moves
and have been there when needed most.*

Preface

During my medical school years, I had the privilege of working in one of the major centers of the world studying autoimmunity. Working in the Immunology Department of the State University of Buffalo School of Medicine, chaired by the late Ernest Witebsky, MD, I was introduced to a new methodology, immunofluorescence, by Ernst H. Beutner, PhD. Immunofluorescence would very significantly impact our specialty of dermatology and the development of immunodermatology.

Immunodermatology had its beginning in the 1930s with the early studies of Sulzberger and co-workers, which showed that sensitized lymphocytes were associated with the clinical expression of contact dermatitis. However, additional interest in immunodermatology did not occur until the late 1950s and early 1960s with the introduction of immunofluorescence.

In late 1964, Ernst Beutner and I reported our initial immunofluorescence findings in patients with pemphigus vulgaris.[1] We reported that patients with pemphigus vulgaris possess circulating autoantibodies directed against intercellular epidermal antigens. This study was followed shortly by a study of pemphigus skin lesions and similar findings in pemphigus foliaceus.[2] In 1967 we reported our findings of tissue fixed and circulating autoantibodies in bullous pemphigoid.[3] This report was followed in 1969 by van der Meer's report[4] of specific IgA deposits in the skin of patients with dermatitis herpetiformis. These early immunofluorescence studies set off an explosive investigative effort over the next three decades that shed light on the diagnosis, classification, pathogenesis, and treatment of the autoimmune bullous skin diseases of humans. This massive research effort by many different investigators has proved to be one of the most exciting and successful investigative efforts in dermatology. I am proud to have been there at the beginning.

The *Atlas of Bullous Disease* provides the reader with a concise, up-to-date review of the bullous skin diseases. Each chapter is organized to include etiology, clinical features, pathology (including immunopathology), how the diagnosis is made, differential diagnoses, and therapy. Major immunologic findings, including immunofluorescent findings, antibody specificity, responsible antigens, and immunogenetics, are featured. Ample illustrations, tables, and diagrams aid the reader in understanding the pathologic events in each of these diseases. Thus the *Atlas of Bullous Disease* is well suited for medical students, residents preparing for board examinations, and practitioners who desire an update, including specific therapies for each of the diseases. A chapter on nonimmunologic acantholytic diseases completes this atlas.

All contributors have considerable expertise in bullous diseases and have provided concise authoritative summaries of each specific disease entity. I am indebted to them for the excellent contributions and to all investigators who have contributed to this field of knowledge.

Robert E. Jordon

References

1. Beutner EH, Jordon RE: Demonstration of skin antibodies in sera of pemphigus vulgaris patients by indirect immunofluorescence staining, *Pro Soc Exp Biol Med* 117:505-510, 1964.
2. Beutner EH, Lever WF, Witebsky E, Jordon RE, Chertock B: Autoantibodies in pemphigus vulgaris: response to an intercellular substance of epidermis, *JAMA* 192:682-688, 1965.
3. Jordon RE, Beutner EH, Witebsky E, et al: Basement zone antibodies in bullous pemphigoid, *JAMA* 200:751-756, 1967.
4. van der Meer JB: Granular deposits of immunoglobulins in the skin of patients with dermatitis herpetiformis, and immunofluorescent study, *Br J Dermatol* 81:493-503, 1969.

Contents

1 **PEMPHIGUS VULGARIS, 1**
   Robert E. Jordon
   Samuel F. Bean

2 **PEMPHIGUS FOLIACEUS, 17**
   Jose M. Mascaro Jr.
   Manish J. Gharia
   Mong-Shang Lin
   Zhi Liu
   Luis A. Diaz

3 **PARANEOPLASTIC PEMPHIGUS, 29**
   Hossein C. Nousari
   Grant J. Anhalt

4 **BULLOUS PEMPHIGOID, 43**
   Javier Alonso-Llamazares
   Margot S. Peters
   Kristin M. Leiferman

5 **CICATRICIAL PEMPHIGOID, 63**
   Neil J. Korman
   Kevin D. Cooper

6 **PEMPHIGOID (HERPES) GESTATIONIS, 75**
   Rachel E. Jenkins
   Martin M. Black

7 **DERMATITIS HERPETIFORMIS, 99**
   Bita Bagheri
   Russell P. Hall III

8 **LINEAR IGA BULLOUS DERMATOSIS, 109**
   Pamela G. Nemzer
   Conleth A. Egan
   John J. Zone

9 **EPIDERMOLYSIS BULLOSA ACQUISITA, 125**
   Edel A. O'Toole
   David T. Woodley

10 **BULLOUS LUPUS ERYTHEMATOSUS, 139**
   Thomas T. Provost

11 **NONIMMUNOLOGIC ACANTHOLYTIC DISEASES, 147**
   Philip R. Cohen

Atlas of Bullous Disease

Pemphigus Vulgaris

Robert E. Jordon
Samuel F. Bean

Pemphigus vulgaris and its variant, pemphigus vegetans, are members of an autoimmune group of blistering skin diseases referred to as the *pemphigus group*. Other members of this disease group are covered in Chapters 2 and 3. Although rare, pemphigus vulgaris may occur in children. Drug-induced pemphigus vulgaris, although less common than drug-induced pemphigus foliaceus, has also been well documented.

Etiology

Like other members of the pemphigus group, pemphigus vulgaris and pemphigus vegetans are autoimmune diseases that affect skin and mucosal surfaces. Patients with both types of pemphigus have autoantibodies that react with desmosome adhesion molecules located on the surfaces of mucosal cells and keratinocytes. These autoantibodies are readily detectable using indirect immunofluorescence (IF) (Figure 1-1, *A*); the pattern of staining on stratified squamous epithelium appears to be intercellular.[3,4,5] More recent studies using epidermal cells grown in tissue culture (Figure 1-1, *B*) have shown that the autoantibodies react with cell surface antigens.[6,11] These autoantibodies are of the immunoglobulin G (IgG) type and may be found in all four IgG subclasses. IgG1 and IgG4 subtypes, however, predominate (Box 1-1). Titers of these autoantibodies often reflect disease activity: high with widespread disease and low when disease activity is minimal. Ample evidence now exists to implicate these autoantibodies as the cause of acantholysis (loss of cohesion of epidermal cells), which is the major histopathologic process in pemphigus.[1,2]

Using direct IF staining, intercellular deposits of both IgG (Figure 1-2, *A*) and complement (Figure 1-2, *B*) are present in early pemphigus vulgaris acantholytic lesions. Direct IF is positive in virtually all cases of pemphigus, if properly performed and if care is taken in selecting an appropriate lesion. Identical findings (Figure 1-3) are present in oral lesions. Intensity of staining is greatest in areas where acantholysis is evident. Thus these autoantibodies are capable of leaving the circulation and reacting with cell surface antigens in vivo.

Pemphigus Antigens

Considerable investigative effort has been focused on the antigens reactive with autoantibodies in all forms of pemphigus. These investigations center primarily on proteins comprising the desmosome complex. Using immunoblotting and immunoprecipitation methodology, a 130-kD desmosome glycoprotein has been identified as the major cell surface antigen in pemphigus vulgaris. An 85-kD protein, identified as plakoglobin, has also been identified by immunoprecipitation and blotting, which is a feature pemphigus vulgaris shares with pemphigus foliaceus. Plakoglobin, a plaque desmosomal protein, forms a complex with the core 130-kD glycoprotein and calcium. Stanley and coworkers[13,15] recently identified this 130-kD protein as desmoglein III, again a major core protein (extracellular) component of desmosomes and adhering junctions (Box 1-1).

Experimental Acantholysis

The major pathologic event in pemphigus vulgaris is the process of acantholysis, resulting in loss of cohesion of individual epidermal cells. Using explants of normal skin and IgG fractions of pemphigus vulgaris patients, Schiltz and coworkers[7] first demonstrated both binding of antibodies and acantholytic changes similar to pemphigus in explanted skin. These changes would occur within 48 to 72 hours. Similar studies have been performed using cultured keratinocytes (both mouse and human) and pemphigus antibodies that have resulted in the loss of cohesion of individual cultured cells. Further studies[9] suggested that this process was mediated by activation of plasmin following release of plasminogen activator from cultured keratinocytes treated with pemphigus antibody. Thus activation of the plasmin system may be one of the factors contributing to the loss of cohesion of epidermal cells, or acantholysis.

Acantholysis has also been induced by passive transfer studies in an experimental animal model (Box 1-1). Using neonatal mice, Anhalt et al[8] showed that daily intraperitoneal injections of pemphigus IgG induced blisters in these animals. The lesions were histopathologically identical to pemphigus, and by direct IF, IgG was

PEMPHIGUS VULGARIS SUMMARY

ETIOLOGY
Pemphigus vulgaris (and vegetans) is an autoimmune bullous skin disease. Autoantibodies are present in sera that react with cell surface antigens, resulting in loss of cohesion of epidermal cells. These antibodies react with a 130-kD desmosomal protein identifed as desmoglein III.

CLINICAL FEATURES
Flaccid blisters rupture, leaving denuded weeping areas of skin. Oral lesions are common and are often the presenting symptom. Common areas for skin lesions include the scalp, chest, upper back, and intertriginous areas.

PATHOLOGY
Suprabasal intraepidermal bulla formation with loss of cohesion of epidermal cells (acantholysis), and an inflammatory infiltrate composed mainly of eosinophils.

DIAGNOSIS
Based on the clinical presentation and characteristic histopathologic and immunopathologic findings.

DIFFERENTIAL DIAGNOSIS
Bullous pemphigoid, epidermolysis bullosa acquisita, erythema multiforme, dermatitis herpetiformis, and linear IgA bullous disease are considered.

TREATMENT
Mainstay of treatment remains high-dose systemic corticosteroids. Immunosuppressive agents may be utilized for steroid sparing and long-term maintenance. Plasmapheresis is useful in selective cases with high antibody titers and extensive disease.

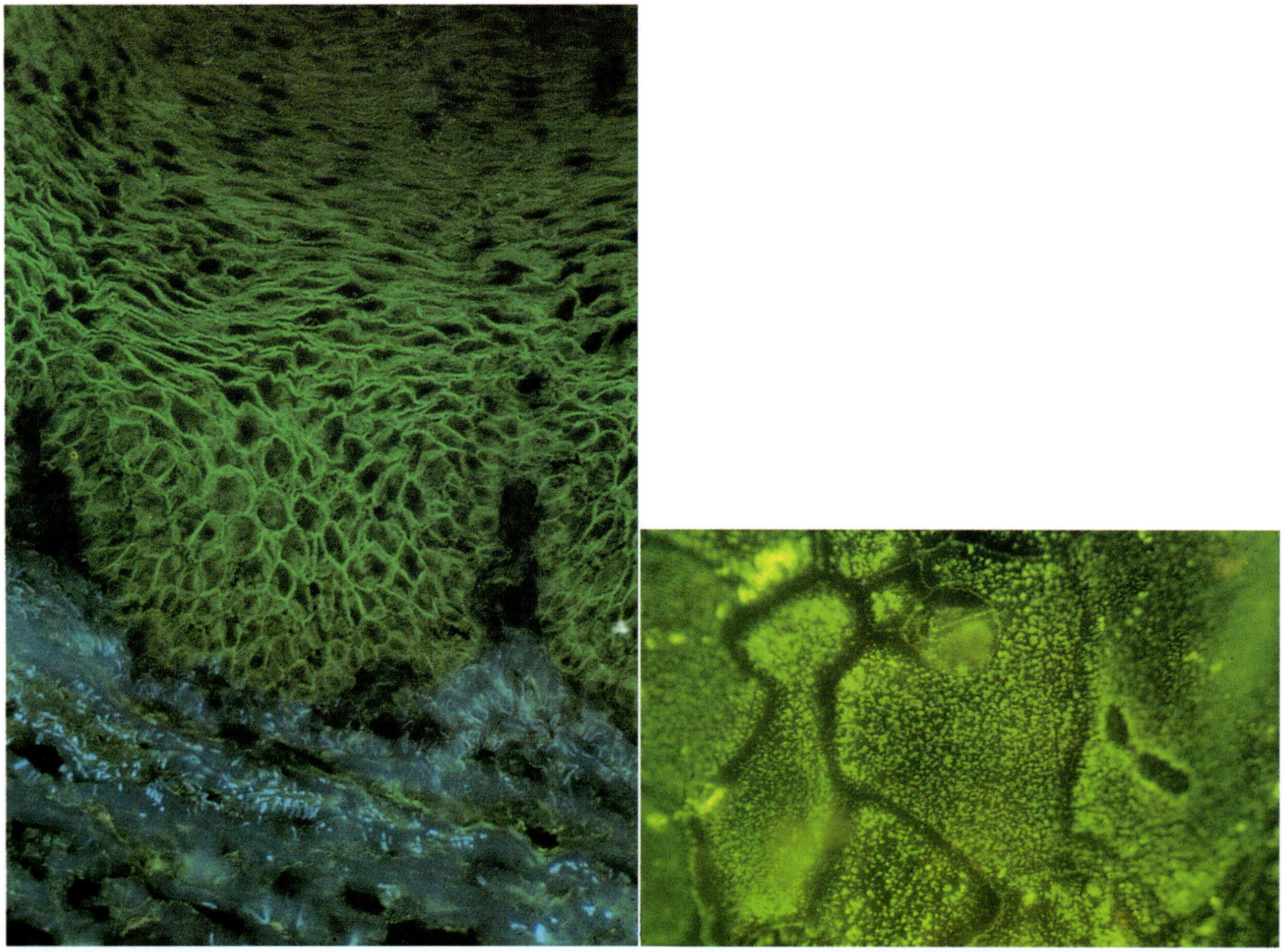

FIGURE 1-1. Indirect IF staining. **A,** Indirect IF staining of monkey esophageal epithelium with pemphigus vulgaris serum and fluorescein isothiocyanate (FITC)-labeled antisera to IgG. Intercellular/cell surface staining is evident. (×250.) **B,** Indirect IF staining of mouse keratinocytes grown in culture, treated with an IgG fraction of pemphigus vulgaris serum and FITC-labeled antiserum to IgG. Granular staining of the cell surfaces is apparent.

BOX 1-1. IMMUNOPATHOLOGIC FINDINGS

HLA ASSOCIATIONS
A10, DR4, Dw10, Dw6

AUTOANTIBODIES
IgG type, react with keratinocyte cell surface antigens. IgG1 and IgG4 subclasses. Antibodies fix complement.

IMMUNOHISTOLOGY
IgG and complement components are found in intercellular/cell surface pattern. Intensity of deposits greatest in areas of acantholysis.

PASSIVE TRANSFER
Acantholysis has been documented in neonatal mice by passively transferring pemphigus IgG fractions and pemphigus IgG affinity purified using recombinant desmoglein 3.

EXPERIMENTAL ACANTHOLYSIS
Using organ culture, acantholysis is induced with pemphigus IgG fractions. Using tissue culture, pemphigus IgG fractions cause epidermal cell detachment. Plasmin and complement activation may amplify this process.

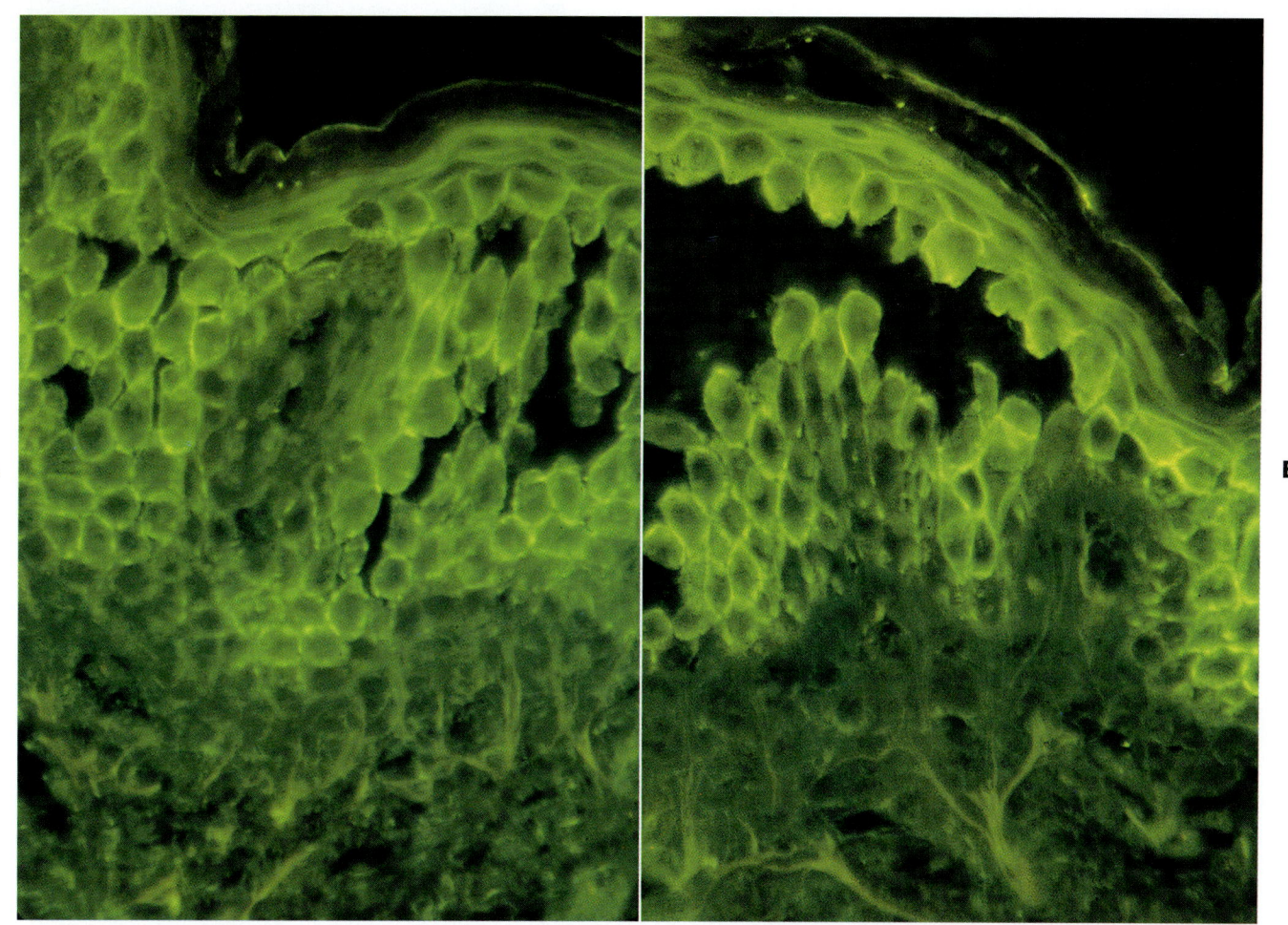

FIGURE 1-2. Direct IF staining of early pemphigus vulgaris skin lesions. **A,** Early acantholytic lesion stained with FTC-labeled antiserum to IgG. Intercellular/cell surface staining is evident. (×500.) **B,** Similar lesion stained with FITC-labeled antiserum to C3. Intracellular/cell surface staining is again evident. (×500.)

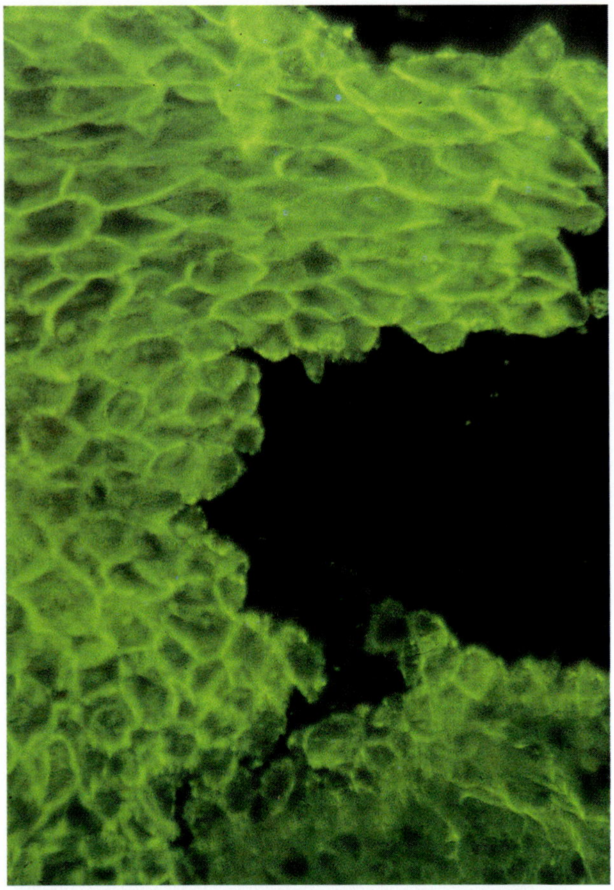

FIGURE 1-3. Direct IF staining of an oral mucosal acantholytic lesion using FITC-labeled antiserum to C3. Intercellular/cell surface staining is evident. (×500.)

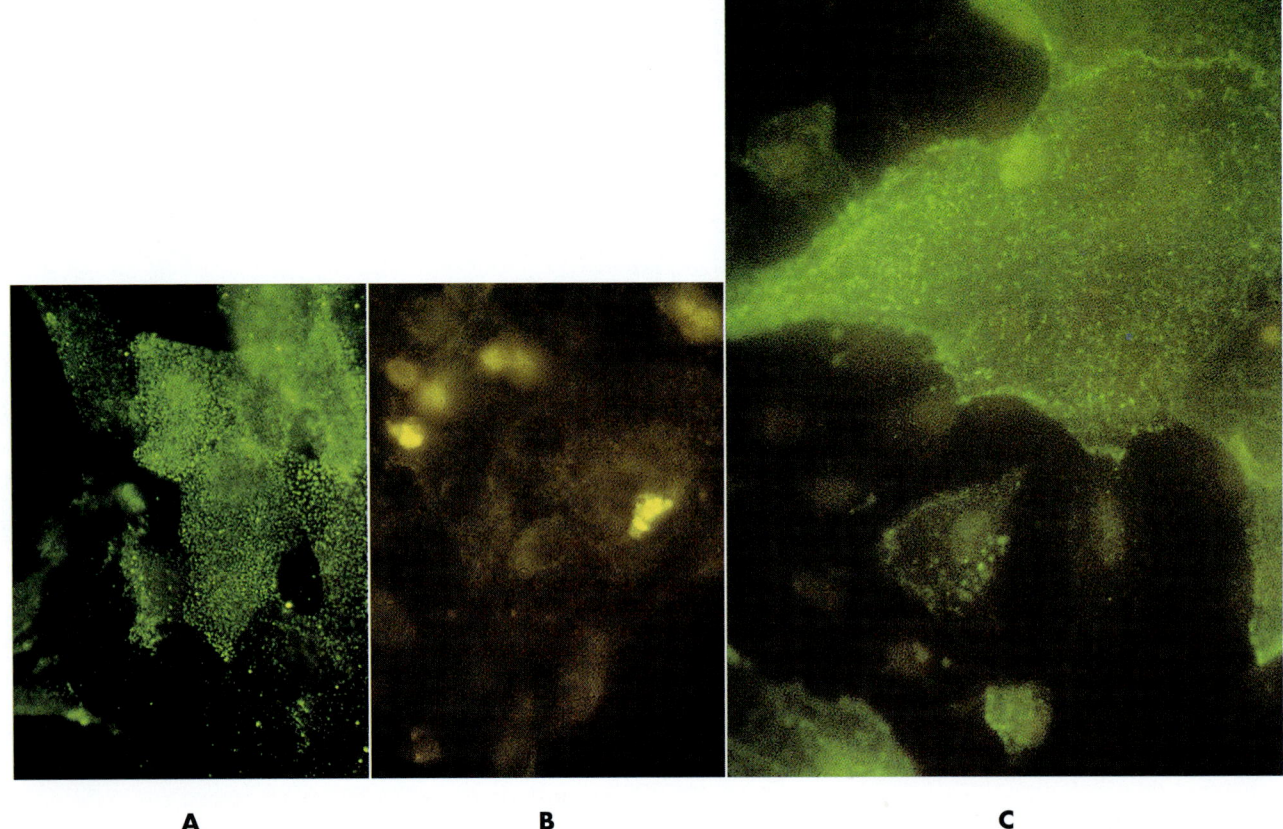

FIGURE 1-4. Complement IF staining of human keratinocytes grown in tissue culture. Cells were treated with an IgG fraction of pemphigus vulgaris serum, a complement source, FITC-labeled anti-C3 (**A** and **B**), and anti-C5b-9 (**C**). **A,** Fixation of C3 to cell surfaces (granular pattern is present). (×500.) **B,** Heat inactivation of the complement source has inhibited C3 staining. (×500.) **C,** Fixation of the membrane attack complex (C5b-9) of complement to cell surfaces. (×500.)

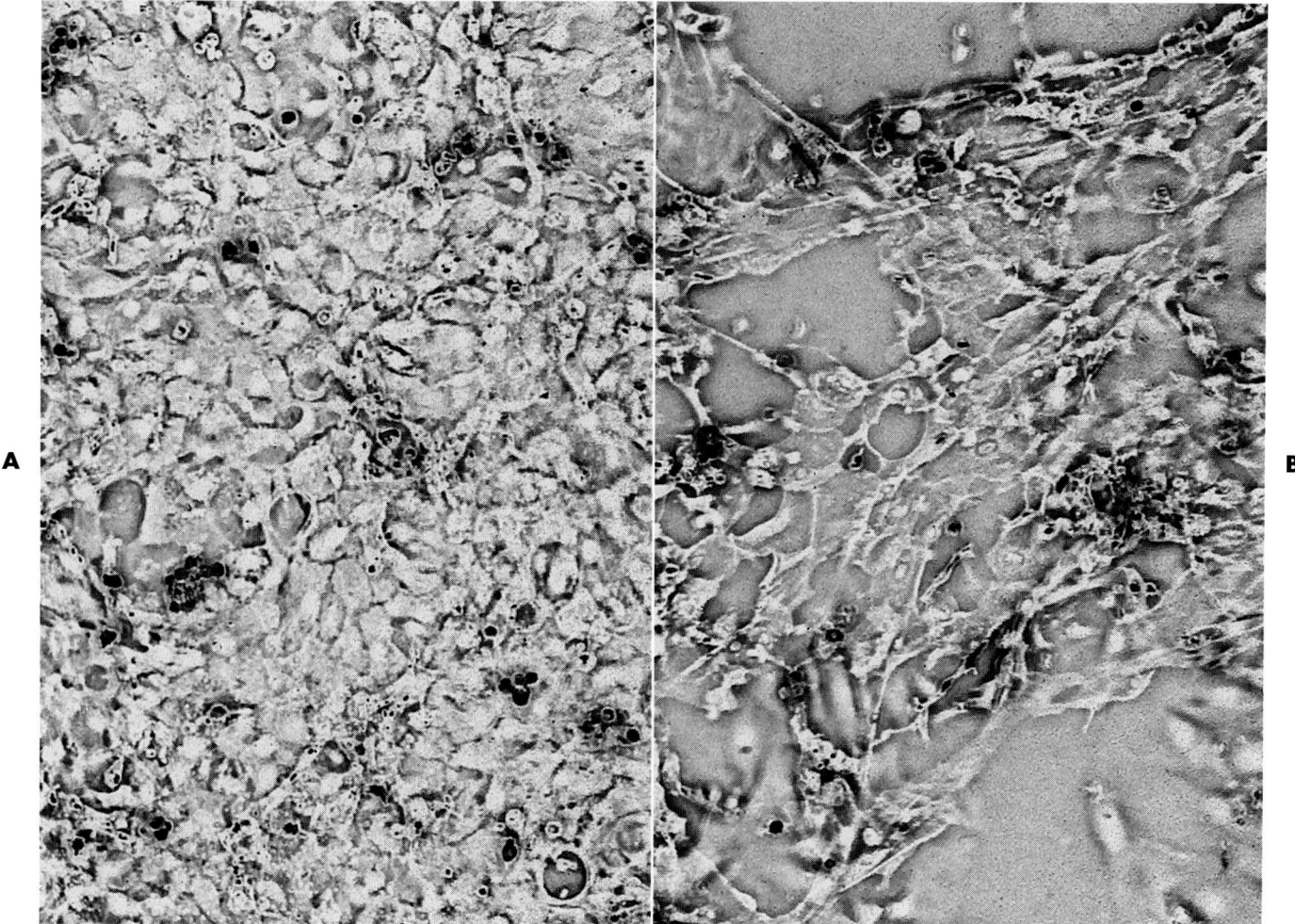

FIGURE 1-5. Human epidermal cell detachment by phase microscopy after 48 hours incubation. **A,** Human keratinocyte monolayer confluency remains intact in the presence of pemphigus vulgaris IgG (1 mg/ml). **B,** Marked detachment occurs when a complement source (AB NHS) is added to pemphigus IgG (1 mg/ml).

bound to the surface of epidermal cells in a pattern identical to pemphigus lesions. Autoantibodies from pemphigus vulgaris patients, affinity purified using recombinant desmoglein 3, have also proved pathogenetic in the mouse model.[15] These findings added further significant proof that anti-desmoglein 3 autoantibodies are the cause of acantholysis in pemphigus vulgaris.

Complement Activation

The complement system may also contribute to the process of acantholysis, although the antibodies alone, in relatively high concentration, are capable of initiating the mechanism. Complement appears to enhance the effects of antibodies on cell detachment and perhaps cell death.

In addition to IgG deposits, a variety of complement components, including classic and alternative pathway components, are present in pemphigus lesions as demonstrated by direct IF staining.[14] These include the terminal components known as the *membrane attack complex*. Pemphigus antibodies have been shown to fix complement in vitro[11] using normal skin and cultured keratinocytes by indirect IF methodology (Figure 1-4, *A* and *B*). Such activation has again been shown to result in assembly of the membrane attack complex or terminal sequence (Figure 1-4, *C*). In other studies, complement has been noted to enhance the effects of pemphigus IgG–mediated cell detachment in tissue culture[12] (Figure 1-5, *A* and *B*). Although pemphigus antibodies are capable of inducing acantholysis in vitro, complement activation appears to enhance this process. Whether complement activation in vivo plays a role in acantholysis and blister formation in pemphigus vulgaris patients remains to be determined.

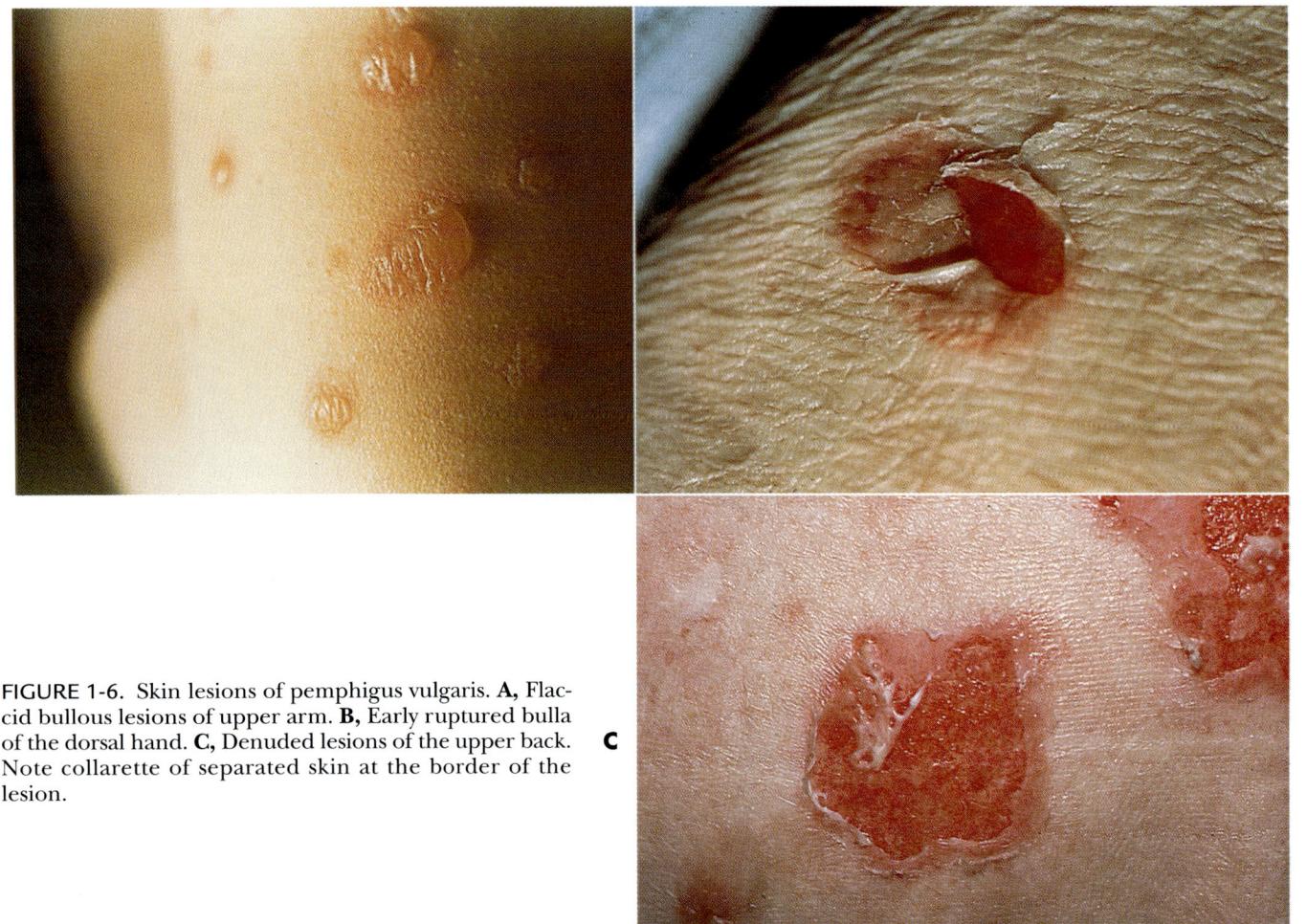

FIGURE 1-6. Skin lesions of pemphigus vulgaris. **A,** Flaccid bullous lesions of upper arm. **B,** Early ruptured bulla of the dorsal hand. **C,** Denuded lesions of the upper back. Note collarette of separated skin at the border of the lesion.

Clinical Features

The characteristic skin lesion of pemphigus vulgaris is a flaccid bulla (Figure 1-6, *A* and Box 1-2).[2] Because of the intraepidermal location, such lesions rupture easily, leaving weeping eroded areas that may extend peripherally (Figure 1-6, *B*). Crusted lesions may be the only clinical evidence of pemphigus. Bullae may arise on normal or erythematous skin. Nikolsky's sign, a dislodging of skin with lateral pressure, is frequently present, especially in widespread active cases. A collarette of tissue (separated skin or scale) is usually present at the borders of the denuded surfaces (Figure 1-6, *C*), a finding that suggests the presence of an acantholytic disease process. Common areas of skin involvement include the scalp, chest, upper back, intertriginous areas, and the umbilicus (Figures 1-7 and 1-8).

BOX 1-2. CLINICAL FEATURES OF PEMPHIGUS VULGARIS

Most common form of pemphigus.
Common in peoples of Jewish or Mediterranean origin.
Skin: Flaccid, bullous lesions; large denuded surfaces.
Common areas of involvement include scalp, chest, upper back, umbilicus, and intertriginous areas.
Mucous membranes: Bullous lesions and erosions of the oral mucosa and gingiva may often precede cutaneous lesions by weeks or months. Lesions may also occur on the vermilion border of lips and conjunctivae and nasal, vaginal, and anal mucosa. Lesions have been described involving the larynx, pharynx, and esophagus.
Lesions are described as tender or painful.
Scarring and pruritus are not prominent features.

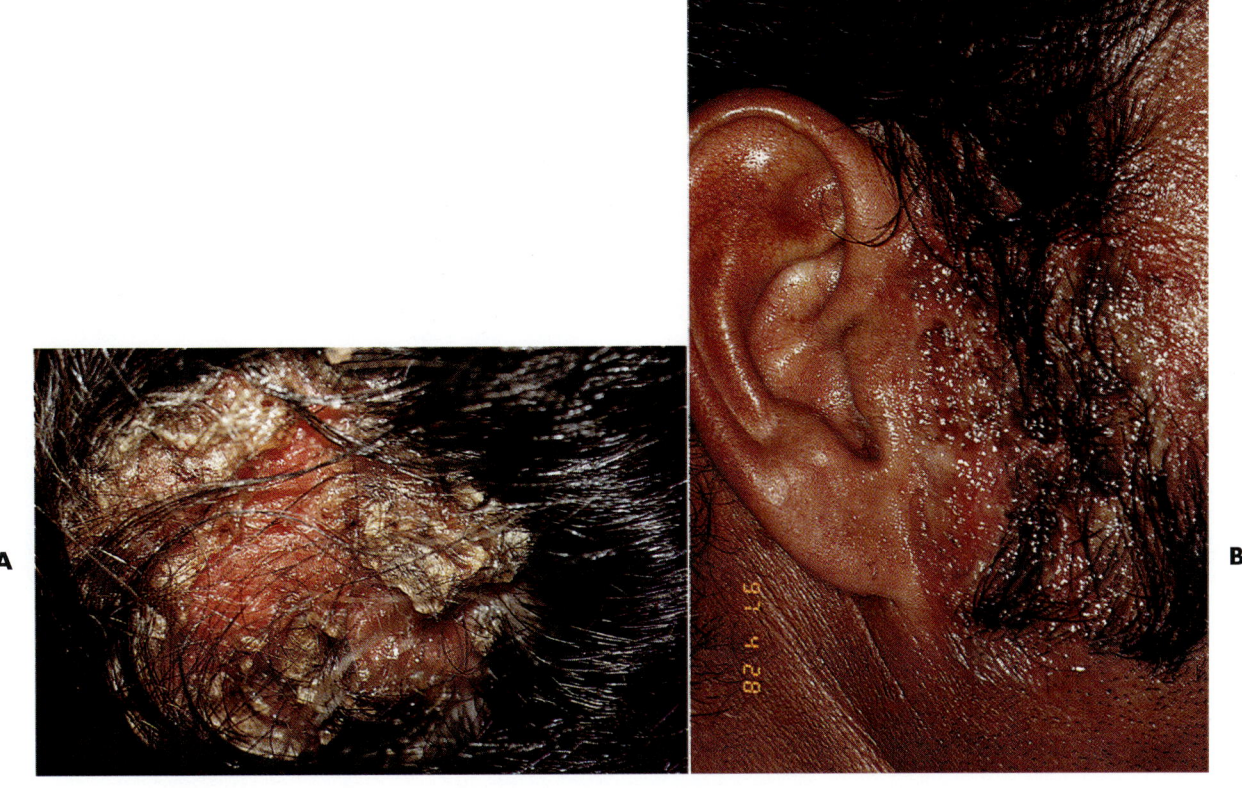

FIGURE 1-7. Hypertrophic crusted lesions of pemphigus vulgaris. **A,** Scalp. **B,** Preauricular "sideburn" area. These lesions are very slow to heal and are often secondarily infected.

FIGURE 1-8. **A,** Weeping bullous lesions of the axillae. **B,** Large denuded lesion of the back. Such lesions are common in patients with extensive pemphigus vulgaris.

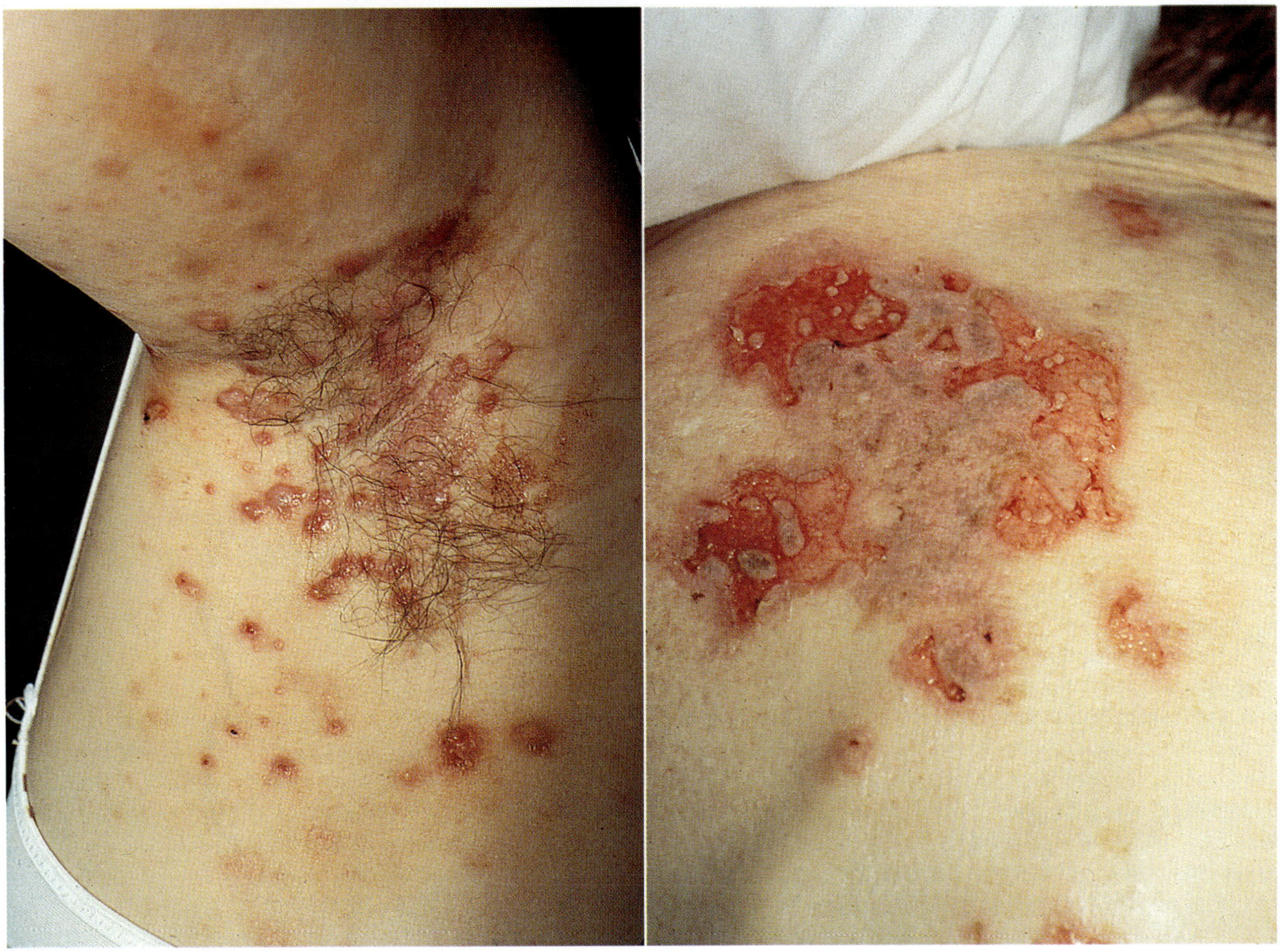

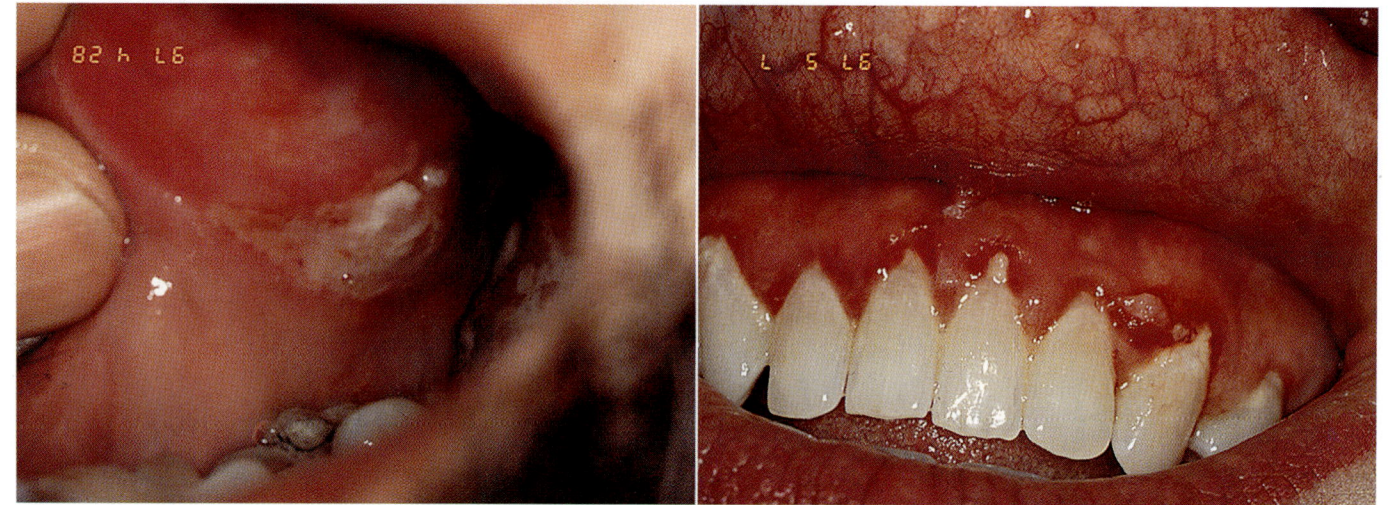

FIGURE 1-9. Pemphigus vulgaris lesions of the oral cavity. **A,** Erosive lesion of the oral cavity. **B,** Superficial, erosive lesions of the gingiva and upper lip. These lesions may be the earliest manifestations of pemphigus vulgaris.

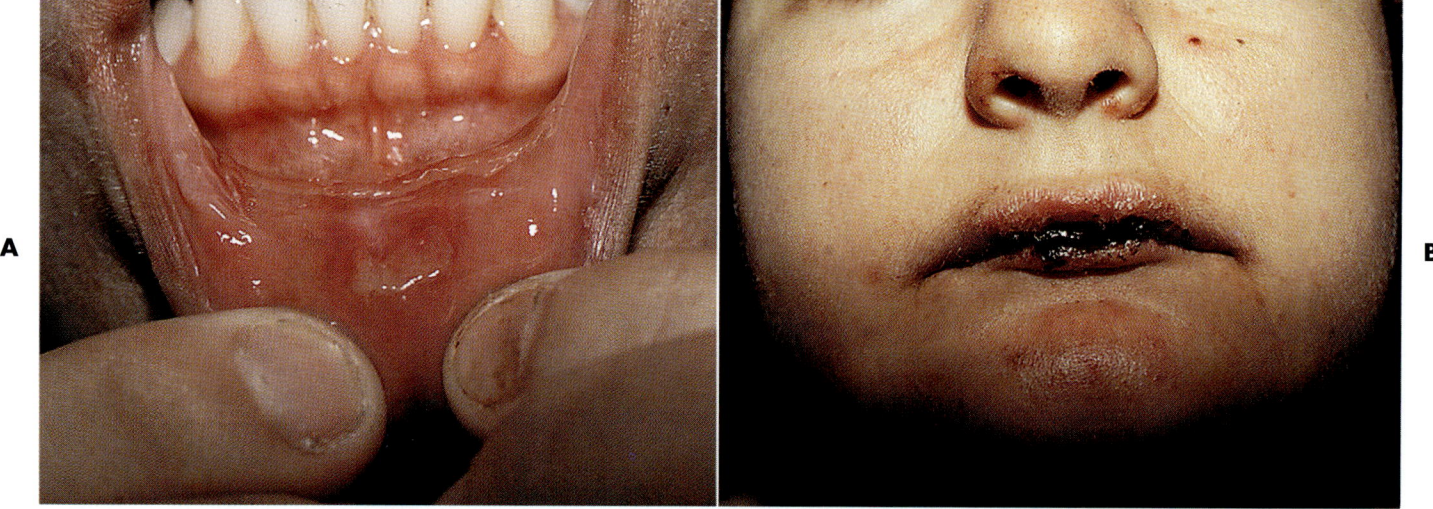

FIGURE 1-10. Pemphigus vulgaris lesions of the lips. **A,** Bullous lesion of the inner lower lip. **B,** Erosive, crusted lesions of the vermilion border of the lips, which is a common site of involvement.

Oral involvement is often the initial manifestation of the disease and occurs at the same time in all patients with pemphigus vulgaris (Box 1-2). Oral lesions may precede cutaneous lesions by several weeks to several months. Unless pemphigus vulgaris is suspected at this stage, the disease is often misdiagnosed. Patients may have pemphigus vulgaris confined to the oral cavity without cutaneous disease. Oral lesions may be so extensive and painful that they interfere with nutrition. Buccal surfaces and the gingiva (Figure 1-9, *A* and *B*) are most often involved. Lesions are commonly present on the hard and soft palates and the vermilion borders of the lips (Figure 1-10, *A* and *B*). The pharynx and larynx may also be involved, resulting in hoarseness. Involvement of the conjunctiva (Figure 1-11, *A*), the tongue (Figure 1-11, *B* and *C*), the esophagus, and the nasal cavity, vagina, and anus are less common.

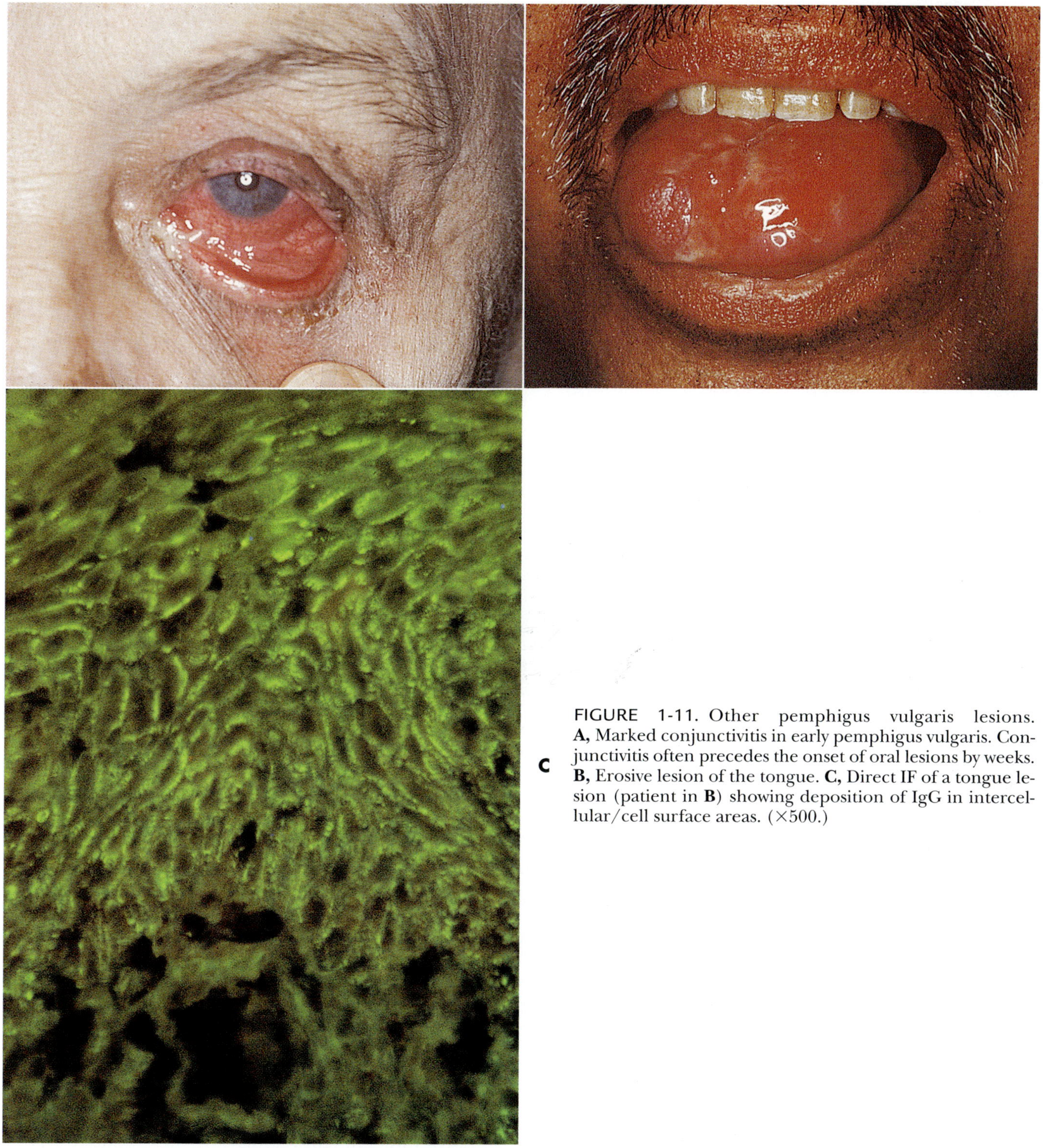

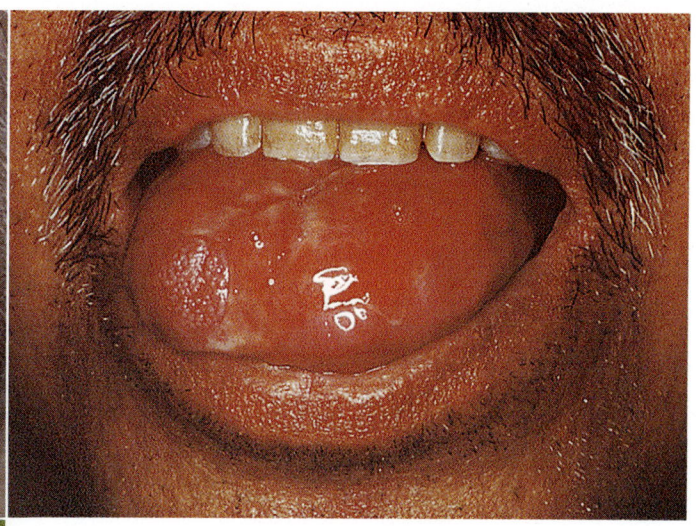

FIGURE 1-11. Other pemphigus vulgaris lesions. **A,** Marked conjunctivitis in early pemphigus vulgaris. Conjunctivitis often precedes the onset of oral lesions by weeks. **B,** Erosive lesion of the tongue. **C,** Direct IF of a tongue lesion (patient in **B**) showing deposition of IgG in intercellular/cell surface areas. (×500.)

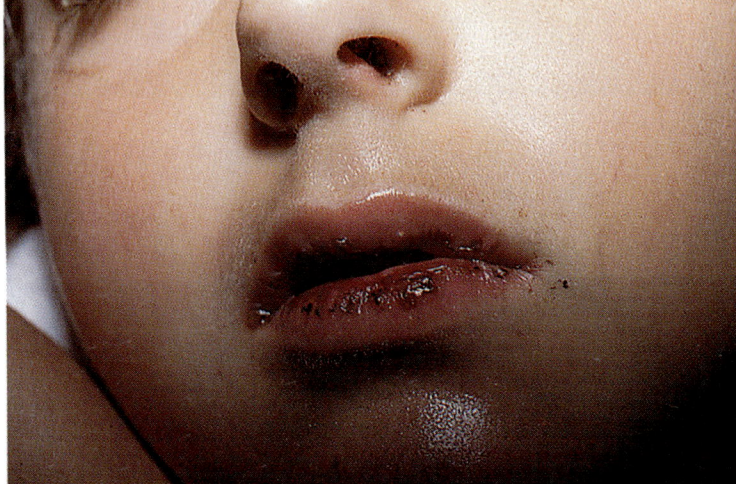

FIGURE 1-12. Childhood pemphigus vulgaris. **A,** Erosive blistering lesions of the lips in a 9-year-old white female. **B,** Erosive lesions of the face, lips, and orbits in a 12-year-old Hispanic male.

Without appropriate therapy, lesions of pemphigus vulgaris tend to heal slowly. Healing lesions may leave hyperpigmentation, but scarring is not a prominent feature. Pruritus is not a common complaint, although patients often describe their lesions as painful.

Pemphigus vulgaris represents the most common form of pemphigus (Box 1-2), although its incidence varies among different populations. It occurs in all races and ethnic groups; it is most common, however, in peoples of Jewish or Mediterranean origin. Onset usually occurs in the fourth through sixth decades of life, but reported cases have been documented in all age groups. Unlike bullous pemphigoid, the disease is rare in the seventh or eighth decades of life. Familial cases of pemphigus vulgaris have been reported, and an increased incidence of HLA-A10, HLA-DR4, HLA-Dw10, and HLA-Dw6, an MLC subtype of DR4, has been shown to confer the highest risk of pemphigus vulgaris in populations of Jewish origin (Box 1-1). Two different nucleotide sequences, one on the DRB1 chain of Dw10, the other on DQB chain of a DQw6 subtype linked to DRw6, predispose Jewish patients to the development of pemphigus vulgaris. Rarely, pemphigus vulgaris may be associated with other autoimmune diseases, such as systemic lupus erythematosus (SLE) and myasthenia gravis. These latter associations, however, are more common in patients with pemphigus foliaceus.

Pemphigus vulgaris is the most common variety of pemphigus that occurs in children, occurring with equal frequency in boys and girls (Figure 1-12, *A* and *B*) and usually occurring in children older than 10 years. Patients with pemphigus vulgaris as young as 2 years of age have been documented. Neonatal pemphigus vulgaris occurs as a result of the passive transfer of antibodies to the fetus and usually resolves within several weeks. In the majority of cases, but not all, the mother has a high titer of circulating autoantibodies.

The course of pemphigus vulgaris is variable. It depends on the extent of the disease, the timeliness of the correct diagnosis, and appropriate therapy at an early stage. The disease may be localized initially, but usually progresses within a few weeks. Unfortunately, the diagnosis may not be suspected until lesions become more widespread, delaying the initiation of appropriate therapy.

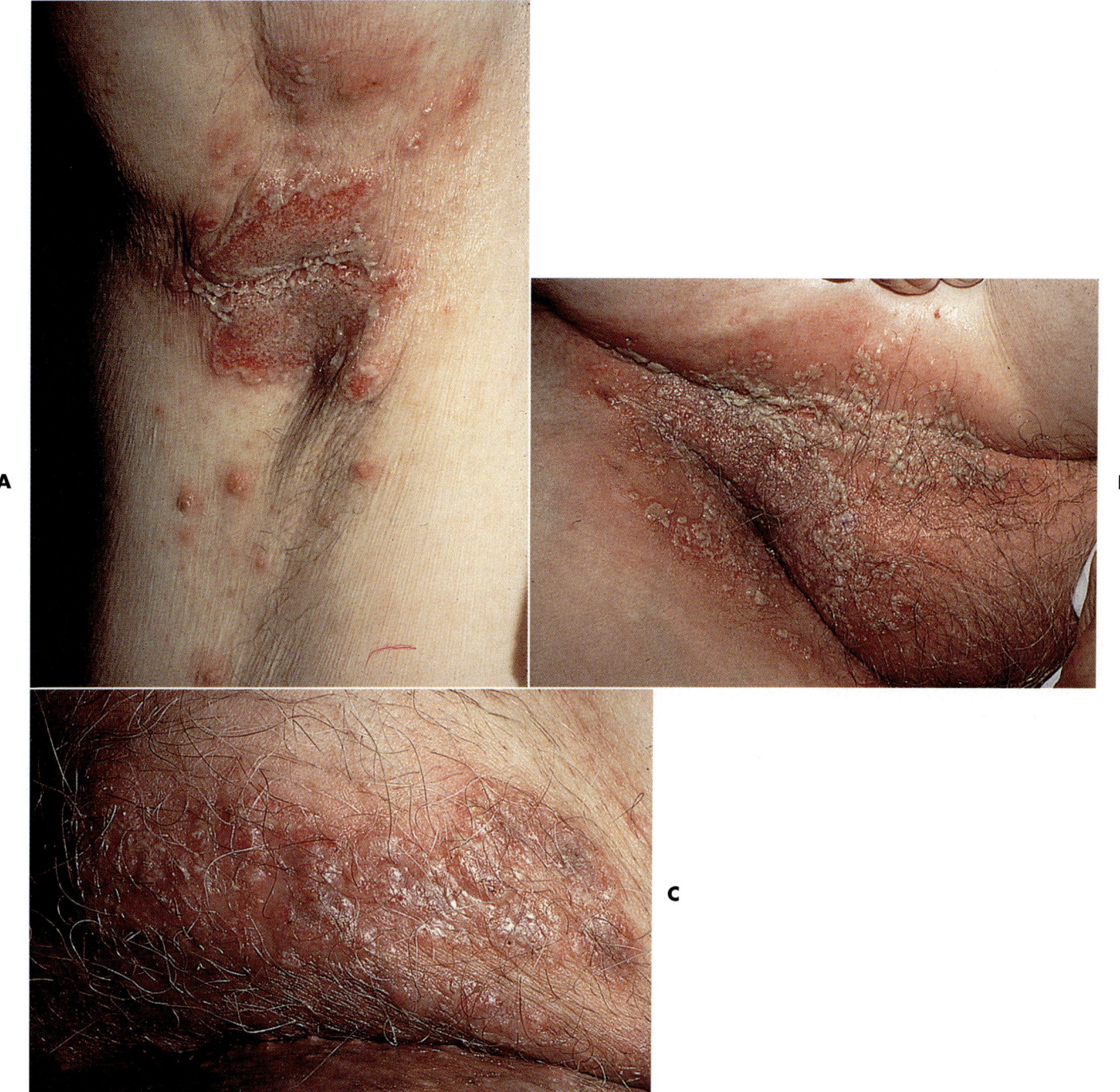

FIGURE 1-13. Skin lesions of pemphigus vegetans. **A,** Erosive hypertrophic lesions of the axilla. **B,** Erosive vegetating lesions with pustules of the groin. Intertriginous areas are commonly involved in pemphigus vegetans. **C,** Lesions of the groin studded with small pustules, which are filled with eosinophils.

Pemphigus vegetans represents a rare variant of pemphigus vulgaris. Two separate types of pemphigus vegetans have been described, the Neumann type whose course is similar to pemphigus vulgaris and a Hallopeau type that is much less severe. Since these types were recognized before the description of acantholysis, only the Neumann type is recognized as pemphigus vegetans.

Lesions of pemphigus vegetans are identical to pemphigus vulgaris in the initial stages of the disease. Painful, flaccid bullae and weeping lesions predominate, but with healing, verrucoid granulating lesions replace denuded areas (Figure 1-13, *A* to *C*). Pustular lesions are often present at the periphery of these verrucoid (vegetating) lesions (Figure 1-13, *C*). Like pem-

BOX 1-3. MEDICATIONS ASSOCIATED WITH DRUG-INDUCED PEMPHIGUS

THIOL GROUP	ANTIBIOTICS	PYRAZOLONE DERIVATIVES	MISCELLANEOUS	
Captopril	Amoxicillin	Aminophenazone	Barbiturates	Levodopa
Gold sodium thiomalate	Ampicillin	Aminopyrine	Benzoin	Lysine acetylsalicylate
Mercaptopropionylglycine	Cefadroxil	Azapropazone	Digoxin	Nifedipine
D-Penicillamine	Ceftazidime	Feprazone	Enalapril	Optalidon
Piroxicam	Cephalexin	Oxyphenbutazone	Heroin	Pentachlorophenol
Thiomazole	Ethambutol		Hydantoin	Phosphamide
Thiopronine	Isoniazid		β-interferon	Progesterone
5-Thiopyridoxine	Penicillin		Interleukin-2	Propranolol
	Rifampin			

phigus vulgaris, oral lesions are common and often the initial manifestation of the disease. Involvement of the vermilion border of the lips is very common. Older cutaneous lesions, particularly in intertriginous areas, become papillomatous and hyperkeratotic, forming characteristic vegetations. The course of pemphigus vegetans is identical to pemphigus vulgaris, necessitating prompt diagnosis and early initiation of therapy.

The occurrence of drug-induced pemphigus is rare but well documented (Box 1-3). Diagnosis is established by a temporal relationship with the drug and typical histologic and IF findings. Although a number of drugs have been reported to cause drug-induced pemphigus, most cases are due to sulfhydryl-containing medications (80%). Captopril and D-penicillamine are the most common offending drugs. In some instances, when the offending drug is discontinued, the disease remits; in other instances, the disease persists. Acantholysis in drug-induced pemphigus may occur because of a direct effect of the drug on the epidermis or as a result of the production of anti-cell surface antibodies in genetically predisposed individuals.

Pathology

Histopathology

Small, early intact blisters should be chosen for histopathologic examination.[2] Histopathologically (Box 1-3), lesions of pemphigus vulgaris show suprabasal intraepidermal bulla formation with marked acantholysis (Figure 1-14, *A* and *B*). This latter finding is a diagnostic hallmark of diseases of the pemphigus group. Lesions of the oral mucosa show identical findings. Basal keratinocytes form the floor of the blister cavity, and a mild inflammatory infiltrate, composed mainly of eosinophils, is usually present. In early lesions, eosinophils often invade the epidermis in clusters. The process is known as *eosinophilic spongiosis*.

Pemphigus vegetans is also characterized by suprabasilar intraepidermal bulla formation with acantholysis (Box 1-4). Again, basal cells form the floor of the blister cavity. Older lesions often manifest pseudoepitheliomatous hyperplasia with papillomatosis and hyperkeratosis (Figure 1-15, *A* and *B*). Intraepidermal abscesses of eosinophils are frequently observed.

Immunopathology

Direct IF studies should be performed in addition to routine histopathology if a diagnosis of either pemphigus vulgaris or pemphigus vegetans is suspected. Ideally, an early, small intact vesicle should be biopsied for direct IF studies. If blisters are no longer present, perilesional skin should be chosen as the biopsy site. Characteristic deposits of IgG and C3 should be present in intercellular/cell surface areas (see Figure 1-2, *A* and *B*), with staining most intense in areas of acantholysis and vesicle formation (Box 1-4). These direct IF findings are now considered to be diagnostic of pemphigus vulgaris and other members of the pemphigus group.

Diagnosis

The diagnosis of pemphigus vulgaris and pemphigus vegetans is based on the clinical presentation (Box 1-2) and typical histopathologic and IF findings (Box 1-4). The presence of flaccid bullae, weeping denuded surfaces, and oral erosions should alert the physician to this diagnosis. Vegetating pustular lesions, particularly in the axillae, groin, and other body folds, suggest the

BOX 1-4. PATHOLOGY

HISTOPATHOLOGY		IMMUNOPATHOLOGY
PEMPHIGUS VULGARIS	*PEMPHIGUS VEGETANS*	IgG and complement deposits in intercellular/cell surface pattern, in both pemphigus vulgaris and vegetans
Suprabasal intraepidermal bullae	Deep suprabasal intrapidermal bulla	
Marked acantholysis present	Acantholysis present	
Major cell infiltrates are eosinophils	Major cell infiltrates are eosinophils	Intensity of staining greatest in areas of acantholysis
	Pseudoepithelomatous hyperplasia	
	Papillomatosis and hyperkeratosis	Absence of such findings questions the diagnosis of pemphigus
	Abscesses of eosinophils	

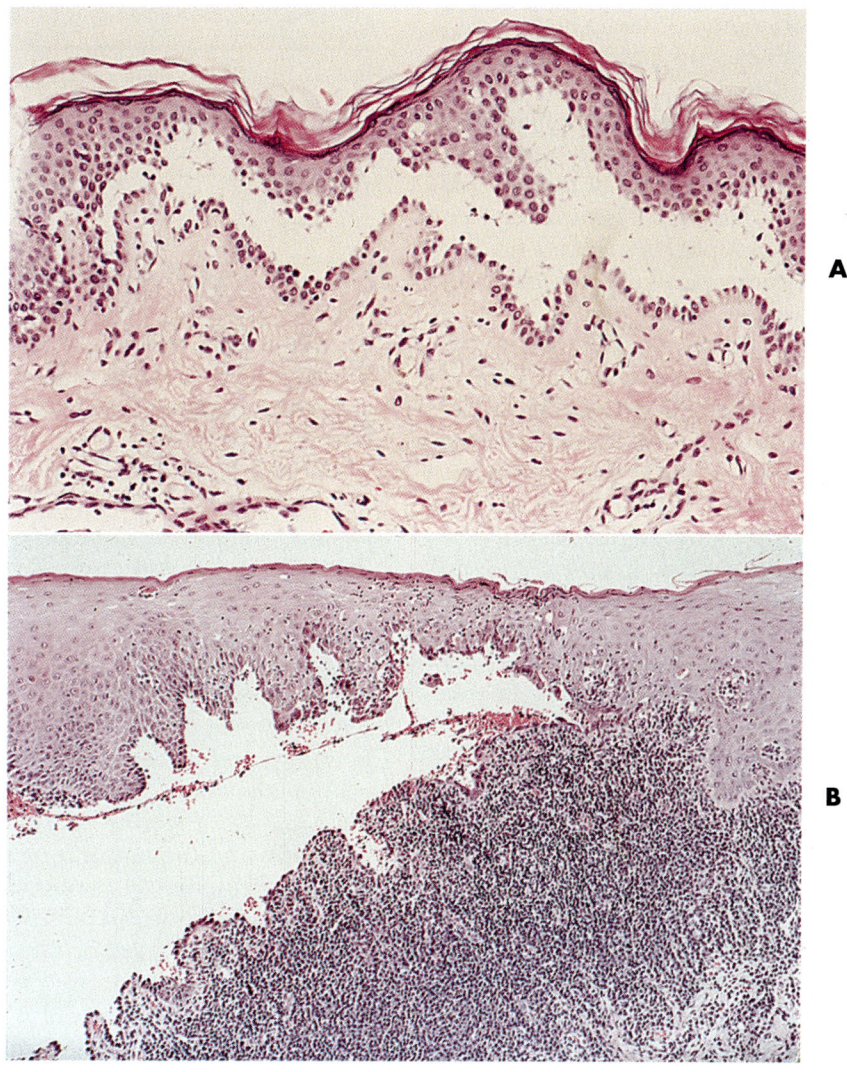

FIGURE 1-14. Histopathology of pemphigus vulgaris. **A,** Early skin lesion demonstrating deep, suprabasal intraepidermal bulla formation with acantholysis and an infiltrate of eosinophils. (×100.) **B,** Early erosive oral lesion showing a deep suprabasilar acantholytic separation of mucosa. An infiltrate of eosinophils and lymphocytes is present. (×100.)

diagnosis of pemphigus vegetans. If pemphigus is suspected, biopsies should be performed for both histopathologic and direct IF study. If performed properly, a diagnosis of pemphigus is established. If direct IF studies are negative, a diagnosis other than pemphigus should be entertained.

Therapy

The mainstay of treatment for patients with pemphigus vulgaris and pemphigus vegetans is systemic corticosteroids. With delineation of the major immunopathologic events in this disease, other forms of therapy, including immunosuppressive medications, are often employed either in combination with steroids or as monotherapy. Combined regimens, using corticosteroids and immunosuppressive agents, have improved the prognosis of the disease (Box 1-5).

During acute episodes, patients with pemphigus vulgaris (and vegetans) may require hospitalization. When active disease is present, no other form of therapy has replaced high-dose systemic steroids. The dose chosen should be high enough to completely suppress further vesicle formation. Most treatment failures are the result of inadequate doses of systemic corticosteroids.

Box 1-5 shows the initial dosages of prednisone utilized, depending on the clinical presentation. If pemphigus vulgaris is confined to the oral cavity, an initial dose of 60 to 80 mg of prednisone is usually sufficient to suppress lesion formation. Once the disease progresses to involve the skin, a higher initial prednisone dose must be chosen. A dosage of 120 to 150 mg of prednisone should be utilized; this dosage should be sufficient to suppress new blister formation. In both instances, prednisone should be administered once a day in a single morning dose to minimize untoward effects. Blood pressure and blood chemistries (particularly blood glucose and electrolytes) should be monitored when prednisone dosage is high. Physicians should be aware of the possible development of infection, including opportunistic organisms, such as gram-negative bacteria, fungi, and tubercle bacilli. Infection should be treated vigorously. Calcium and vitamin D supplements are also recommended when using high-dose, long-term prednisone therapy.

With cessation of new blister formation, the prednisone dose may be reduced at regular intervals (2 to 3 weeks) with careful clinical monitoring. Once a dose level of 60 mg per day is achieved, further reductions should be more gradual. Decreasing pemphigus antibody titers are helpful in gauging the response to treatment, but decreasing clinical activity is the most important parameter. At a dosage of 60 mg of prednisone daily, further reductions can be made on alternate days in an attempt to change to alternate-day therapy. This maintenance therapy can further reduce the untoward side effects of long-term prednisone administration. If

BOX 1-5. PEMPHIGUS VULGARIS THERAPY

INITIAL
Prednisone
Oral disease only: 60-80 mg daily
Skin and oral: 100-200 mg daily
MAINTENANCE
Prednisone: Alternate day therapy
STEROID-SPARING AGENTS
Azathioprine: 50-150 mg daily
Cyclophosphamide: 100-200 mg daily
Methotrexate: 25-35 mg weekly
Cyclosporine: 6-8 mg/kg daily
OTHER THERAPIES
Gold intramuscular: 25-50 mg weekly
Dapsone (Pemphigus vegetans): 50-100 mg daily
Plasmapheresis:* Weekly

*Used in combination with prednisone in high titer cases. Cyclophosphamide given after procedure to prevent antibody rebound.

patients remain controlled on alternate-day therapy, they may be treated with prednisone alone rather than in combination with other immunosuppressive agents. The alternate-day dose of prednisone should be gradually reduced to the lowest possible level, while still maintaining control.

Because of the requirement of long-term use of high-dose daily corticosteroids in the treatment of both pemphigus vulgaris and pemphigus vegetans, alternative therapies to minimize steroid side effects are employed. A variety of steroid-sparing agents, including immunosuppressive drugs, are available. In the acute stages, however, they are of little value and should not be used in place of corticosteroids. Immunosuppressive agents, in particular, should not be started until prednisone has been tapered to between 80 and 60 mg per day. Such agents take about 3 to 4 weeks to have an effect; their main use is for steroid sparing and maintenance therapy, reducing the amount of prednisone required for control over a shorter period of time. In many instances, prednisone may be discontinued once control has been established; the patient may be maintained on the steroid-sparing immunosuppressive agent alone.

Several immunosuppressive agents may be employed. Methotrexate, either orally or intramuscularly, has been used in doses of 25 to 35 mg per week after tapering high-dose prednisone to about 60 mg per day. Folinic acid (Leucovorin) 0.5 mg/kg may be administered 1 to 2 hours after intramuscular methotrexate to minimize side effects. Cyclophosphamide (Cytoxan) may also be used for maintenance therapy. Dosages of 100 to 200 mg daily may be given initially, followed by reduction to 100 mg daily within 2 to 3 weeks for maintenance. Cy-

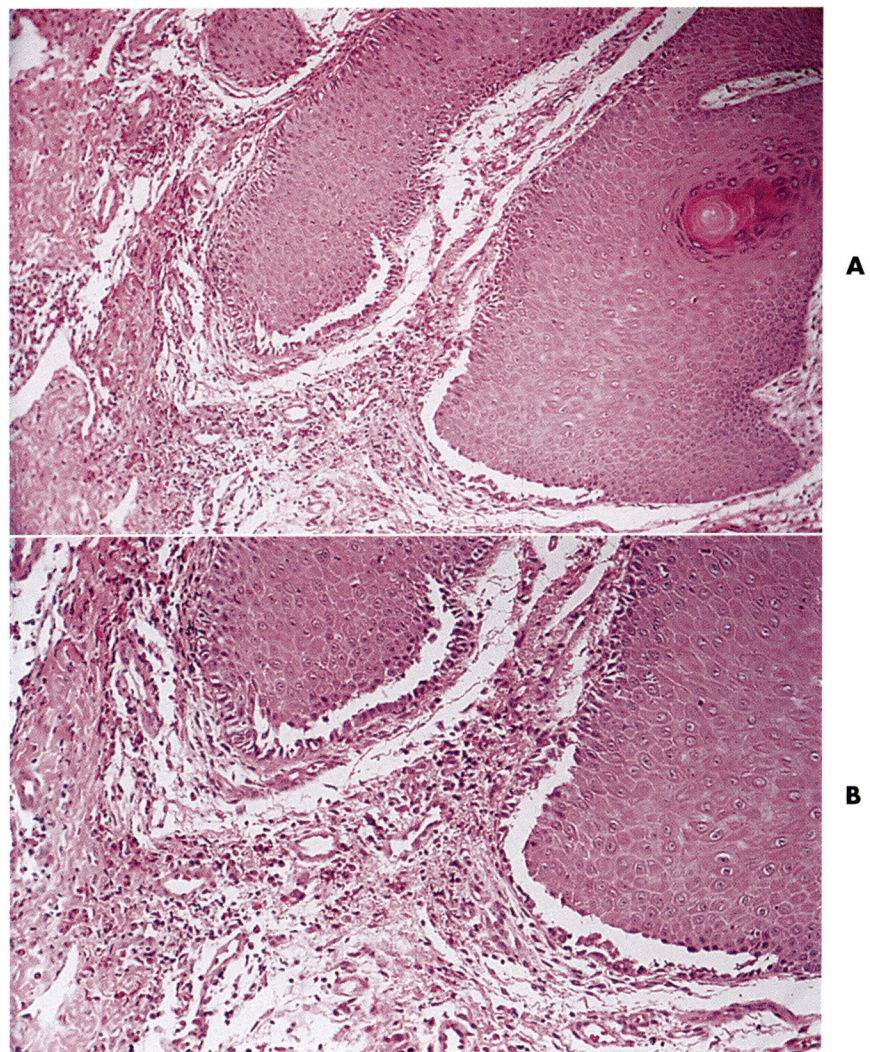

FIGURE 1-15. Histopathology of pemphigus vegetans. **A,** Hypertrophic lesion. Suprabasilar separation is noted at the base of the lesion. (×100.) **B,** Higher power of same lesion showing suprabasilar intraepidermal separation and acantholysis. Eosinophils are present in the infiltrate. (×250.) *Courtesy Philip R. Cohen, MD, University of Texas Medical School, Houston, Texas.)*

closporine has been utilized successfully in selected patients with pemphigus vulgaris but mainly as a steroid-sparing agent, with a divided daily dosage of 6 to 8 mg/kg per day given orally. Since cyclosporine administration may result in significant nephrotoxicity, long-term maintenance therapy is not advised.

Our favorite steroid-sparing agent is azathioprine (Imuran). Azathioprine may be administered in dosages of 50 to 150 mg daily after the initial response to prednisone and the reduction of high-dosage prednisone. After 3 to 4 weeks of azathioprine, the prednisone dosage may be significantly reduced or changed to alternate-day usage, or in some instances, discontinued.

Untoward effects of these immunosuppressive agents include hematopoietic depression, hepatotoxicity, renal toxicity, and an increased incidence of malignancy. Careful monitoring of blood elements and chemistries at regular intervals is advised, and a vigil must be maintained for the development of secondary infection.

An additional steroid-sparing regimen, other than immunosuppressives, is chrysotherapy. Although reported to be efficacious without concomitant corticosteroid therapy, this approach is most often used in combination with prednisone. Gold must be administered intramuscularly, since the oral form is not effective. A test dose of 10 mg of gold sodium thiomalate is administered, followed by 25 mg 1 week later. Thereafter 50 mg per week is given until clinical improvement is noted or toxicity develops, or a total of 1 gm of gold has been administered without effectively lowering the corticosteroid dose. Gold sodium thiomalate, 50 mg every 2 to 4 weeks, is administered as maintenance therapy. Toxicity, including severe skin reactions, may develop.

In patients with prednisone-resistant pemphigus and high titers of pemphigus antibodies, plasmapheresis also may be an efficacious approach. Plasma exchange tends to work best when used in combination with systemic steroids and immunosuppressives. Concomitant use of immunosuppressives, such as Cytoxan, after plasmapheresis is thought to prevent the occurrence of antibody rebound. Not all patients, however, respond to plasmapheresis.

Other therapeutic approaches reported to be of some value include dapsone, mycophenolate mofetil, pulse IV corticosteroids, and extracorporeal photochemotherapy. All have been found to be effective in selected patients. Dapsone may be more useful in patients with pemphigus vegetans. Oral antibiotics should be administered when necessary to treat secondary infection.

REFERENCES

1. Civatte A: Diagnostic histopathologique de la dermatite polymophe douloreuse ou maladie de Duhring-Brocq, *Ann Dermatol Syphilig* 3:1-30, 1943.
2. Lever WF: Pemphigus, *Medicine* 32:1-123, 1953.
3. Beutner EH, Jordon RE: Demonstration of skin antibodies in sera of pemphigus vulgaris patients by indirect immunofluorescence staining, *Proc Soc Exp Biol Med* 117:505-510, 1964.
4. Beutner EH, Lever WF, Witebsky E, et al. Autoantibodies in pemphigus vulgaris: Response to an intercellular substance of epidermis, *JAMA* 192:682-688, 1965.
5. Beutner EH, Jordon RE, Chorzelski TP: The immunopathology of pemphigus and bullous pemphigoid, *J Ivest Dermatol* 51:63-80, 1968.
6. Diaz LA, Marcello CL: Pemphigoid and pemphigus antigens in cultured epidermal cells, *Br J Dermatol* 98:631-637, 1978.
7. Schiltz JR, Michel B, Papay R: Pemphigus antibody interaction with human epidermal cells in culture: A proposed mechanism for pemphigus acantholysis, *J Clin Invest* 62:778-788, 1978.
8. Anhalt GL, Labib RS, Voorhees JJ, et al: Induction of pemphigus in neonatal mice by passive transfer of IgG from patients with the disease, *N Engl J Med* 306:1189-1196, 1982.
9. Hashimoto K, Shafron KM, Webber PS, et al: Anti-cell surface pemphigus autoantibody stimulates plasminogen activator activity of human epidermal cells. A mechanism for the loss of cohesion and blister formation, *J Exp Med* 157:259-272, 1983.
10. Stanley JR, Koulu L, Thivolet C: Distinction between epidermal antigens binding pemphigus vulgaris and pemphigus foliaceus autoantibodies, *J Clin Invest* 74:313-320, 1984.
11. Kawana S, Geoghegan WD, Jordon RE: Complement fixation by pemphigus antibody. II. Complement enhanced detachment of epidermal cells, *Clin Exp Immunol* 61:517-525, 1985.
12. Doubleday CW, Geoghegan WD, Jordon RE: Complement fixation by pemphigus antibody. IV. Enhanced epidermal cell detachment in the absence of human plasminogen, *J Lab Clin Med* 111:28-34, 1988.
13. Eyre RW, Stanley JR: Identification of pemphigus vulgaris antigen extracted from normal human epidermis and comparison with pemphigus foliaceus antigen, *J Clin Invest* 81:807-812, 1988.
14. Xia P, Jordon RE, Geoghegan WD: Complement fixation by pemphigus antibody. V. Assembly of the membrane attack complex on cultured human keratinocytes, *J Clin Invest* 82:1939-1947, 1988.
15. Amagai M, Karpati S, Prussick R, et al: Autoantibodies against the amino-terminal cadherin-like binding domain of pemphigus vulgaris antigen are pathogenic, *J Clin Invest* 90:919-926, 1992.

2

Pemphigus Foliaceus

Jose M. Mascaro Jr
Manish J. Gharia
Mong-Shang Lin
Zhi Liu
Luis A. Diaz

Epidemiology and Etiology

Subcorneal blisters and pathogenic antiepidermal autoantibodies characterize the nonendemic and endemic forms of pemphigus foliaceus. The endemic form is also known as fogo selvagem, which in Portuguese means "wild fire." The major advances in pemphigus foliaceus are depicted in Figure 2-1, including the initial description of pemphigus foliaceus by Cazenave in 1844[1] and of fogo selvagem by Paes-Leme in 1903.[2] Although pemphigus foliaceus can occur worldwide, fogo selvagem is endemic to certain subtropical regions of rural Brazil (Figure 2-2). Clusters of cases of an endemic fogo selvagem-like disease have also been reported in other parts of Latin America. The majority of fogo selvagem cases in Brazil originate from endemic areas irrigated by the Araguaia, Tocantins, Parana, and Paraguay rivers and their tributaries.[3] The endemic areas tend to be agriculturally developing regions (Figure 2-3) that are heavily infested with a variety of biting insects. A case-controlled study indicated that exposure to one of these insects, the black fly (family *Simuliidae*), may be a relevant etiologic factor of fogo selvagem.[4] However, individuals developing fogo selvagem are exposed to many other factors in their native environment, hence elucidating a single cause is a formidable task.

Strong epidemiologic evidence suggests that fogo selvagem is precipitated by an environmental factor in genetically predisposed individuals. Due to the scarcity of patients, few immunogenetic studies have been performed on the nonendemic form of pemphigus foliaceus. In fogo selvagem, however, several studies documented the familial nature of the disease and the increased frequency of certain HLA alleles in these patients. In a series of 2,686 patients with fogo selvagem, 18% were familial cases, and 93% of these familial cases represented genetically related family members[5] (Box 2-1). Recent studies demonstrated that Amerindian populations of Brazil with a high prevalence of fogo selvagem express certain HLA-DRB1 alleles, such as DRB1* 0201, 0404, 1402, and 1406, with a relative risk as high as 14.[6-9] Interestingly, these alleles all share the same amino acid sequence (residues 67 to 74) at the third hypervariable region of the DRB1 gene, i.e., the sequence LLEQRRAA[10] (Figure 2-4). This "shared epitope hypothesis," which was originally proposed for rheumatoid arthritis,[11] may also confer susceptibility in patients with fogo selvagem.

Pathogenesis

In 1964, Beutner and Jordon first reported the presence of circulating antibodies to the epidermal intercellular spaces (ICS) of the skin in the sera of patients with pemphigus, thus demonstrating that pemphigus is an autoimmune disease.[12] The pathogenicity of fogo selvagem autoantibodies has been demonstrated by passive-transfer experiments.[13] In these studies, the IgG fraction from the serum of patients with fogo selvagem induced blistering within 24 hours when injected intraperitoneally into neonatal Balb/c mice (Figure 2-5). Histologic examination of lesional skin of these animals revealed typical acantholytic blisters located in the granular cell layer of the epidermis (Figure 2-6), as seen in human pemphigus foliaceus. Direct immunofluorescence (IF) examination of the mouse skin showed deposits of human IgG autoantibodies and mouse C3 in the ICS (Figure 2-7). Indirect IF testing of the mouse serum showed circulating human autoantibodies in

---

This work was supported in part by U.S. Public Health Service Grants R37-AR32081, R01-AR32599 (LAD), R29-AI44223 (ZL), and T32-AR07577 (MJG) from the National Institutes of Health and a VA Merit Review Grant (LAD). This work was also supported by Fellowship awards (JMM and MSL) and a Career Development Award (ZL) from the Dermatology Foundation.

PEMPHIGUS FOLIACEUS SUMMARY

EPIDEMIOLOGY AND ETIOLOGY

The etiology of both nonendemic and endemic forms of pemphigus foliaceus is unknown, but epidemiologic evidence suggests an environmental precipitating factor in the endemic form, fogo selvagem.

PATHOGENESIS

Both forms of pemphigus foliaceus are IgG autoantibody-mediated diseases. These antiepidermal autoantibodies recognize a desmosomal glycoprotein, desmoglein 1 (Dsg1).

CLINICAL FEATURES

The clinical hallmark in both forms of pemphigus foliaceus is a superficial vesicle that easily ruptures, leaving areas of denuded skin. Nikolsky's sign is positive, and the disease may be localized or generalized, producing exfoliative erythroderma. Mucosal involvement is not seen in these patients.

PATHOLOGY

The vesicles in both forms of pemphigus foliaceus are intraepidermal and located in the subcorneal region of the epidermis.

DIAGNOSIS

Clinical, histologic, immunologic, and epidemiologic criteria are unique to pemphigus foliaceus. These diagnostic criteria are similar for both forms of pemphigus foliaceus, except for the epidemiology of fogo selvagem, which is typical for this endemic form of the disease.

TREATMENT

Systemic corticosteroids and immunosuppressive agents are the drugs of choice to treat patients with pemphigus foliaceus. In some patients, plasmapheresis may be useful.

DIFFERENTIAL DIAGNOSIS

The following disorders must be differentiated from pemphigus foliaceus: pemphigus vulgaris, impetigo, staphylococcal scalded skin syndrome, atypical pustular psoriasis, seborrheic dermatitis, and discoid lupus erythematosus.

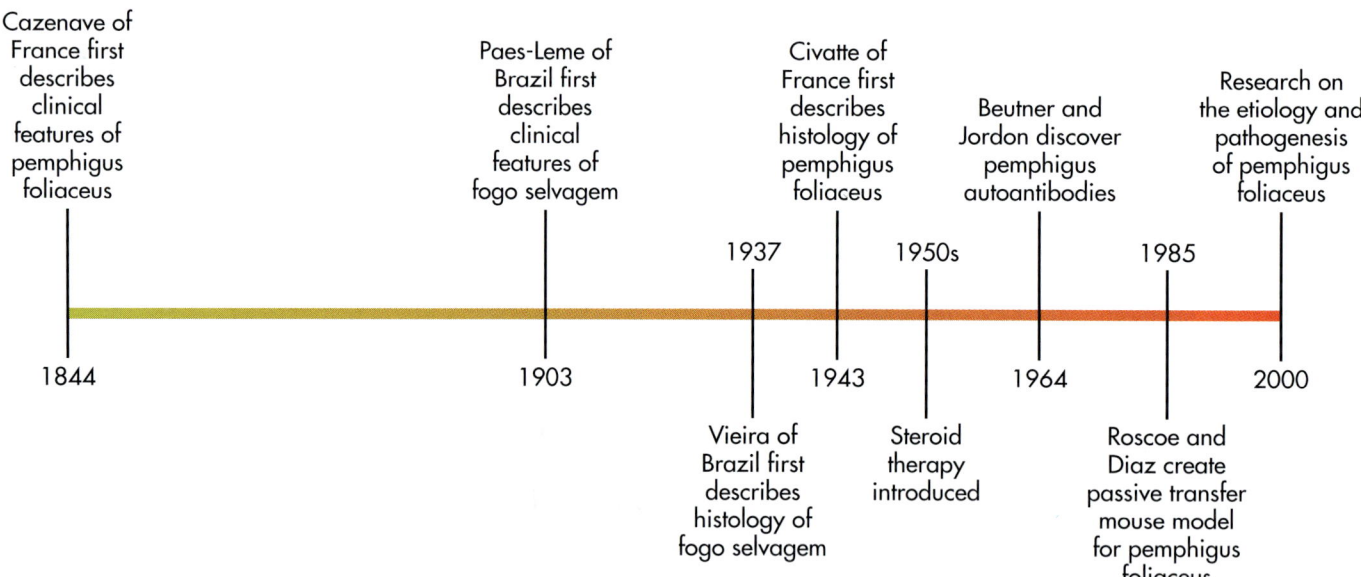

FIGURE 2-1. Major advances in pemphigus foliaceus.

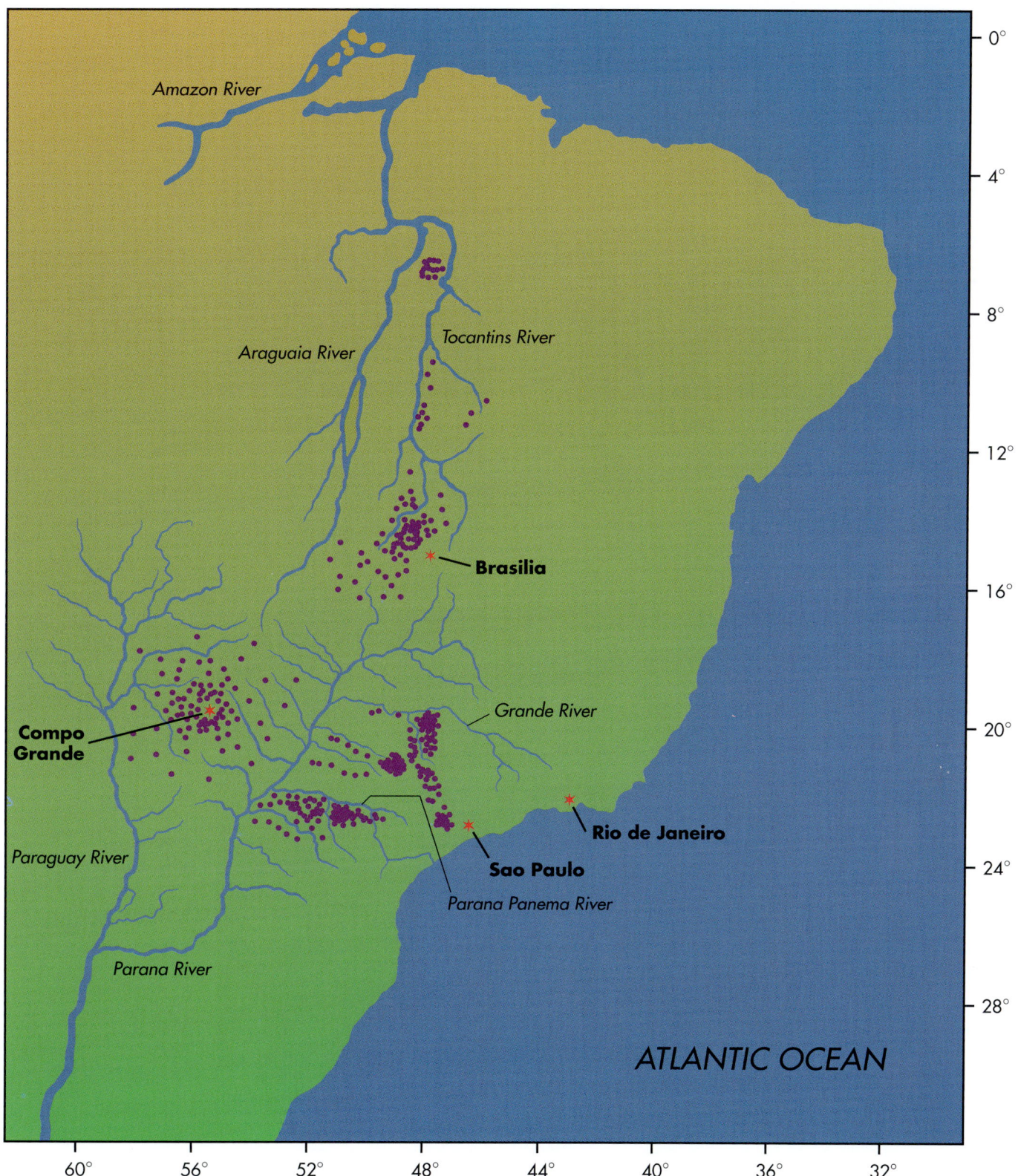

FIGURE 2-2. Pemphigus foliaceus can occur worldwide, but in certain regions of Brazil there is the endemic form, fogo selvagem. At the present time the Brazilian states of Goias, Minas Gerais, Mato Grosso do Sul, and Mato Grosso have the greatest number of cases of fogo selvagem. The geographic distribution of patients *(black dots)* follows areas drained by tributaries of the Tocantins and Parana rivers. The number of black dots (cases) is an approximate representation of the geographic origin of individual cases. *(From Diaz LA, Sampaio SA, Rivitti EA, et al: J Invest Dermatol 92:4-12, 1989.*

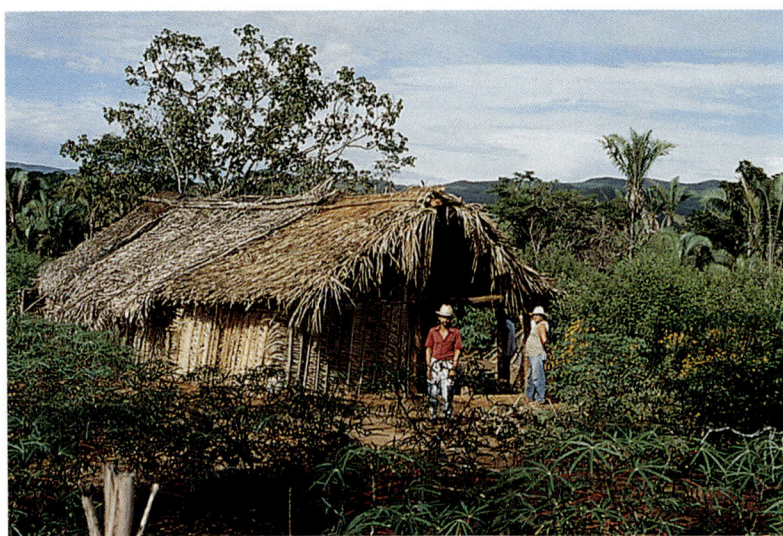

FIGURE 2-3. Fogo selvagem occurs in areas of Brazil where land is being developed for agriculture. A native Brazilian with fogo selvagem (in red) stands in front of his rustic home surrounded by the typical environment of an endemic area. These homes are usually close to either a small river or creek. These watering areas are heavily infested with blood-sucking insects, some of which may play a role in fogo selvagem.

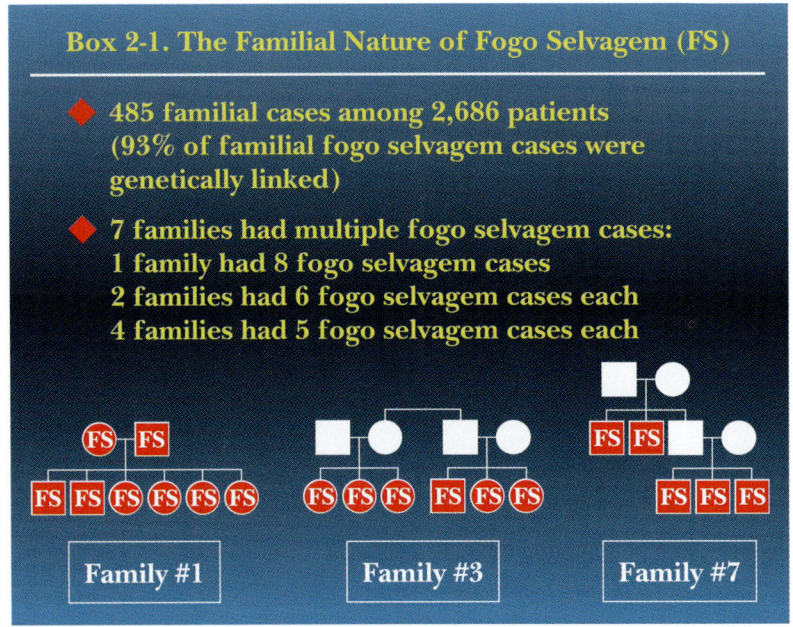

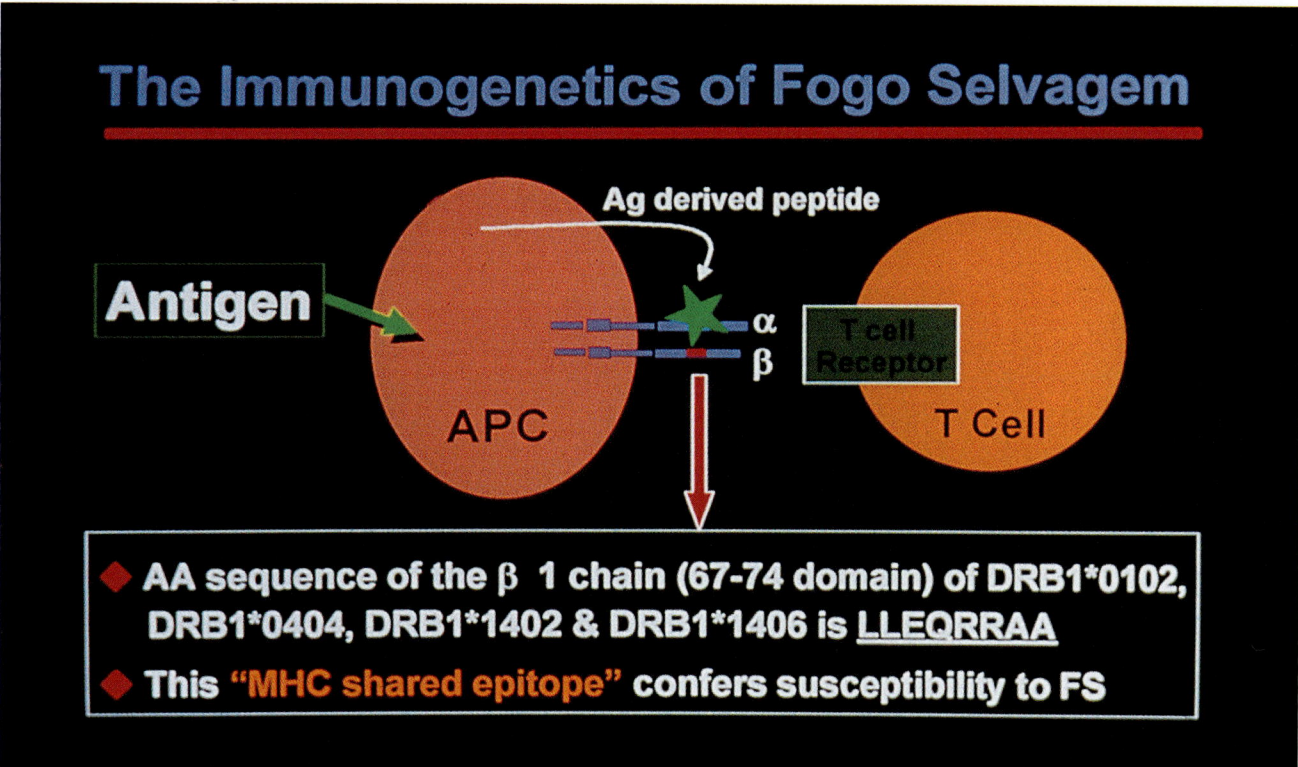

FIGURE 2-4. A relatively large number of cases of fogo selvagem affect genetically related family members. Three families are presented to document the familial nature of fogo selvagem. Immunogenetic evaluation of these patients reveals a strong association of the disease with class II HLA alleles. A common amino acid sequence is shared by these alleles in the third hypervariable region of the beta chain, which may confer susceptibility to fogo selvagem.

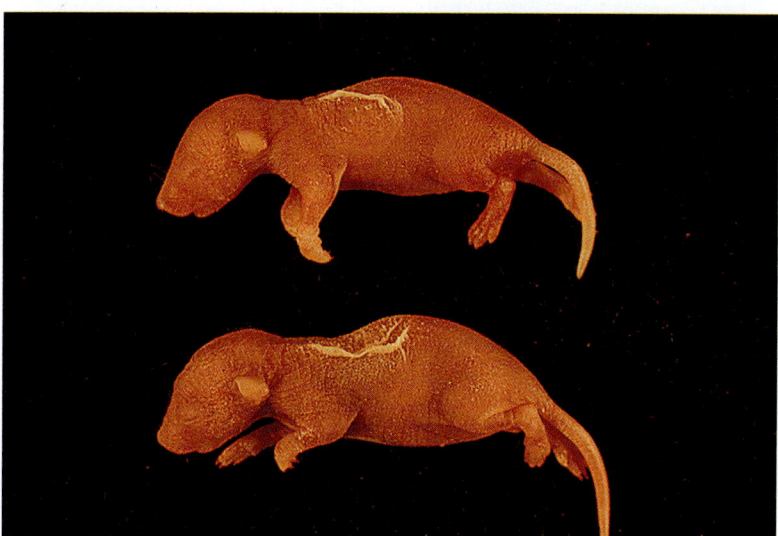

FIGURE 2-5. The pathogenicity of fogo selvagem autoantibodies has been demonstrated by passive-transfer experiments. Here, IgG antibodies from sera from patients with fogo selvagem were injected intraperitoneally in neonatal Balb/c mice causing blisters within 24 hours of injection.

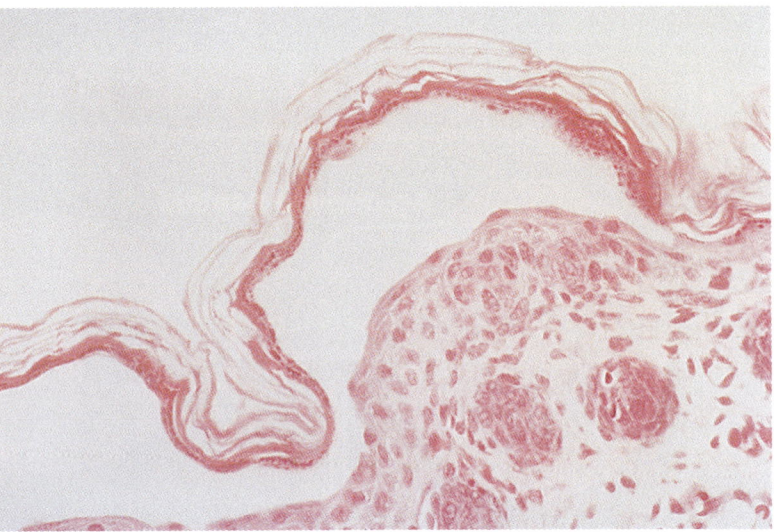

FIGURE 2-6. Histologic examination of lesional skin from the passive-transfer model shows typical acantholysis within the granular layer of the epidermis, identical to human pemphigus foliaceus histology.

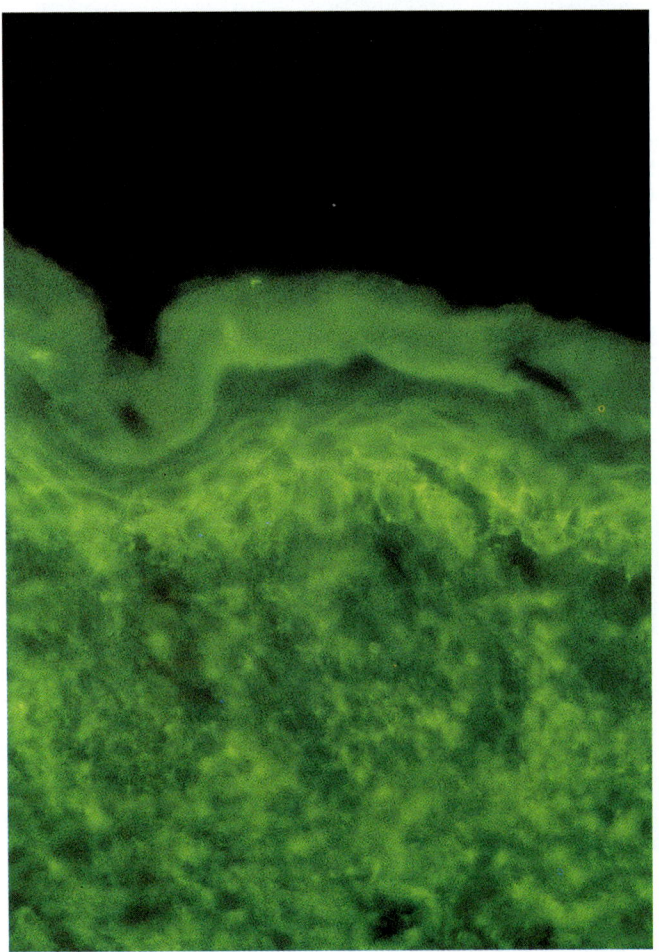

FIGURE 2-7. Direct IF of perilesional skin from the passive-transfer model shows deposits of human IgG antibodies and mouse C3 in the intercellular spaces of the epidermis.

titers that correlated well with the epidermal disease seen in these animals.

The intercellular cell-to-cell adhesion organelles, known as desmosomes, are the target of pemphigus foliaceus autoantibodies. These autoantibodies specifically recognize Dsg1, a desmosomal core glycoprotein of 160-kD molecular weight[14] (Figure 2-8). Dsg1 has been cloned, sequenced, and shown to be a transmembrane glycoprotein belonging to the cadherin family of cell-adhesion molecules.[15] The gene encoding Dsg1 has been mapped to chromosome 18.[16] The extracellular domain of Dsg1, against which autoantibodies are directed, shares with the rest of the cadherins an extracellular domain with three pairs of calcium-binding sites. These sites appear to be crucial in homophilic cell-to-cell adhesion in the epidermis. The intracellular domain of Dsg1 interacts with the keratinocyte cytoskeleton.

Immunoprecipitation and enzyme-linked immunosorbent assays (ELISA) have been developed to test for pemphigus foliaceus autoantibodies. Full length recombinant Dsg1 was produced in a baculovirus expression system for ELISA studies.[17] Tryptic fragments of Dsg1 have also been extracted from bovine muzzle epithelium and radiolabeled with I^{125} for use in immunoprecipitation studies. The soluble Dsg1 glycopeptides of varying molecular weights (80, 60, 45 kD) were recognized by all pemphigus foliaceus sera and 50% of pemphigus vulgaris sera tested.[18] A 66-kD soluble fragment of Dsg1 was recently generated, representing the ectodomain of this molecule, using a baculovirus expression system. This fragment, after radiolabeling with I^{125}, immunoprecipitates when incubated with sera from a patient with pemphigus foliaceus (Figure 2-9). These newer techniques

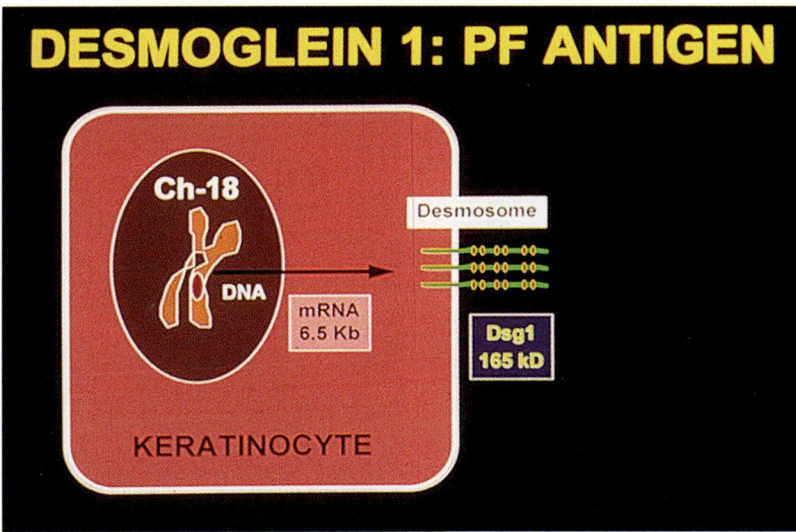

FIGURE 2-8. In pemphigus, the antiepidermal autoantibodies are directed against desmosomal antigens. Desmosomes are intercellular organelles that play an essential role in cell-to-cell adhesion. In pemphigus foliaceus, autoantibodies specifically recognize the desmosomal core glycoprotein desmoglein 1 (Dsg1), which is encoded on chromosome 18.

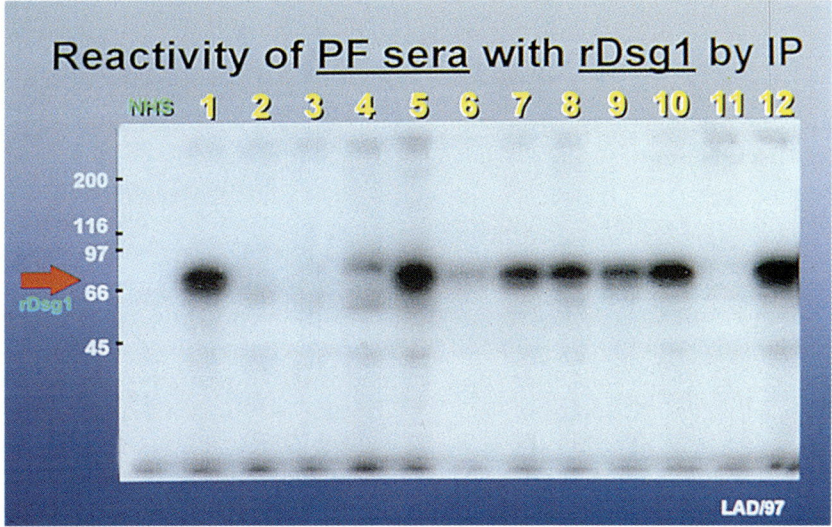

FIGURE 2-9. Immunoprecipitation studies, using the extracellular domain of recombinant Dsg1 produced in a baculovirus expression system, demonstrate that antibodies from sera from a patient with fogo selvagem all recognize the 66-kDa ectodomain of this molecule. The Dsg1 peptide was radiolabeled with radioactive I^{125}.

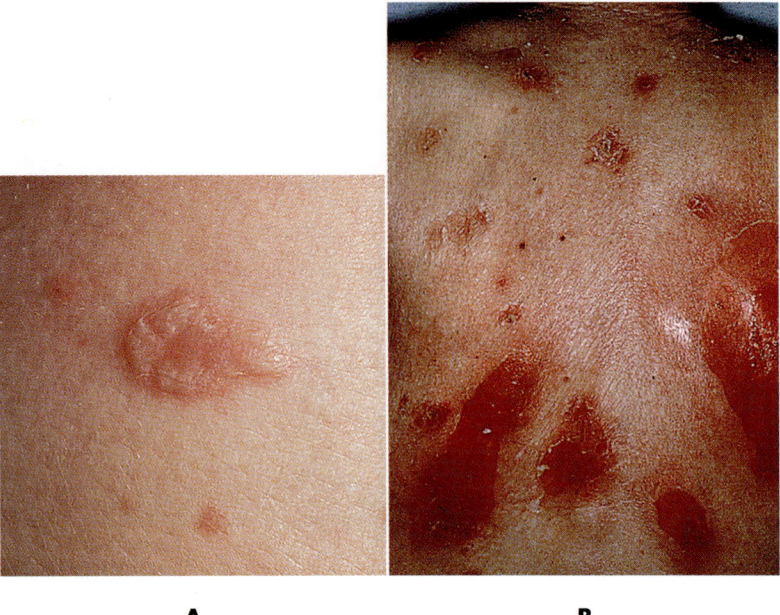

A **B**

FIGURE 2-10. The primary cutaneous lesions in pemphigus foliaceus are superficial blisters that rupture easily, leaving denuded areas of skin. These lesions may occur all over the body, but they are usually most prominent on the face, neck, and trunk (the so-called seborrheic areas). In some patients the lesions can generalize and cause an exfoliative erythroderma. **A**, Intact blisters. **B**, Denuded lesions.

are highly sensitive in detecting pemphigus foliaceus autoantibodies and may be a useful addition to IF studies in diagnosing this disease.

Clinical Features

Both the endemic and nonendemic forms of pemphigus foliaceus have similar clinical features. The primary lesion is a superficial vesicle (Figure 2-10, *A*) that ruptures easily, leaving superficially denuded areas of skin (Figure 2-10, *B*). These lesions are localized in the seborrheic areas of the face and trunk. The scalp is often involved, exhibiting verrucous plaques. After a few weeks or months of evolution the disease may progress to involve large areas of the body, producing an exfoliative erythroderma that is characterized by confluent superficial erosions with exudative crusting (Figure 2-11, *A*). Mucosal blisters and erosions are not observed in these patients; this feature distinguishes pemphigus foliaceus from pemphigus vulgaris. There are rare cases of fulminant pemphigus foliaceus in which the patient develops a rampant widespread bullous eruption within a short period of time (Figure 2-11, *B*). Patients with this severe form of pemphigus foliaceus require hospitalization to prevent dehydration, electrolyte imbalances, and superimposed infections. During active disease, Nikolsky's sign (removal of normal-appearing perilesional epidermis when shearing forces are applied) is a typical finding.

In the localized variant of pemphigus foliaceus (Figure 2-12), round or oval keratotic plaques with a yellow-brown surface are distributed within the seborrheic areas of the face and trunk. This form of pemphigus foliaceus has been mistakenly called *Senear-Usher syndrome* because of its close resemblance to lupus erythematosus. These patients however, have no evidence of lupus erythematosus on skin biopsies or by serologic studies. These lesions can also become generalized, producing multiple keratotic plaques and nodular lesions.

Histopathology

The French dermatologist, Civatte, described the classic histologic features of pemphigus foliaceus in 1943.[19] He noted that unlike pemphigus vulgaris, where blisters occur just above the basal cell layer of epidermis, pemphigus foliaceus forms blisters at the level of the stratum granulosum. However, it was the Brazilian dermatologist, Vieira, who first described these findings in patients with fogo selvagem in 1937.[20] Unfortunately this report remained unknown because it was written in Portuguese.

The chief histologic feature of both endemic and nonendemic forms of pemphigus foliaceus is the pres-

FIGURE 2-11. **A,** Exfoliative erythroderma in a patient with endemic pemphigus foliaceus. **B,** Extensive crusted lesions on legs of patient with nonendemic pemphigus foliaceus.

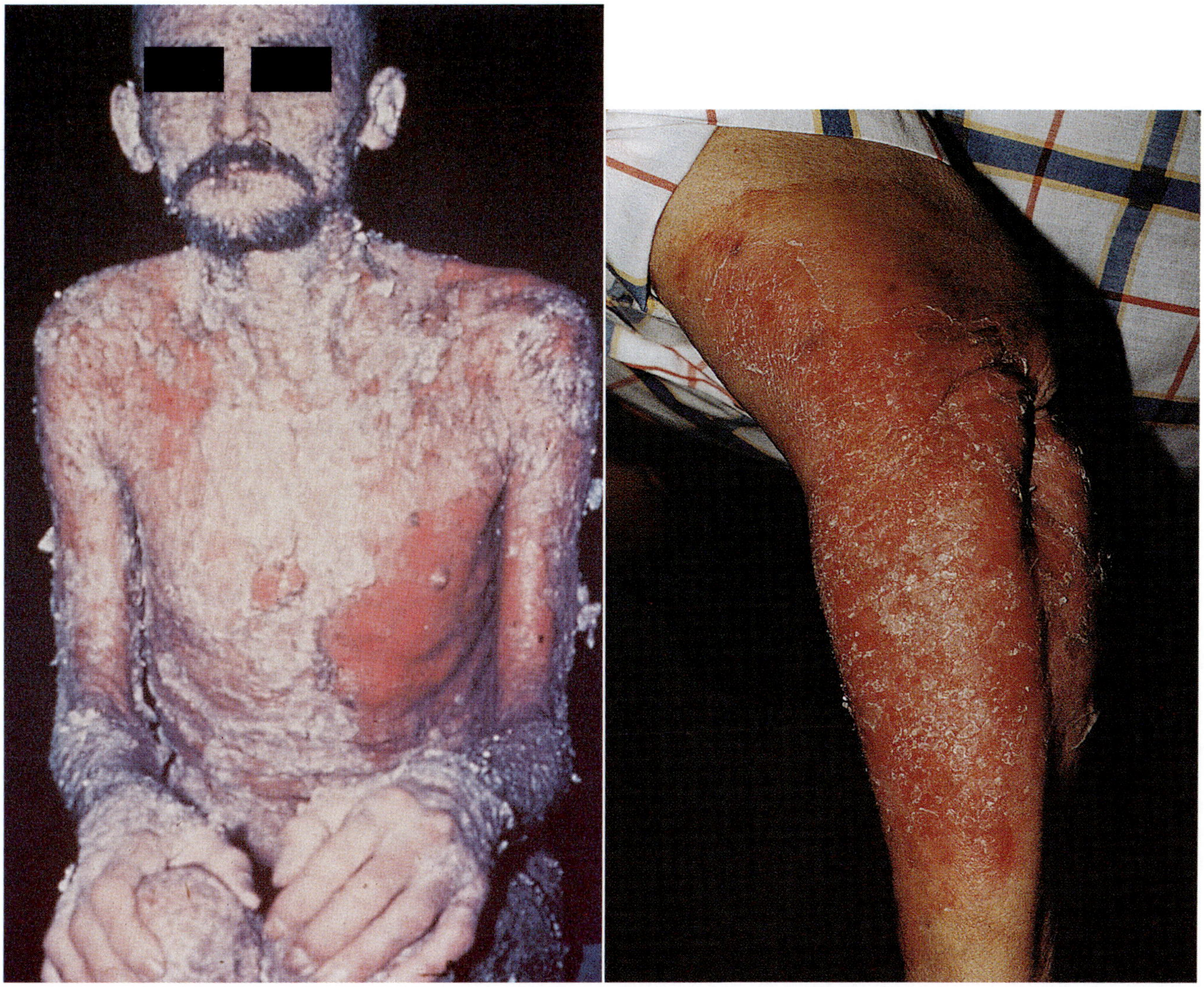

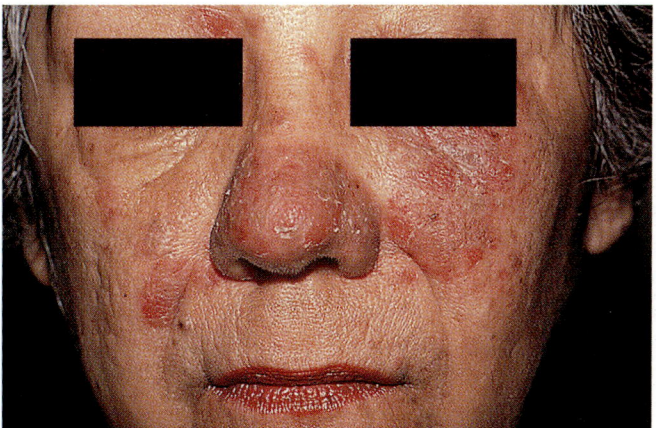

FIGURE 2-12. Facial lesions on patient with nonendemic pemphigus foliaceus.

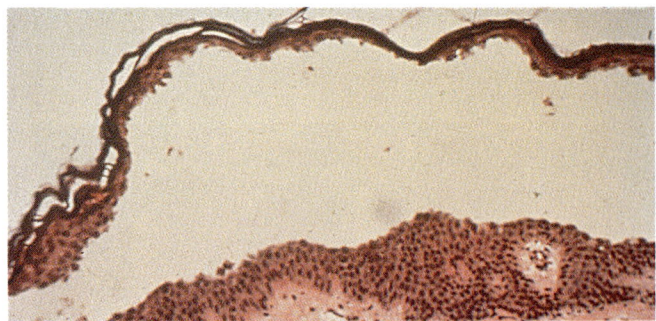

FIGURE 2-13. This photo demonstrates the classic separation within the granulosa layer of the epidermis, resulting in a subcorneal blister.

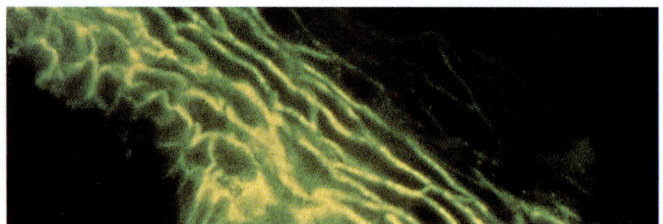

FIGURE 2-14. Indirect IF techniques first demonstrated that patients with pemphigus foliaceus have circulating antibodies directed against the epidermis. Antibodies from the patient are directed against antigenic sites within the epidermis of a normal human skin sample.

ence of vesicles located in the subcorneal region of the epidermis (Figure 2-13). The acantholytic process occurs immediately above, within, or below cells of the stratum granulosum. Although light microscopy reveals acantholysis in the subcorneal layer, electron microscopy (EM) reveals acantholysis affecting keratinocytes in all layers of the epidermis. The cell detachment is visible (with EM) on the lateral surfaces of cells of the basal layer and extends outward toward the stratum spinosum and granulosum. The cell detachment is complete at the level of the granular cell layer. The stratum corneum forms the roof of the vesicle, and the stratum spinosum forms the floor.

Some of the vesicles in pemphigus foliaceus skin lesions may occasionally be filled with neutrophils. In rare situations, eosinophilic spongiosis may be present in some biopsies early or late in the disease.[21] In cases where eosinophilic spongiosis is detected in biopsies of clinically infiltrated inflammatory plaques, the term *pemphigus herpetiformis* has been applied.[22]

Diagnosis

Fogo selvagem may be differentiated from nonendemic pemphigus foliaceus by the epidemiologic features previously mentioned. The absence of oral lesions distinguishes both forms of pemphigus foliaceus from pemphigus vulgaris. Histologic examination helps distinguish early stages of pemphigus foliaceus from other bullous diseases. Subcorneal vesicles favor the diagnosis of pemphigus foliaceus, whereas suprabasilar vesicles are more diagnostic of pemphigus vulgaris, when viewed by light microscopy. Furthermore, direct IF studies of patient's skin biopsies show deposits of IgG in the ICS (Figure 2-14) and indirect IF examination of the patient's serum reveals circulating pemphigus foliaceus autoantibodies. As shown in Table 2-1, fogo selvagem autoanti-

Table 2-1. *Pemphigus Autoantibodies in Fogo Selvagem*

Subjects		Mean Indirect IF Titer
Patients (n: 196)	Localized (n: 31)	160
	Generalized (n: 98)	640
	Unknown form (n: 67)	320
Relatives (n: 138)	Parents (n: 32)	Negative*
	Siblings (n: 57)	Negative
	Offspring (n: 43)	Negative
	Uncles/aunts (n: 2)	Negative
	Cousins/nephews (n: 4)	Negative
Cohabitants (n: 13)	In-laws, other	Negative
Normal controls (n: 38)	Endemic areas	Negative
Normal controls (n: 44)	Nonendemic areas	Negative

*Sera tested at dilutions 1:20, 1:40, and 1:80.

bodies are disease specific and the titers roughly correlate with the extent and activity of the disease.[23] The IF staining pattern produced by pemphigus foliaceus and pemphigus vulgaris serum on squamous epithelium is indistinguishable.

In subepidermal blistering diseases, such as bullous pemphigoid, Herpes gestationis, and linear IgA disease, Nikolsky's sign is negative and serologic studies reveal different autoantibody systems.

Currently, immunoprecipitation and ELISA techniques employing recombinant forms of Dsg1 are sensitive and accurate in detecting autoantibodies in the sera of patients with pemphigus foliaceus. These tests also roughly correlate with the activity and extent of disease and with the titers of autoantibodies in the patient serum.

Therapy

Systemic corticosteroids are the first line of therapy for all forms of pemphigus foliaceus. Before the use of steroids, fewer than 10% of patients with fogo selvagem went into spontaneous remission and 40% died within the first 2 years. Approximately 50% of patients presented with a chronic disease characterized by periodic exacerbations, eventually leading to death. With the advent of steroids the mortality dropped to a current rate of less than 10%.[24] Other immunosuppressive agents, such as azathioprine, cyclophosphamide, and plaquenil, have been used in combination with corticosteroids with good results. Plasmapheresis is a less commonly used modality of treatment. Deaths most commonly occur today as a result of delay in treatment or as a result of complications, such as bacterial or viral infections.

REFERENCES

1. Cazenave P: Pemphigus chronique, general forme rare do pemphigus foliace, *Ann Mal Peu* 1:208-210, 1844.
2. Paes-Leme C: Contribuicao ao estudo do Tokelau, Rio de Janeiro, Brazil, 1903, Tese Facultade de Medicina.
3. Sampaio SA, Rivitti EA, Aoki V, et al: Brazilian pemphigus foliaceus, endemic pemphigus foliaceus, or fogo selvagem (wild fire), *Derm Clinics* 12(4):765-776, 1994.
4. Lombardi C, Borges DC, Chaul F, et al: Environmental risk factors in endemic pemphigus foliaceus (fogo selvagem), *J Invest Dermatol* 98:847-850, 1992.
5. Auad A: Penfigo Foliaceo Sul-Americano no Estado de Goias, *Rev Patol Trop* 1:293-346, 1972.
6. Petzl-Erler ML, Santamaria J. Are HLA class II genes controlling susceptibility and resistance to Brazilian pemphigus foliaceus (fogo selvagem)? *Tissue Antigens* 33:408-411, 1989.
7. Moraes JR, Moraes ME, Fernandez-Vina M, et al: HLA antigens and risk for development of pemphigus foliaceus (fogo selvagem) in endemic areas of Brazil, *Immunogenetics* 33:388-391, 1991.
8. Cerna M, Fernandez-Vina M, Friedman H, et al: Genetic markers for susceptibility to endemic Brazilian pemphigus foliaceus (Fogo Selvagem) in Xavante Indians, *Tissue Antigens* 42:138-140, 1993.
9. Friedman H, Campbell I, Rocha-Alvarez R, et al: Endemic pemphigus foliaceus (fogo selvagem) in native Americans from Brazil, *J Am Acad Dermatol* 32:949-956, 1995.
10. Moraes ME, Fernandez-Vina M, Lazaro A, et al: An epitope in the third hypervariable region of the DRB1 gene is involved in the susceptibility to endemic pemphigus foliaceus (fogo selvagem) in three different Brazilian populations, *Tissue Antigens* 49:35-40, 1997.
11. Gregersen PK, Silver J, Winchester RJ: The shared epitope hypothesis. An approach to understanding the molecular genetics of susceptibility to rheumatoid arthritis, *Arthritis Rheum* 30:1205-1212, 1987.
12. Beutner EH, Jordon RE: Demonstration of skin antibodies in sera of pemphigus vulgaris patients by indirect immunofluorescent staining, *Proc Soc Exptl Biol Med* 117:505-510, 1964.
13. Roscoe JT, Diaz LA, Sampaio SAP, et al: Brazilian pemphigus foliaceus autoantibodies are pathogenic to BALB/c mice by passive transfer, *J Invest Dermatol* 85:538-541, 1985.
14. Koulu L, Kusumi A, Steinberg MS, et al: Human autoantibodies against a desmosomal core protein in pemphigus foliaceus, *J Exp Med* 160:1509-1518, 1984.
15. Wheeler GN, Parker AE, Thomas CL, et al: Desmosomal glycoprotein DG1, a component of intercellular desmosome junctions, is related to the cadherin family of cell adhesion molecules, *Proc Natl Acad Sci USA* 88:4796-4800, 1991.
16. Buxton RS, Wheeler GN, Pidsley SC, et al: Mouse desmocollin (Dsc3) and desmoglein (Dsg1) genes are closely linked in the proximal region of chromosome 18, *Genomics* 21(3):510-516, 1994.
17. Ishii K, Amagai M, Hall RP, et al: Characterization of autoantibodies in pemphigus using antigen-specific enzyme-linked immunosorbent assays with baculovirus-expressed recombinant desmogleins, *J Immun* 159:2010-2017, 1997.
18. Olague-Alcala M, Giudice GJ, Diaz LA: Pemphigus foliaceus sera recognize an N-terminal fragment of bovine desmoglein-1, *J Invest Dermatol* 102:882-885, 1994.
19. Civatte A: Diagnostic histopathologique de la dermatite polymorphe douloureuse ou maldie de Duhring-Brocq, *Ann Dermatol Symph* 3:1-30, 1943.
20. Vieira JP: Novas contribuicoes ao estudo do pemphigo foliaceo (fogo selvagem) no estado de Sao Paulo, Sao Paulo, Brazil, 1937, Empresa Grafica da Revista dos Tribunais.
21. Hoss DM, Shea CR, Grant-Kels JM: Neutrophilic spongiosis in pemphigus, *Arch Dermatol* 132:315-318, 1996.
22. Santi CG, Maruta CW, Aoki V, et al: Pemphigus herpetiform is rare clinical expression of nonendemic pemphigus foliaceus, fogo selvagem, and pemphigus vulgaris, *J Am Acad Dermatol* 34:40-46, 1996.
23. Squiquera HL, Diaz LA, Sampaio SA, et al: Serologic abnormalities in patients with endemic pemphigus foliaceus (fogo selvagem), their relatives, and normal donors from endemic and non-endemic areas of Brazil, *J Invest Dermatol* 91:189-191, 1988.
24. Bystryn JC, Steinman NM: The adjuvant therapy of pemphigus. An update, *Arch Dermatol* 132(12):1518-1519, 1996.

Paraneoplastic Pemphigus

Hossein C. Nousari
Grant J. Anhalt

Etiology

Paraneoplastic pemphigus is an autoimmune mucocutaneous blistering disease that occurs in the context of an occult or known neoplasm.[1] This syndrome meets the following criteria for pemphigus:
1. Acantholysis of mucocutaneous lesions
2. Pemphigus-like antibodies that bind the cell surface of stratified squamous epithelia
3. Pathogenic antibodies, which on transfer into neonatal mice produce acantholytic skin lesions that are indistinguishable from those of pemphigus vulgaris.[1]

Paraneoplastic pemphigus autoantibodies bind other epithelial and nonepithelial tissues that express desmoplakins.[1] The neoplasms associated with paraneoplastic pemphigus fall broadly into the following two categories: B cell neoplasms and thymoma or thymoma-like tumors (e.g., Castleman's disease) (Figure 3-1). Castleman's disease is a rare lymphoproliferative disorder that can be associated with other autoimmune phenomena such as myasthenia gravis and autoimmune cytopenias.[2] Two variants of this disease have been described; one is a localized form (hyaline vascular) and the other a variant that behaves like a lymphoma (multicentric plasma cell).

No definite correlation exists between tumor burden and the activity of the autoimmune disease in cases associated with malignancies.[3] However, if an associated benign tumor is surgically excised, the disease generally improves substantially or goes into complete remission. The etiology of the syndrome is still speculative. Antitumor immune responses may cross-react with normal constitutive proteins of epithelia. This cross-reaction explains the concurrence of apparent humoral- and cell-mediated cytotoxicity involving the epithelium. Treatment with cytokines may induce paraneoplastic pemphigus.[4] Interestingly, patients with Castleman's disease have elevated interleukin (IL)-6,[5] which is a cytokine that has been implicated in the pathogenesis of certain autoimmune diseases. Therefore dysregulated cytokine production by tumor cells may also drive the induction of autoimmunity, raising the possibility of complex neoplasm-immune system interactions.

Clinical Features

Stomatitis remains a constant feature of the disease, and in no cases to date has this been absent. The stomatitis in paraneoplastic pemphigus consists of debilitating and refractory erosions and ulcerations that affect all surfaces of the oropharynx and characteristically extend onto and involve the vermilion of the lips (Figures 3-2 to 3-4). Occasionally, oral lesions are the only manifestation of the disease.[6] The stomatitis is resistant to conventional immunosuppresive therapy. Erosions of other mucosal surfaces can also be observed.[7] The cutaneous lesions of paraneoplastic pemphigus are quite variable and appear to change in the individual patient, according to the stage of the disease. The blisters on the extremities are sometimes quite tense, resembling those seen in bullous pemphigoid (Figure 3-5). A vesicobullous eruption mimicking erythema multiforme may also be seen (Figures 3-6 and 3-7). Lesions on the trunk are sometimes arcuate, resembling those seen in linear IgA bullous disease (Figure 3-8). Despite this heterogeneity, all show acantholytic blistering in histopathology. It has also been observed that lichenoid eruptions are very common and may be the only cutaneous sign of the disease,[8] or may develop in previously blistering lesions. These lesions consist of infiltrated erythematous papules and plaques. In the chronic form of the disease and after treatment, this lichenoid eruption may predominate over blistering on the cutaneous surface (Figure 3-9). Both blisters and lichenoid lesions affecting the palms and the soles are common and help to distinguish this disease from pemphigus vulgaris in which lesions of the palms and soles are very unusual. In addition, some individuals with chronic lichenoid skin lesions also have painful ulcerative paronychial lesions.

Respiratory involvement in paraneoplastic pemphigus has been recently recognized as a severe and usually fatal complication of the disease. This complication is manifested by progressive dyspnea, suggestive of diagnoses such as bronchiolitis obliterans, respiratory distress syndrome, respiratory infections, or pulmonary

PARANEOPLASTIC PEMPHIGUS SUMMARY

ETIOLOGY
Paraneoplastic pemphigus is an autoimmune mucocutaneous blistering disease that occurs in the context of an occult or known neoplasm. Autoantibodies against desmosomal and hemidesmosomal proteins are serologic markers of the syndrome.

CLINICAL FEATURES
A severe stomatitis that characteristically involves the vermilion of the lips is the most consistent clinical finding. Cutaneous involvement can be polymorphic, including vesiculobullous and lichenoid eruptions.

PATHOLOGY
Suprabasilar acantholysis in mucosal and blistering lesions and an interface or lichenoid dermatitis in chronic and nonblistering lesions are seen. Direct IF of perilesional specimens shows IgG and C3 deposition on epithelial cell surfaces and along the BMZ.

DIAGNOSIS
Indirect IF evaluation of patients' sera using murine bladder as a substrate reveals IgG binding epithelial cell surfaces. Demonstration of autoantibodies against the paraneoplastic pemphigus complex through immunoprecipitation. This complex consists of antigens with molecular weight of 250 kD (desmoplakin I), 230 kD (bullous pemphigoid antigen 1), 210 kD (desmoplakin II), 210 kD (envoplakin), 190 kD (periplakin), and 170 kD (unidentified).

DIFFERENTIAL DIAGNOSIS
Pemphigus vulgaris, linear IgA bullous disease, bullous and cicatricial pemphigoid, erythema multiforme, lichen planus, chemotherapy-induced mucositis, and herpes simplex virus infection.

THERAPY
Prognosis is ominous. Therapy includes surgical removal of excisable benign neoplasms or combination prednisone/cyclosporine for disease associated with lymphoreticular malignancies.

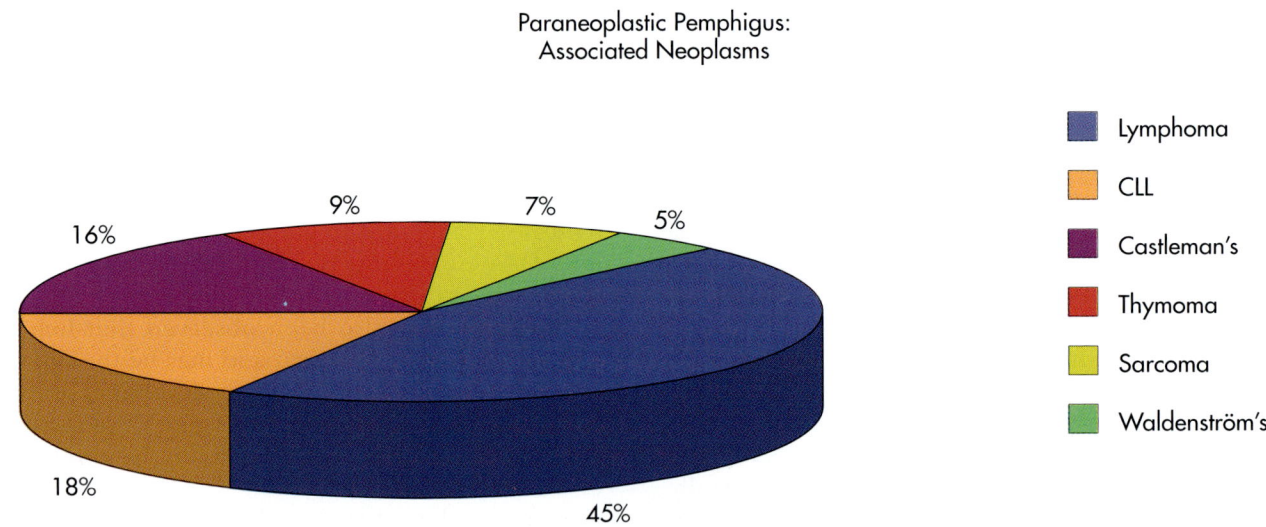

FIGURE 3-1. Tumors associated with paraneoplastic pemphigus. *CLL*, Chronic lymphocytic leukemia.

Chapter 3 *Paraneoplastic Pemphigus* 31

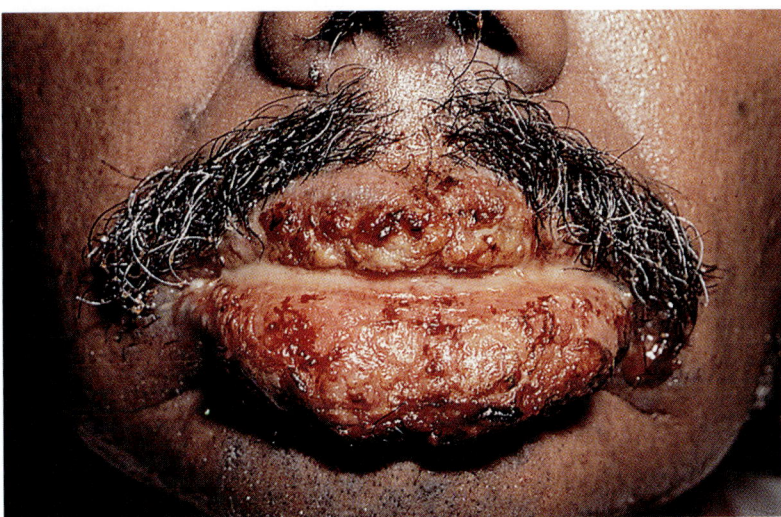

FIGURE 3-2. Extensive crusted erosions involving the vermilion of the lips in a patient presenting with lymphoma-associated paraneoplastic pemphigus.

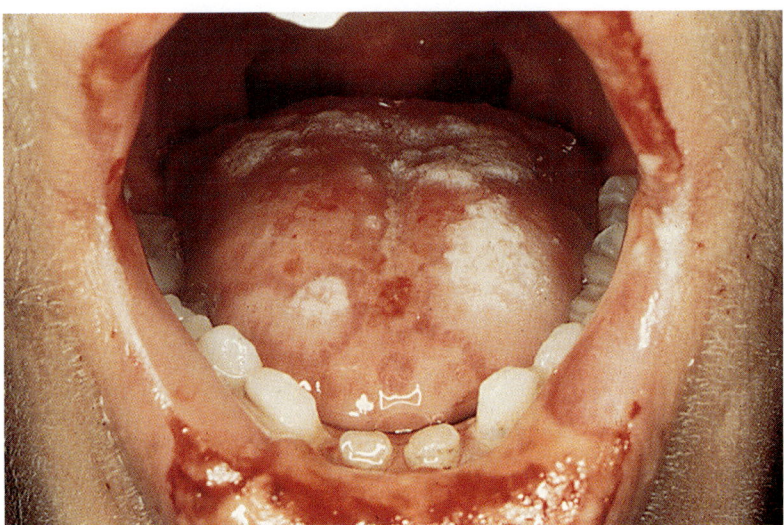

FIGURE 3-3. Stomatitis involving labial mucosa in a patient with paraneoplastic pemphigus.

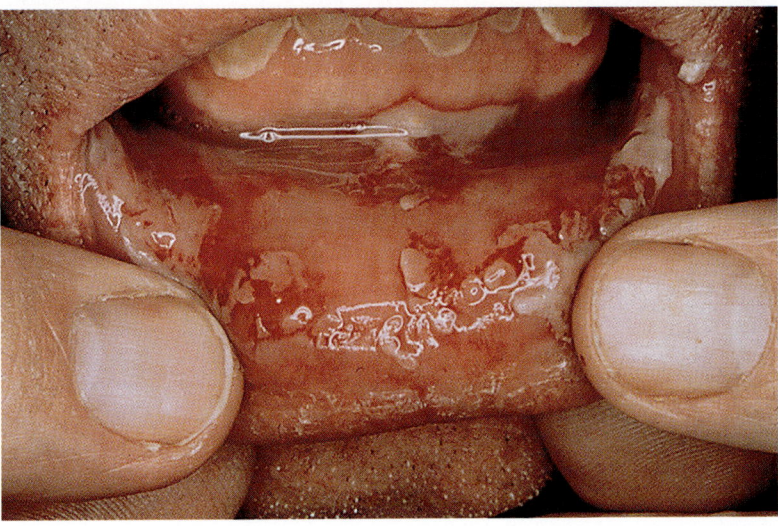

FIGURE 3-4. Erosive stomatitis with tongue involvement in paraneoplastic pemphigus.

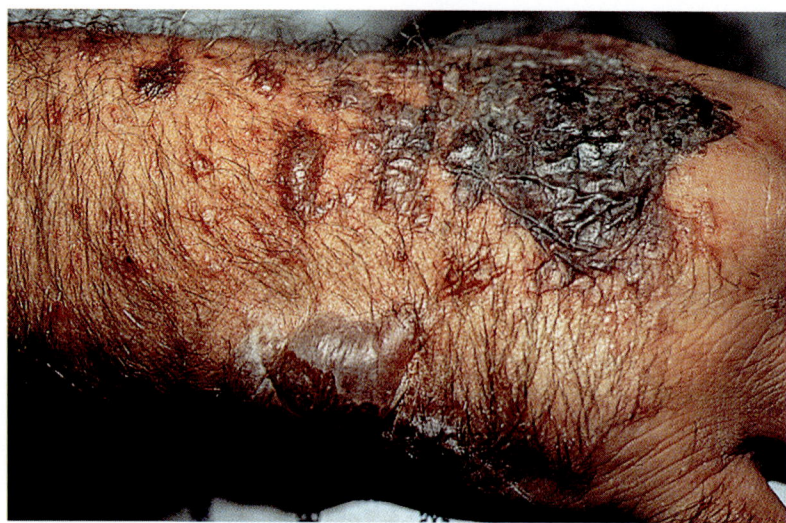

FIGURE 3-5. Bullous pemphigoid-like eruption of a hand in paraneoplastic pemphigus.

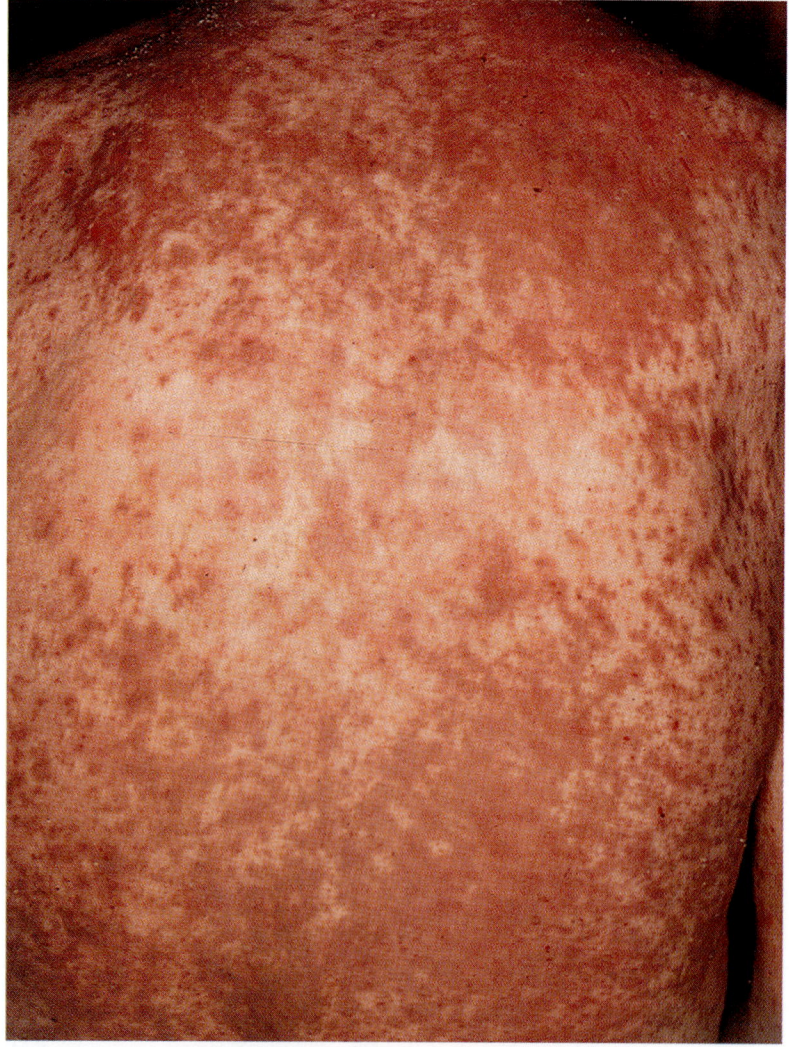

FIGURE 3-6. Erythema multiforme-like eruption on the back of a patient with paraneoplastic pemphigus.

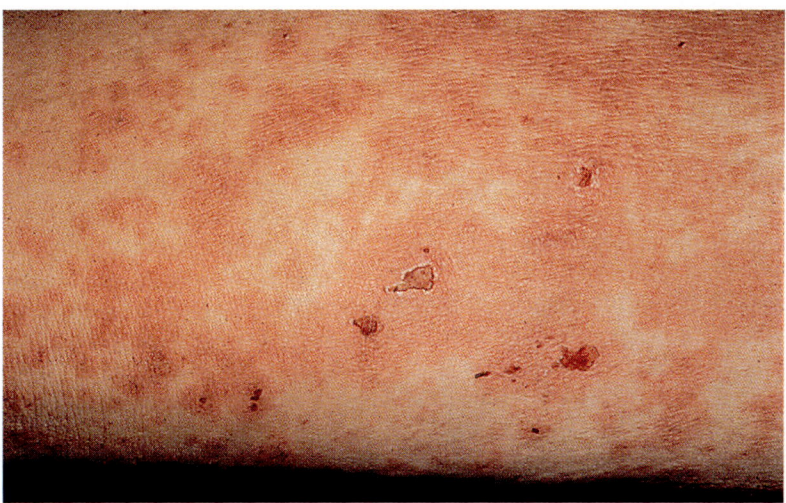

FIGURE 3-7. Erythema multiforme-like eruption on the forearm of a patient with paraneoplastic pemphigus.

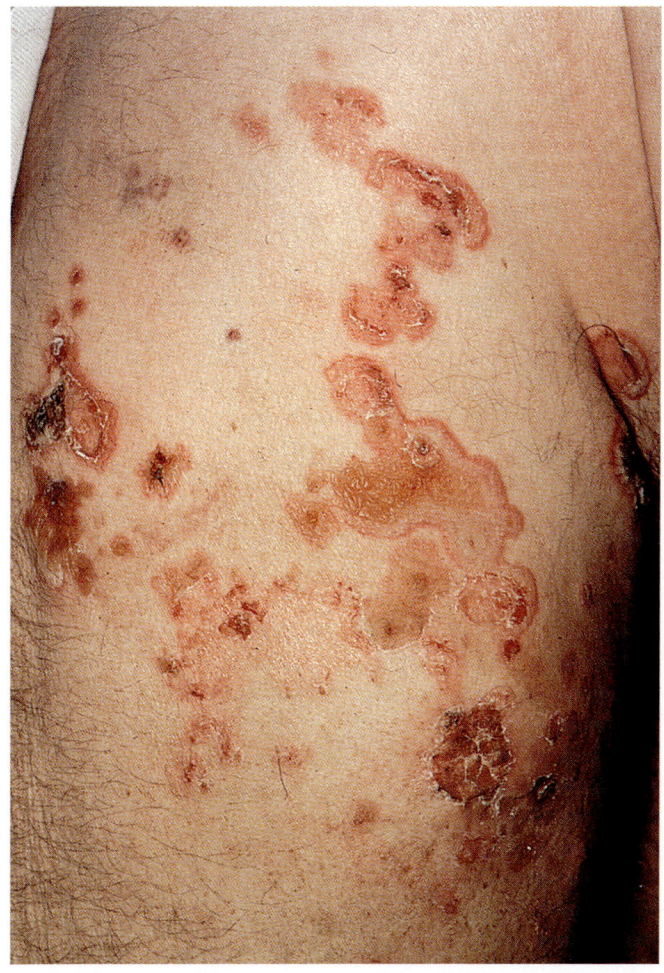

FIGURE 3-8. Circinate blisters mimicking linear IgA bullous disease on the thigh of patient with paraneoplastic pemphigus.

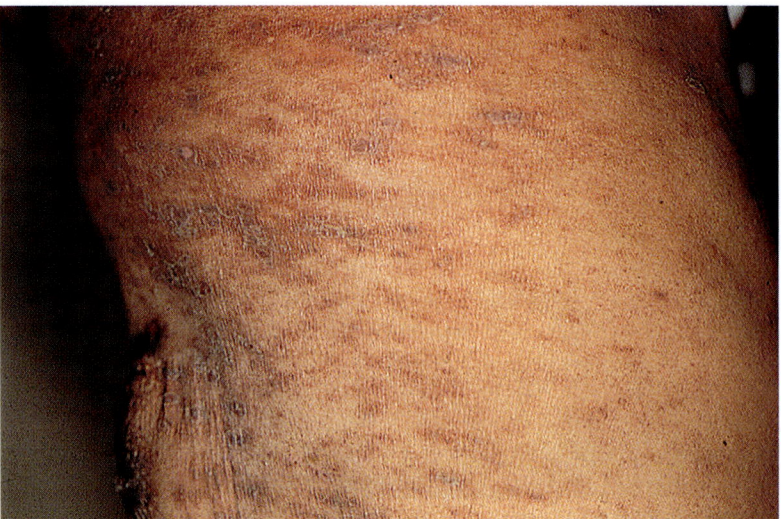

FIGURE 3-9. Lichen planus-like eruption on the arm of patient with paraneoplastic pemphigus.

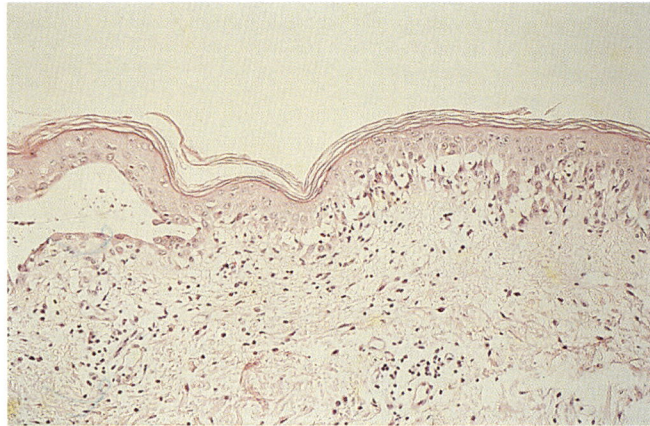

FIGURE 3-10. Suprabasilar acantholysis in a skin biopsy of patient with paraneoplastic pemphigus.

toxicity due to chemotherapy or radiotherapy.[2,3] Endobronchial examination with biopsies from perilesional areas for routine histopathology and immunofluorescence (IF) evaluation should be performed in patients with progressive respiratory symptoms.

Pathology

Histopathologic examination of paraneoplastic pemphigus lesions are as variable as the clinical features of the disease.[9] The stomatitis is severe and extensive, and biopsies from ulcerative lesions often yield nonspecific inflammatory changes. If perilesional mucosal samples are obtained, these biopsies should show suprabasilar acantholysis.

Similarly, biopsies from intact cutaneous blisters reveal suprabasilar acantholysis (Figure 3-10). Unlike other forms of pemphigus, there may be significant inflammatory infiltrates in early lesions. Nonblistering lesions can show individual keratinocyte necrosis with lymphocytic infiltration into the epidermis. These findings are similar to those seen in erythema multiforme or graft versus host disease. In addition, vacuolar interface change with sparse lymphocytic infiltrate of the basilar epithelium can be seen and resembles changes seen in cutaneous lupus erythematosus. The lichenoid skin lesions show areas of dense lymphocytic infiltrate in the upper dermis and individual lymphocytes infiltrating into the epithelium with occasional individual cell necrosis. The histopathologic variability of this disease may be related to the heterogeneous antitumor immune response. It is speculated that both humoral- and cell-mediated immunity play a role in the pathogenesis of the mucocutaneous lesions of paraneoplastic pemphi-

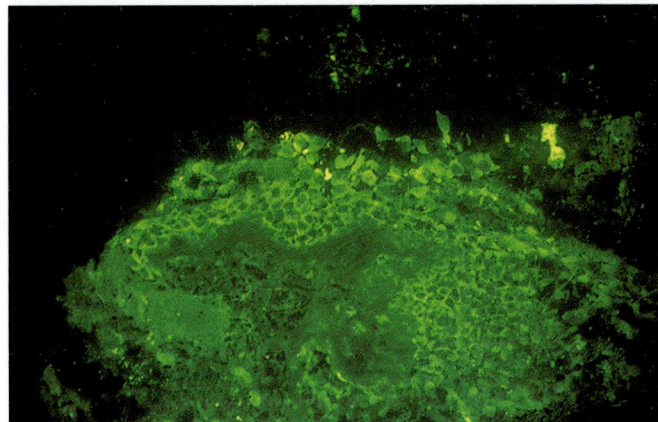

FIGURE 3-11. Direct IF shows linear IgG and patchy deposition on the epithelial cell surfaces and at the BMZ in oral mucosa biopsy of a patient with paraneoplastic pemphigus.

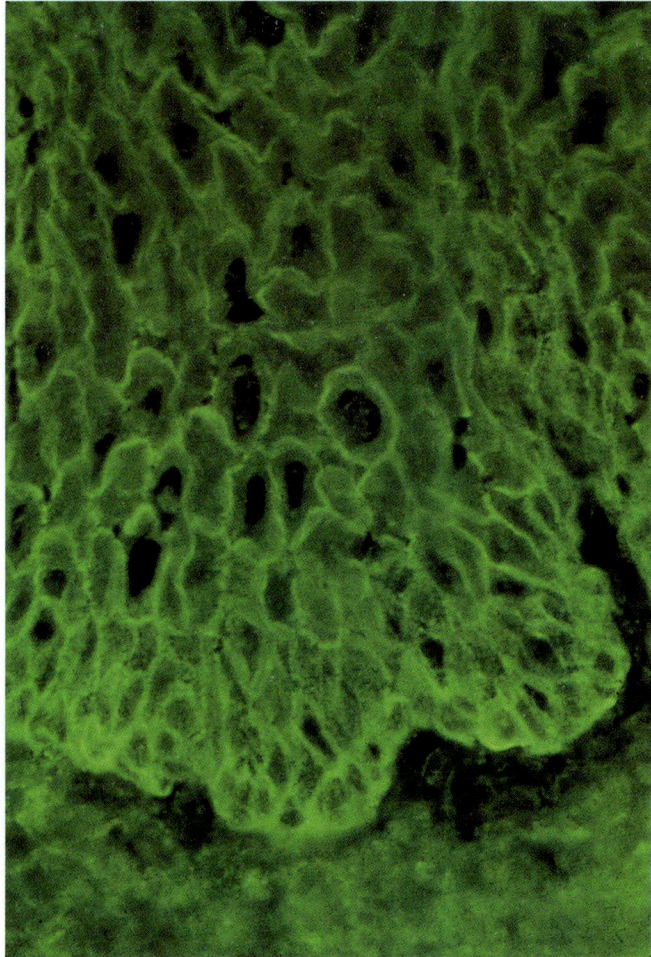

FIGURE 3-12. Indirect IF on monkey esophagus showing binding of paraneoplastic pemphigus autoantibodies to the cell surface and also along the basilar surface of the basal epithelial cells.

gus. This immunity is a unique feature of paraneoplastic pemphigus; humoral-mediated immunity is almost exclusively responsible for the mucocutaneous lesions in pemphigus vulgaris or pemphigus foliaceus.

Passive transfer of autoantibodies from patients with paraneoplastic pemphigus into neonatal mice induces acantholytic cutaneous and oral lesions. Ultrastructural examination of skin lesions of these mice reveals suprabasilar acantholysis and detachment of apical and lateral sides of basal cells of the skin and esophagus, which are findings identical to those seen in pemphigus vulgaris. In acantholytic cells, keratin tonofilaments detach from their insertion into the desmosomes, with subsequent rounding up and clumping of the cytoskeleton in a perinuclear distribution. The lichenoid or vacuolar interface changes that suggest cell-mediated autoimmunity are not induced by immunoglobulin injections. Specifically, only suprabasilar acantholysis without cellular infiltration is seen. No other internal organs are involved, and there is no lymphocytic–mediated cell damage.

Direct IF examination of perilesional biopsy specimens shows immunoglobulin G (IgG) and occasionally C3 deposition on the epithelial cell surfaces. Occasionally, granular/linear IgG and C3 is also found at the basement membrane zone (BMZ) (Figure 3-11). The incidence of false-negative direct IF findings in paraneoplastic pemphigus seems to be higher than in other forms of pemphigus. This incidence could be due to the intracellular location of the paraneoplastic pemphigus antigens and the frequent absence of clinically uninvolved mucosal area where a perilesional biopsy could best be obtained.

Indirect IF evaluation of the sera of patients with paraneoplastic pemphigus reveals the presence of circulating IgG antibodies that bind the cell surfaces of stratified squamous epithelium of monkey esophagus in a pattern that is indistinguishable from that observed in pemphigus vulgaris or foliaceus. However, indirect IF can also show linear immunostaining along the lamina propria (Figure 3-12) and an intense cytoplasmic background fluorescence. Because paraneoplastic pemphigus sera have autoantibodies against proteins of the plakin family, indirect IF performed in desmoplakin-rich tissues reveals a unique immunostaining pattern. For instance, these sera bind to murine bladder epithelium (Figure 3-13), intercalated discs of myocardium (Figure 3-14), and surfaces of hepatocytes (Figure 3-15). The most useful tissue to demonstrate the presence of anti-desmoplakin antibodies is murine blader epithelium. Direct IF evaluation of endobronchial biopsy specimens of patients with paraneoplastic pemphigus that have respiratory involvement reveals IgG deposition on the epithelial cell surfaces and also along the lamina propria.

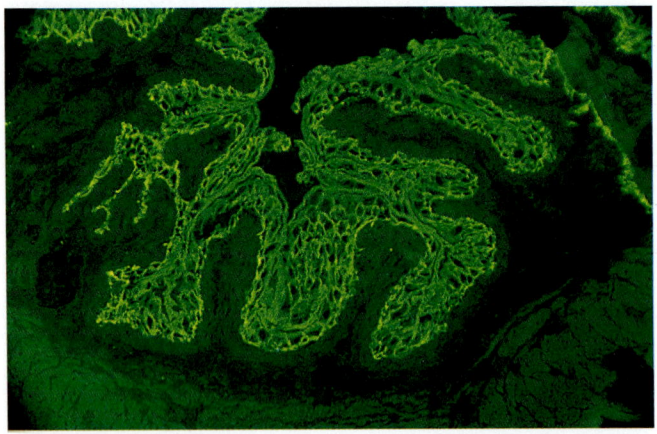

FIGURE 3-13. Indirect IF of paraneoplastic pemphigus autoantibodies on murine bladder showing the typical fluorescent pattern caused by reactivity with desmoplakins in this tissue.

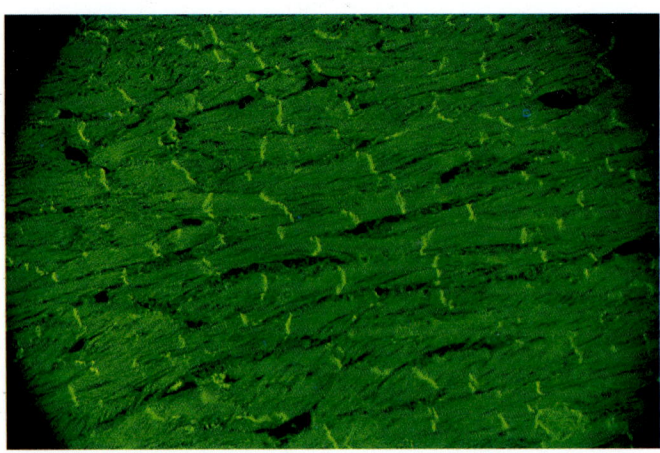

FIGURE 3-14. Indirect IF on murine myocardium showing reactivity with desmoplakins in the intercalated discs.

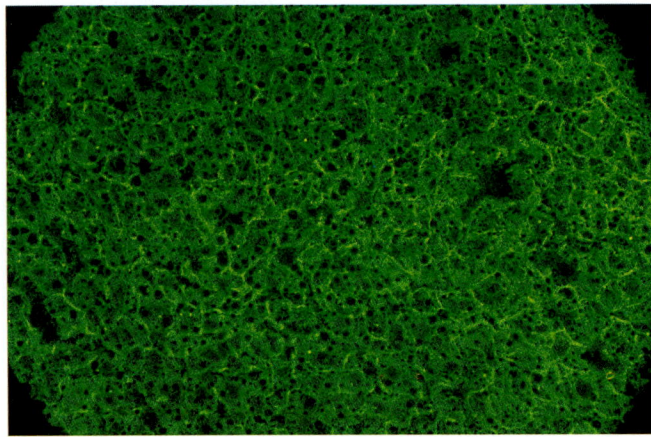

FIGURE 3-15. Indirect IF on murine liver showing reactivity with hepatocyte desmosomes.

BOX 3-1. PARANEOPLASTIC PEMPHIGUS: DIAGNOSTIC CRITERIA

- Mucosal ulcerations and blisters and polymorphous skin lesions in the context of an underlying neoplasm
- Histologic findings of vacuolar interface change, keratinocyte necrosis, and intraepidermal acantholysis
- Deposition of IgG and C3 on epidermal cell surfaces and variably also along the BMZ
- Serum autoantibodies that bind to the cell surfaces of monkey esophagus and also to urinary bladder epithelium
- Serum autoantibodies that recognize antigens of 250 kD, 230 kD, 210 kD, 190 kD, and 170 kD by immunochemical techniques such as immunoprecipitation

Diagnosis

Significant observations have been made since the original diagnostic criteria of the disease (Box 3-1). First, it has been noted that not all patients with paraneoplastic pemphigus fulfill each of these criteria completely. For instance, the cutaneous lesions observed in this disease may be very polymorphic. Blistering lesions may not occur on the skin in some patients. Multiple and repeated mucocutaneous biopsies are sometimes necessary to demonstrate acantholysis in histopathology. Circulating autoantibodies are readily detected, but direct IF of affected skin can occasionally be negative. The diagnosis can currently be established by the following:

1. Characteristic clinical findings are present, including intractable stomatitis.

Table 3-1. *Differentiation of Paraneoplastic Pemphigus from Pemphigus Vulgaris through Indirect IF*

Indirect IF	Monkey esophagus	Murine bladder
Paraneoplastic pemphigus	Positive	Positive
Pemphigus vulgaris	Positive	Negative

2. Biopsy of lesional and perilesional skin shows acantholysis or the other histologic features previously described.
3. IgG autoantibodies bound to the cell surface of affected epithelium are demonstrated. Note that in perilesional biopsies, false negative direct IF results are more common than in pemphigus vulgaris, and repeated biopsies may be necessary to establish the diagnosis. A combination of both cell-surface and BMZ deposition of IgG and complement components may be seen, resulting from the cross-reactivity of autoantibodies with desmoplakins and the BP230 antigen.
4. Circulating IgG "pemphigus-like" autoantibodies should be found in the serum. Circulating antibodies of pemphigus vulgaris can be distinguished from those in paraneoplastic pemphigus by using nonstratified squamous epithelia as a substrate for indirect IF.[1,10] The rationale for this test is based on the knowledge that patients with paraneoplastic pemphigus have autoantibodies that are reactive with the desmoplakins, which are desmosomal plaque proteins that are present in all epithelia and in some nonepithelial structures such as the intercalated discs of myocardium. On the contrary, pemphigus vulgaris and pemphigus foliaceus antigens (desmogleins 3 and 1, respectively) are expressed only in stratified squamous epithelia. Therefore if serum is tested by indirect IF on monkey esophagus (stratified squamous epithelia) and rodent urinary bladder epithelium (transitional epithelia), the anti-desmoplakin antibodies from patients with paraneoplastic pemphigus react with desmoplakins present in both substrates. Sera from patients with pemphigus vulgaris and pemphigus foliaceus is positive on monkey esophagus but does not react with bladder epithelium where desmogleins are not present (Table 3-1). This test is imperfect, and both false-positive and false-negative results do occur. The sensitivity and specificity of this serologic test is estimated at 75% and 83%, respectively.

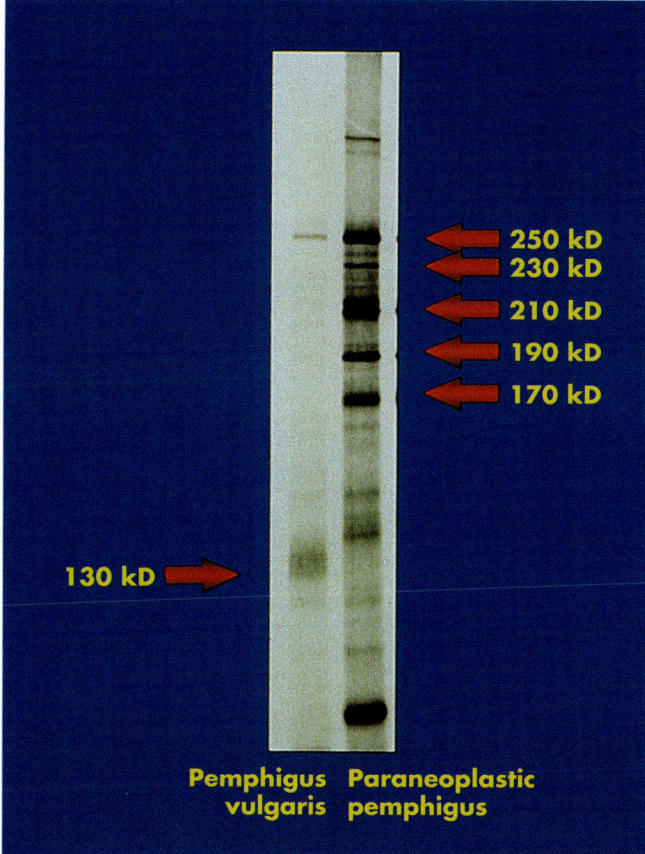

FIGURE 3-16. Immunoprecipitation, showing the differentiation of pemphigus vulgaris from paraneoplastic pemphigus. Pemphigus vulgaris antibodies recognize only the 130-kD desmoglein 3 molecule, whereas paraneoplastic pemphigus antibodies recognize the characteristic high molecular weight antigen complex, consisting of related proteins of the plakin family and the still unidentified 170-kD antigen.

5. The "gold standard" for diagnosis is identification of the characteristic antigen complex by serum autoantibodies, as shown by immunoprecipitation.[1,10] This test defines the antigen specificity of the reactivity at the molecular level and clearly differentiates the antibodies reacting with 130-kD pemphigus vulgaris antigen from the complex of high molecular weight antigens recognized by patients with paraneoplastic pemphigus (Figure 3-16). Immunoprecipitation for detection of these paraneoplastic pemphigus autoantibodies is a very specific and sensitive test; however, it is rather expensive, involves the use of radioisotopes, and has very limited availability at the present time. Western immunoblotting can be substituted for immunoprecipitation but has limitations. In immunoblotting, the only antigens that are reliably detected are 210-kD (envoplakin) and 190-kD

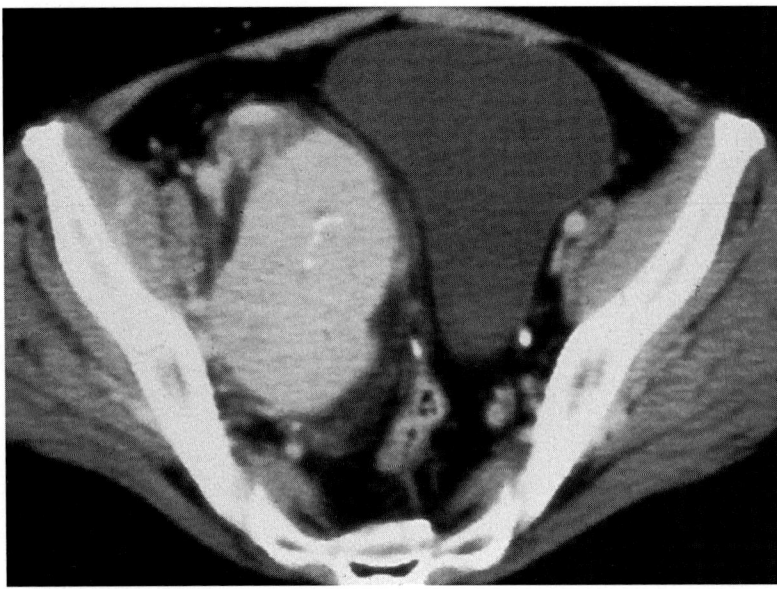

FIGURE 3-17. CT of the pelvis showing an occult retroperitoneal tumor in a patient with paraneoplastic pemphigus.

BOX 3-2. **MOLECULAR WEIGHTS AND ANTIGENS OF THE PARANEOPLASTIC PEMPHIGUS COMPLEX**

250 kD:	desmoplakin I
230 kD:	bullous pemphigoid antigen 1
210 kD:	desmoplakin II (upper band of doublet)
	envoplakin (lower band of doublet)
190 kD:	periplakin
170 kD:	unidentified

(periplakin) polypeptides.[11] The other bands are not detected, presumably because they are denatured in the immunoblotting procedure.

Affected patients have polyclonal IgG autoantibodies against a unique complex of high molecular weight antigens (250 kD, 230 kD, 210 kD, 190 kD, and 170 kD)[16] (Box 3-2). The autoantibody specificity of the disease is remarkably consistent. The 250-kD antigen represents desmoplakin I, a desmosomal plaque protein. The 210-kD antigen is commonly seen as a doublet band, in which the slower migrating band corresponds to desmoplakin II, a related desmosomal plaque protein, and the faster migrating band is envoplakin, a precursor of the epidermal cornified envelope cell that also belongs to the family of plakin proteins.[12] The 230-kD antigen is the bullous pemphigoid antigen 1 (BPAG1, BP230 kD), a major hemidesmosome plaque protein that has approximately 30% homology with desmoplakin I. The 190-kD antigen has been recently identified as another protein of the "plakin family," called *periplakin*.[13] The definitive identity of the 170-kD antigen remains unknown. Autoantibodies against the 170-kD antigen are present in almost all paraneoplastic pemphigus sera.[16] This antigen may be a novel epidermal adhesion molecule and may be very important in the actual pathogenesis of blistering, but proof is lacking.

The majority of paraneoplastic pemphigus cases occur in patients with a known neoplasm. However, in about a third of the cases, there are no known neoplastic lesions at the time the mucocutaneous eruption develops. Since only a small number of lymphoreticular malignancies are associated with the syndrome, investigations for occult lesions can be directed and efficient. In cases with associated occult lymphoma, malignancies are usually found in periaortic, abdominal, or retroperitoneal lymph nodes. Chronic lymphocytic leukemia (CLL) is always associated with abnormal circulating B cells. Castleman's disease in its localized form usually arises as a solitary tumor in the chest, abdominal retroperitoneal space, or occasionally behind or around the urinary bladder (Figure 3-17). Diffuse Castleman's disease has a similar distribution to abdominal lymphomas. Castleman's disease is essentially the only neoplasm found in patients with paraneoplastic pemphigus under the age of 20 years (Figure 3-18). Thus this neoplasm is highly suspect in this patient population. Thymomas are found usually in the anterior mediastinum, and Waldenström's macroglob-

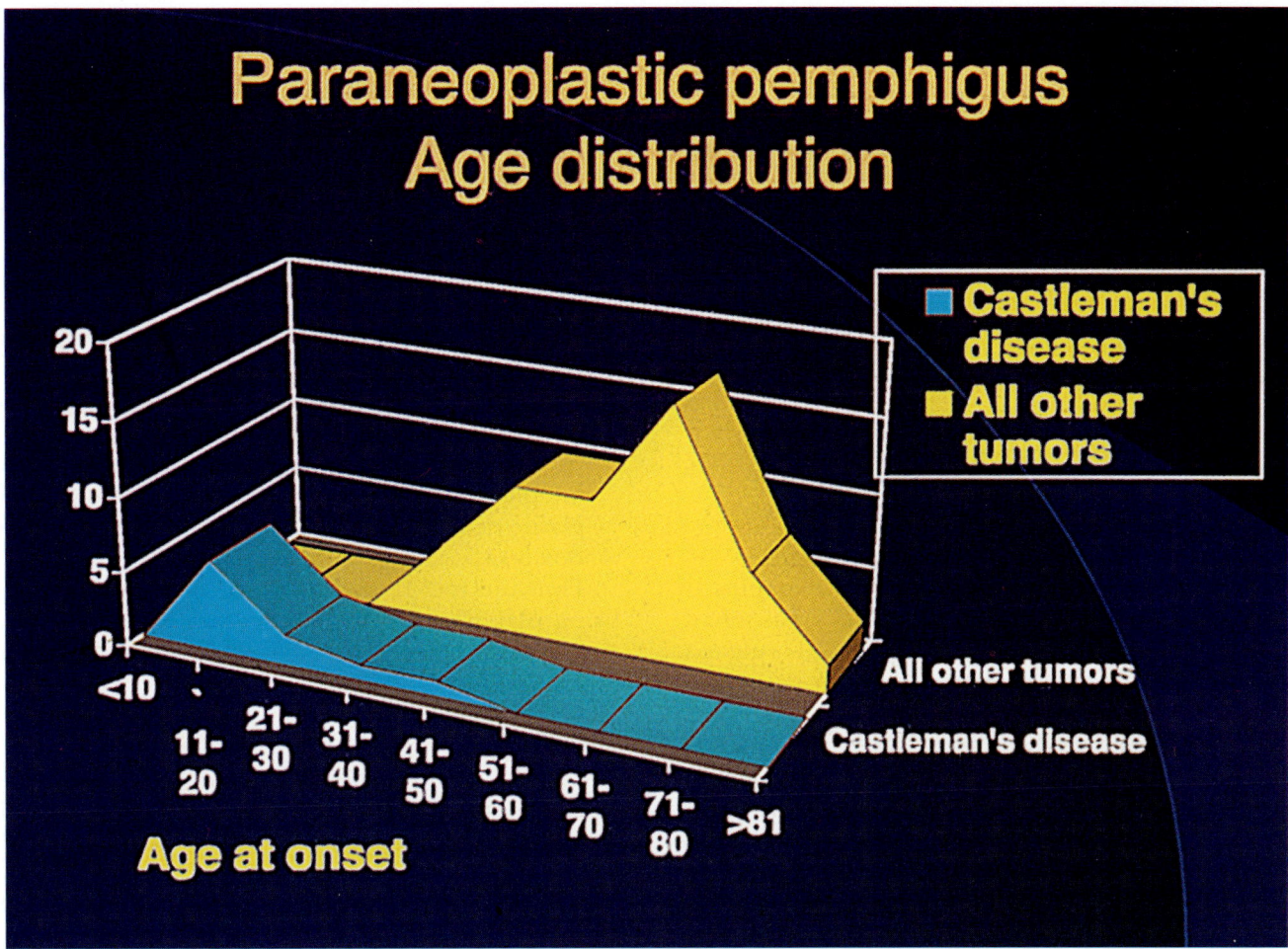

FIGURE 3-18. Incidence of tumors associated with paraneoplastic pemphigus by age groups. Castleman's disease occurs almost exclusively in patients with paraneoplastic pemphigus under the age of 30. In older age groups, CLL and non-Hodgkin's lymphoma are the predominant associated neoplasms.

ulinemia is detected by finding a monoclonal increase in serum IgM. Finally, the three cases of sarcomas associated with paraneoplastic pemphigus have all been located in the abdominal retroperitoneal cavity[2] and may be true follicular dendritic cell sarcomas, which arise from the antigen-presenting follicular cells of abdominal lymph nodes. The most frequently effective examinations are computed tomography (CT) scans of chest, abdomen, and pelvis, peripheral blood smears, and serum gamma-globulin measurements. The short list of potentially associated neoplasms makes the investigation of such cases relatively quick and efficient (Box 3-3), and at present there is no indication for doing other invasive tests, e.g., gastrointestinal tract endoscopy, imaging of other body areas, or more expensive imaging tests such as magnetic resonance imaging (MRI).

BOX 3-3. RECOMMENDED INVESTIGATIONS FOR SUSPECT PARANEOPLASTIC PEMPHIGUS

- Biopsy skin or mucosa for H&E, direct IF*; serum for indirect IF
- Serum for immunoprecipitation (most reliable laboratory test)
- CBC, LDH, chemistry panel, serum protein electrophoresis
- Examination of liver, spleen, lymph nodes
- CT of chest, abdomen, and pelvis

H&E, Hematoxylin-eosin; *CBC*, complete blood count; *LDH*, lactate dehydrogenase.
*Some false-negative results with direct IF expected.

> **BOX 3-4. INITIAL DIAGNOSES APPLIED TO PATIENTS WITH PARANEOPLASTIC PEMPHIGUS**
>
> Pemphigus vulgaris
> Erythema multiforme/toxic epidermal necrolysis
> Atypical pemphigus foliaceus
> Chemotherapy-induced mucositis
> Herpes simplex virus stomatitis
> Lichen planus or lichenoid eruptions
> Cicatricial and bullous pemphigoid
> Linear IgA bullous disease

Differential Diagnoses

Before the definition of the paraneoplastic pemphigus syndrome by immunochemical techniques, cases had been assigned diagnoses such as pemphigus vulgaris associated with a neoplasm, concomitant erythema multiforme and pemphigus, and concomitant lichen planus and pemphigus vulgaris. Other diagnoses applied include the coexistence of pemphigus and pemphigoid, pemphigus erythematosus, atypical pemphigus foliaceus, stomatitis due to chemotherapy, persistent herpes simplex virus infection, linear IgA bullous disease, and cicatricial pemphigoid (Box 3-4). Paraneoplastic erythema multiforme has been reported; in retrospect, many of these cases may have been misdiagnosed cases of paraneoplastic pemphigus. Erythema multiforme is usually an acute event or a chronic but relapsing and remitting disease. Thus chronic persistent erythema multiforme major would be the variant that could mimic paraneoplastic pemphigus clinically. However, this form of erythema multiforme is extremely rare and associated with chronic herpes simplex virus or Epstein-Barr virus infection in immunocompromised patients. Viral cultures, immunohistochemistry, and polymerase chain reaction readily diagnose herpes virus infection in biopsies. In a group of patients with erythema multiforme major, autoantibodies against desmoplakins have been identified, but antibodies against other components of the paraneoplastic pemphigus complex were not found.[14] These patients were immunocompetent with no underlying malignancy or demonstrable herpes virus infection.

Adequate perilesional specimens for direct evaluation and conventional indirect IF for circulating antibodies would distinguish and differentiate the majority of autoimmune–mediated blistering diseases from paraneoplastic pemphigus with a high degree of accuracy. However, pemphigus vulgaris is the most important diagnosis to rule out, since its clinical and immunohistochemical features can be very similar to paraneoplastic pemphigus. Clinical signs that would raise the suspicion of paraneoplastic pemphigus include the following:

1. "Oral pemphigus" with severe stomatitis involving the vermilion of the lip (can be seen in pemphigus vulgaris but is rather uncommon)
2. "Pemphigus vulgaris" in unusual age groups (very young or elderly patients)
3. "Pemphigus vulgaris" refractory to conventional therapy
4. "Pemphigus vulgaris" characterized by polymorphic and especially lichenoid cutaneous lesions
5. "Pemphigus vulgaris" in patients with preexisting neoplasms known to be associated with paraneoplastic pemphigus such as lymphoma and CLL (see Box 3-1).

Thus indirect IF evaluation of these patient's sera using plakin-rich tissues and confirmation with immunoprecipitation should be performed in these clinical scenarios.

Therapy

The majority of patients with benign thymoma or localized Castleman's disease (hyaline vascular type) who had these tumors surgically excised experienced either substantial improvement or complete remission of the disease.[2]

In patients with malignant neoplasms, there is no consensus regarding a therapeutic regimen that is consistently effective. The majority of patients with malignancies die in a period of 1 month to 2 years after diagnosis, either from complications of the syndrome or from its treatment. The causes of death in patients with paraneoplastic pemphigus have been attributed to multiple factors, including sepsis, gastrointestinal bleeding, "multiorgan failure," and respiratory failure. Paraneoplastic pemphigus autoantibodies reacting against plakins of the respiratory epithelium may be responsible in some cases of respiratory failure[3]; respiratory involvement is an ominous prognostic sign. Some long-term survivors have been reported, but this is an unusual event.

Oral corticosteroids produce only partial improvement. Cutaneous lesions respond more quickly, but the stomatitis is generally refractory to any form of therapy. Many other agents have been used on an anecdotal basis with inconsistent results (Box 3-5). Some patients may respond to a combination of prednisone and cyclosporine.[15] Intravenous cyclophosphamide, either by conventional pulse dosing or ablative high-dose infusion, seems to be a promising form of treatment.

BOX 3-5. THERAPY OF PARANEOPLASTIC PEMPHIGUS

- Excision of surgically amenable tumors, e.g., Castleman's disease (hyaline vascular and localized forms of the plasma cell type), thymomas, sarcomas
- Prednisone (0.5 to 1 mg/kg/day), alone or in conjunction with cyclosporine (5 mg/kg/day)
- Intravenous cyclophosphamide: conventional pulse (500-750 mg/dose) or ablative high-dose infusion (200 mg/kg given as 50 mg/kg/day for 4 consecutive days)
- Additional, variably effective therapies include oral cyclophosphamide, azathioprine, dapsone, plasmapheresis, immunoapheresis, photopheresis, intravenous immunoglobulins

References

1. Anhalt GJ, Kim S-C, Stanley JR, et al: Paraneoplastic pemphigus. An autoimmune mucocutaneous disease associated with neoplasia, *N Engl J Med* 323:1729-1735, 1990.
2. Anhalt GJ: Paraneoplastic pemphigus, *Adv Dermatol* 12:77-96, 1997.
3. Fullerton SH, Woodley DT, Smoller B, et al: Paraneoplastic pemphigus with immune deposits in bronchial epithelium, *JAMA* 267:1550-1502, 1992.
4. Kirsner RS, Anhalt GJ, Kerdel FA: Treatment with alpha interferon associated with the development of paraneoplastic pemphigus, *Br J Dermatol* 132:474-478, 1995.
5. Beck JT, Hsu SM, Wijdenes J, et al: Alleviation of systemic manifestations of Castleman's disease by monoclonal anti-interleukin-6 antibody, *N Engl J Med* 330:602-605, 1994.
6. Bialy-Golan A, Brenner S, Anhalt GJ: Paraneoplastic pemphigus: Oral involvement as the sole manifestation, *Acta Derm Venereol (Stockh)* 76:253-254, 1996.
7. Meyers SJ, Varley GA, Meisler DM, et al: Conjunctival involvement in paraneoplastic pemphigus, *Am J Ophthalmol* 114:621-624, 1992.
8. Stevens SR, Griffiths CE, Anhalt GJ, et al: Paraneoplastic pemphigus presenting as a lichen planus pemphigoides-like eruption, *Arch Dermatol* 129:866-869, 1993.
9. Horn TD, Anhalt GJ: Histologic features of paraneoplastic pemphigus, *Arch Dermatol* 128:1091-1095, 1991.
10. Helou J, Allbritton J, Anhalt GJ: Accuracy of indirect immunofluorescent testing in the diagnosis of paraneoplastic pemphigus, *J Am Acad Dermatol* 32:441-447, 1995.
11. Hashimoto T, Amagai M, Watanabe K, et al: Characterization of paraneoplastic pemphigus autoantigens by immunoblot analysis, *J Invest Dermatol* 104:829-834, 1995.
12. Kim S-C, Kwon YD, Lee IJ, et al: cDNA cloning of the 210 kDa paraneoplastic pemphigus antigen reveals that envoplakin is a component of the antigen complex, *J Invest Dermatol* 109:365-369, 1997.
13. Mahoney MG, Aho S, Uitto J, et al: The members of the plakin family of proteins recognized by paraneoplastic pemphigus antibodies include periplakin, *J Invest Dermatol* 111(2):308-313, 1998.
14. Foedinger D, Anhalt GJ, Boecskoer B, et al: Autoantibodies to desmoplakin I and II in patients with erythema multiforme, *J Exp Med* 181:169-179, 1995.
15. Stahle-Bacdahl M, Hedblad M-A, Skoglund C, et al: Paraneoplastic pemphigus: A report of two patients responding to cyclosporin, *Eur J Dermatol* 5:671-675, 1995.
16. Oursler JR, Labib RS, Ariss-Abdo L, et al: Human autoantibodies against desmoplakins in paraneoplastic pemphigus, *J Clin Invest* 89:1775-1782, 1992.

Bullous Pemphigoid

Javier Alonso-Llamazares
Margot S. Peters
Kristin M. Leiferman

Etiology

Bullous pemphigoid is an autoimmune blistering disorder in which antibodies with specificity for antigens of hemidesmosomal proteins in stratified squamous epithelia[1] circulate in the peripheral blood and bind to basement membrane zone (BMZ). Although the definitive etiopathogenesis is not known, various aspects of the disease have been elucidated over the last half-century (Table 4-1). In 1953, Lever[2] defined the major groups of bullous diseases according to clinical and histologic parameters. Blister formation in bullous pemphigoid was related to detachment of the basal epidermal cells from the BMZ. Twelve years later, on the basis of immunofluorescence (IF) studies, Beutner et al reported the detection of circulating antibodies directed against the epidermal BMZ, and Jordon et al[3] demonstrated the presence of IgG and C3 bound to the dermal-epidermal junction in skin from patients with this disease. Subsequently, immunoelectron microscopic studies localized the site of autoantibody binding in bullous pemphigoid to the hemidesmosomal plaques of basal keratinocytes.

Immunoprecipitation and immunoblotting techniques on extracts of cultured basal keratinocytes have been used to further characterize the target antigen(s) for the autoantibodies in this disorder. Although marked antigenic heterogeneity has been observed using bullous pemphigoid sera in immunoblotting studies, most patients have circulating antibodies to a 230-kD protein, the major bullous pemphigoid antigen, BP230, a component of the hemidesmosomal plaque. Approximately 30% of sera also recognize a 180-kD protein, the minor bullous pemphigoid antigen, BP180, a transmembrane glycoprotein attached to the hemidesmosomal plaque.[4] Recently, cloning of both the 230-kD and 180-kD proteins has been accomplished, allowing a better understanding of the structure and function of the dermal-epidermal junction. In addition, experimental studies using passive transfer of rabbit antibodies to BP180 into neonatal BALB/c mice have reproduced the macroscopic morphologic changes and microscopic histologic findings of dermal-epidermal separation that characterize this condition.[5] However, what provokes the onset of the disease is unknown and the mechanism of blister formation is still not understood. A flow diagram of the hypothetic etiopathogenesis of bullous pemphigoid is shown in Figure 4-1.

The presence of antibody alone in either the acquired human disease or in animal models of bullous pemphigoid does not result in blister formation. Complement deposition is found at the BMZ, and its detection contributes to diagnosis of the disease. Activation of the classic complement pathway with alternative pathway amplification occurs at the BMZ, and the membrane-attack complex (C5 to C9) has been demonstrated in lesions. Immunoglobulin subclass typing has shown that immunoglobulin G4 (IgG4) is the most common type found both in serum and tissue from patients with bullous pemphigoid, although other immunoglobulin subclasses may be found. Paradoxically, this immunoglobulin does not have complement-fixing activity, and its significance, as well as the role of complement, in the disease is also unclear.[5,6]

In the murine model of bullous pemphigoid in which neonatal BALB/c mice were injected with rabbit anti-BP180 IgG,[5] histologic examination of lesions showed subepidermal vesicle formation with focal neutrophil infiltration in blister cavities and in the dermis near blisters. Lesion formation in this model has been shown to depend on complement activation and neutrophil recruitment; infiltrating neutrophils are activated via molecular interaction between the Fc receptor and the tissue-bound IgG. The release of neutrophil elastase appears to mediate the BMZ separation leading to subepidermal blister formation. Systemic treatment of BALB/c mice with neutralizing antibodies to interleukin-1 (IL-1) or IL-6 blocks the pathogenic effects of the anti-BP180 IgG, suggesting that IL-1 and IL-6 are inflammatory mediators important for subepidermal blister formation in this animal model.

BULLOUS PEMPHIGOID SUMMARY

ETIOLOGY
Bullous pemphigoid is an acquired immunobullous disease of unknown etiology. Autoantibodies are produced primarily to two BMZ antigens with molecular weights of 230 kD (major bullous pemphigoid antigen in >90% of patients) and 180 kD (minor bullous pemphigoid antigen in approximately 30% of patients), which are protein components of hemidesmosomal plaques of basal keratinocytes.

CLINICAL FEATURES
Tense blisters and urticarial plaques with a predisposition for flexural areas develop on skin of elderly patients; mucosa may also be involved but not as debilitating or severe as in pemphigus.

PATHOLOGY
Subepidermal bullae contain an inflammatory cell infiltrate characterized by eosinophils, which are also found along the BMZ, within the epidermis (eosinophilic spongiosis) and in the dermis.

DIAGNOSIS
Immunohistopathogic studies, including direct IF of tissue showing linear BMZ deposition of IgG and C3 and indirect IF demonstrating the presence of circulating BMZ. IgG antibodies that bind to the epidermal component of salt-split human skin are needed to support the clinical diagnosis.

TREATMENT
Topical glucocorticoids may suffice for localized disease, sulfones or antibiotics may be used for limited disease, and systemic glucocorticoids alone or combined with nonsteroidal immunosuppressive agents are indicated for extensive disease.

DIFFERENTIAL DIAGNOSIS
Epidermolysis bullosa acquisita, linear IgA bullous dermatosis, dermatitis herpetiformis, and bullous LE are among the diagnostic considerations.

Table 4-1. *Historical Perspective of Bullous Pemphigoid*

AUTHOR(S)	YEAR(S)	DISCOVERY
Lever WF	1953-1965	Clinical and histologic descriptions differentiate pemphigoid and pemphigus
Beutner E, Jordon RE, et al	1965-1967	Demonstration of autoantibodies in circulation and bound to the dermal-epidermal junction
Stanley JR et al	1981	Characterization of the 230-kD bullous pemphigoid antigen by immunoprecipitation
Mutasim DF et al	1985	Ultrastructural localization of bullous pemphigoid antigen to the hemidesmosomal plaque
Labib RS et al	1986	Identification of the 180-kD bullous pemphigoid antigen by immunoblotting
Stanley JR et al	1988-1993	Cloning of complementary DNA for human 230-kD bullous pemphigoid antigen
Giudice GJ, Diaz LA, et al	1990-1992	Cloning of complementary DNA for human 180-kD bullous pemphigoid antigen
Liu Z et al	1993-1995	Animal model of bullous pemphigoid developed and investigated

An *in vitro* model for bullous pemphigoid, using normal human skin tissue incubated with bullous pemphigoid sera, complement, and peripheral blood leukocytes, demonstrated that dermal-epidermal separation did not occur without the presence of leukocytes. Granulocyte involvement in blister formation is additionally supported by the findings of increased eosinophil granule proteins and neutrophil myeloperoxidase in blister fluid and in sera from patients with bullous pemphigoid. Hypogranulated mast cells, intact and degenerating eosinophils, and macrophages have been observed in areas beneath the epidermal BMZ in human bullous pemphigoid lesions; epidermal basal cell and lamina densa separation was associated with macrophage and eosinophil accumulation at the dermal-epidermal junction and migration through the basal lamina. In these studies, the presence of peroxidase-positive lysosomes and granules from eosinophils and neutrophils along the lamina lucida suggests that they contributed to separation. As the activities of products from granulocytes have been defined, their presence adds further support for their involvement in the disease process. For example, a 92-kD gelatinase produced by eosinophils cleaves the extracellular domain of BP180 and has been identified at the site of blister formation in bullous pemphigoid. Analyses of eosinophil infiltration in developing lesions of bullous pemphigoid showed degenerating eosinophils with deposition of eosinophil granule proteins in areas of BMZ separation, as well as eosinophils migrating into developing blister cavities, adhering to

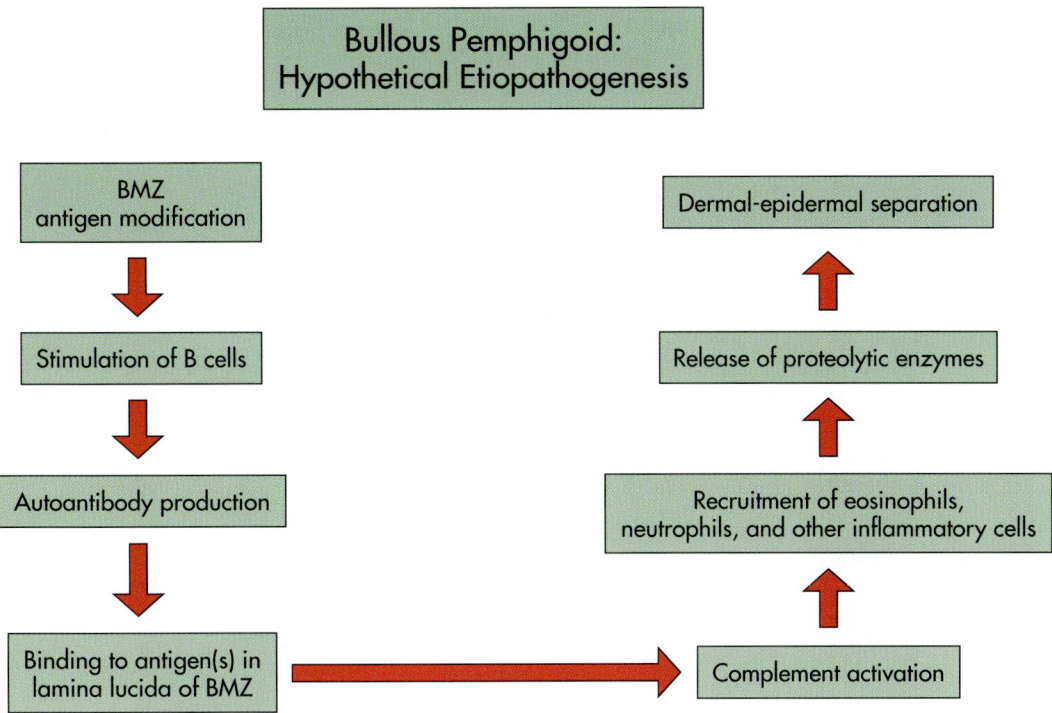

FIGURE 4-1. Diagram showing the hypothetical etiopathogenesis of bullous pemphigoid.

basal cells and releasing granule products onto basal cells.[7] Eosinophils localized at the BMZ in areas of blister formation showed an activated phenotype associated with degranulation onto basal keratinocytes.

Bullous pemphigoid blister fluids contain high concentrations of eosinophil granule proteins. Major basic protein, comprising the core of the specific eosinophil granule, is a potent cytostimulant and toxin that is active on many mammalian cells. Eosinophil-derived neurotoxin and eosinophil cationic protein, found in the granule matrix, are ribonucleases with potent biological effects; both of these proteins cause superficial ulceration when injected into guinea pig skin. Blister fluid is able to activate esoinophils as judged by a change in density and enhancement of cytotoxic potential with augmentation of cell-surface receptors and receptor-linked oxidative metabolism. Blister fluid from bullous pemphigoid lesions has also been found to stimulate eosinophil colony formation and to enhance eosinophil survival in culture. The survival enhancement was inhibited by antibodies to IL-3 and IL-5 with some but less inhibition by antibodies to granulocyte macrophage–colony stimulating factor (GM-CSF). IL-3, IL-5 and GM-CSF have significant effects on eosinophilopoiesis, survival in culture and activation with increased surface receptor expression, including IgG receptors, and enhanced function. Previous studies showed that IL-6 and tumor necrosis factor (TNF)-α were increased in bullous pemphigoid blister fluid but the source of the cytokines has not been identified. Eosinophils synthesize and secrete various cytokines, including TNF-α, GM-CSF, IL-1α, IL-3, IL-6, and possibly IL-5, indicating that they are equipped to participate in the ongoing inflammation. Peripheral blood eosinophilia is observed in almost half of bullous pemphigoid patients and elevated serum IgE levels are found in up to two thirds of patients.[1] In one study, serum IgE levels were found to correlate with disease activity.

Although the specific etiology of bullous pemphigoid is not yet delineated, increasingly an essential role for leukocytes, particularly eosinophils,[7] is implicated in the mechanism of blister formation.

Clinical Features

Presentation Characteristics

Bullous pemphigoid is a disease that typically develops in the elderly, although it may occur in younger adults and has been reported in neonates and children. There is neither gender nor racial predilection, and specific genetic factors related to HLA associations have not been identified.[1] Lesions consist of widespread tense bullae (Figure 4-2), which may be large and located predominantly on flexural surfaces, including abdomen, inner thighs, groin, axillae, and less commonly the head and neck areas. Blisters usually develop on erythematous or urticarial skin (Figure 4-3) but may also arise in normal-appearing skin (Figure 4-4). In contrast to pem-

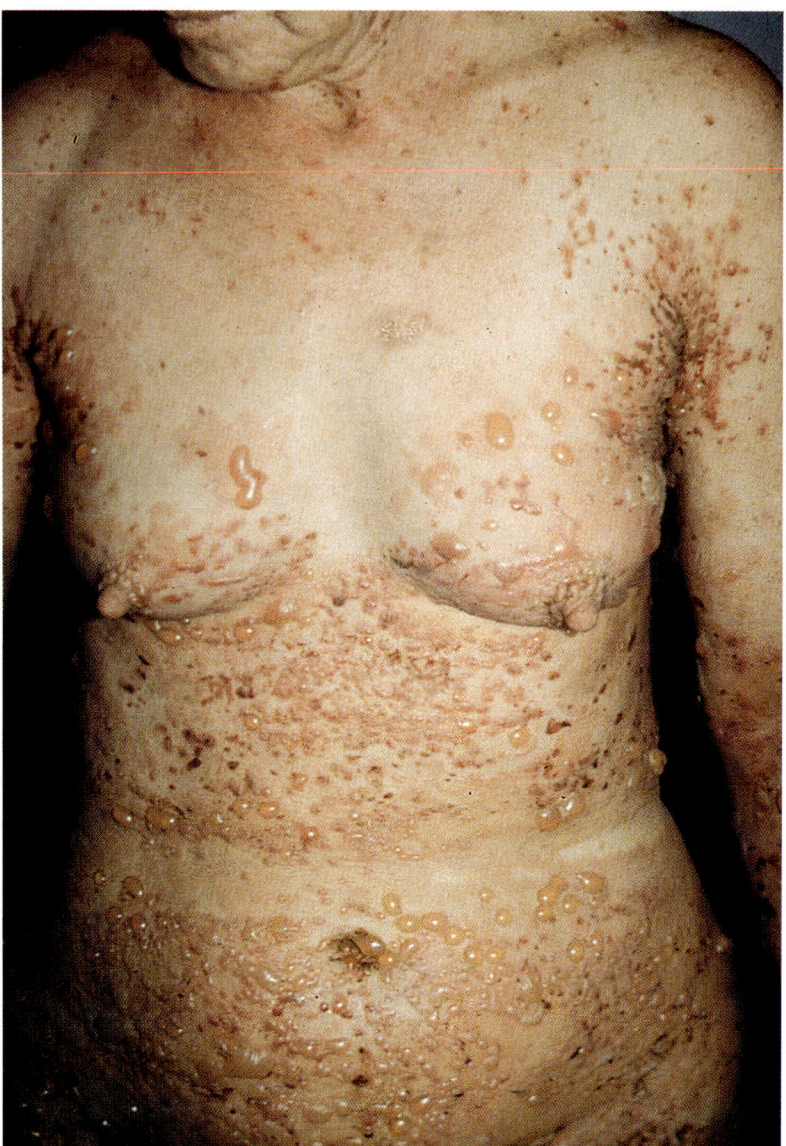

FIGURE 4-2. Generalized tense bullae in patient with bullous pemphigoid.

phigus, bullae rupture rather than extend on traumatization (Nikolsky's sign is negative). Therefore erosions are common (Figure 4-5). If healing is uncomplicated, lesions resolve and leave only postinflammatory pigmentary changes. The absence of scarring or milia is helpful in differentiating this disorder from cicatricial pemphigoid, epidermolysis bullosa acquisita, and porphyria cutanea tarda.[8]

Pruritus is a common feature at presentation, and some patients may present with prodromal eruptions consisting of pruritic urticarial (Figure 4-6) or eczematous lesions (Figure 4-7) that may last for months or even years before the appearance of blisters.[9] A forme fruste of bullous pemphigoid may occur more commonly than expected in which an elderly patient presents with unexplained chronic, generalized pruritus and on physical examination, only excoriations are observed. The typical prodromal eruption consisting of urticarial lesions is not present. Follow-up evaluations show that some of these patients have developed bullous lesions but others have had pruritus as the only clinical manifestation of the disease.

In contrast to pemphigus vulgaris and cicatricial pemphigoid, oral lesions in bullous pemphigoid are uncommon at presentation. Thereafter oral mucosal involvement develops in 10% to 40% of patients. Mucosal lesions of bullous pemphigoid are usually limited to the gingiva (Figure 4-8) and transiently to the oropharynx (Figure 4-9). Anogenital mucosa may also be involved (Figure 4-10).[1,8]

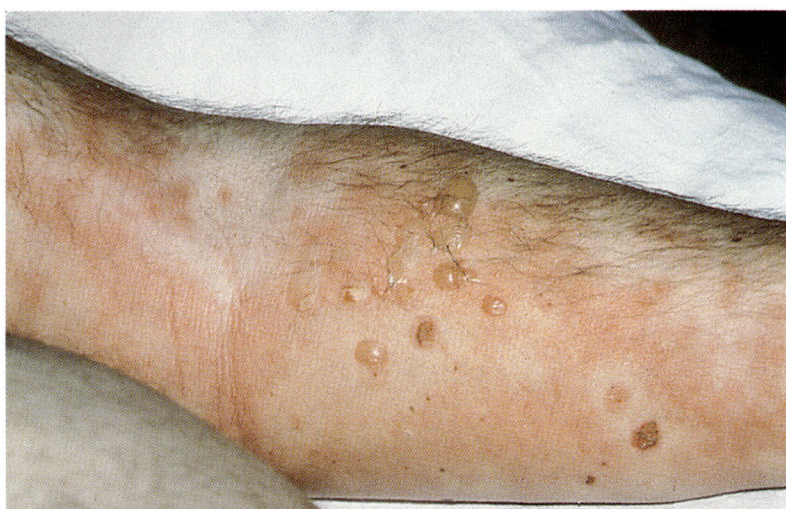

FIGURE 4-3. Tense blisters in bullous pemphigoid arising on erythematous and urticarial bases.

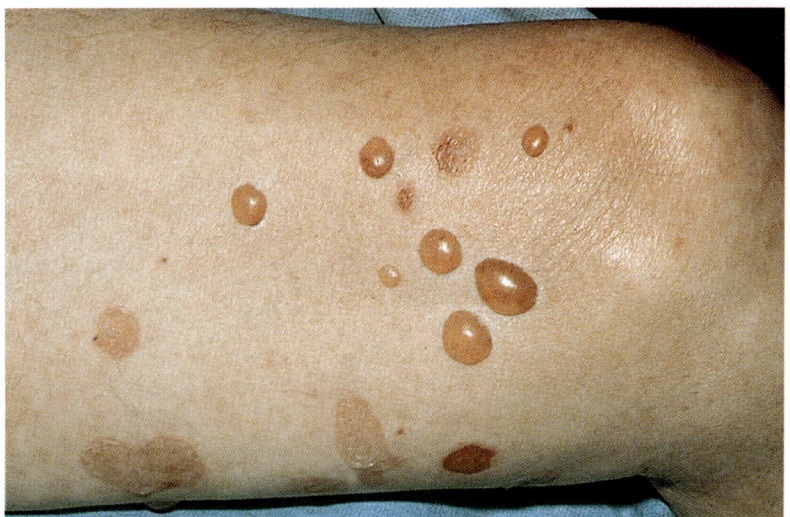

FIGURE 4-4. Tense blisters in bullous pemphigoid arising on normal-appearing skin.

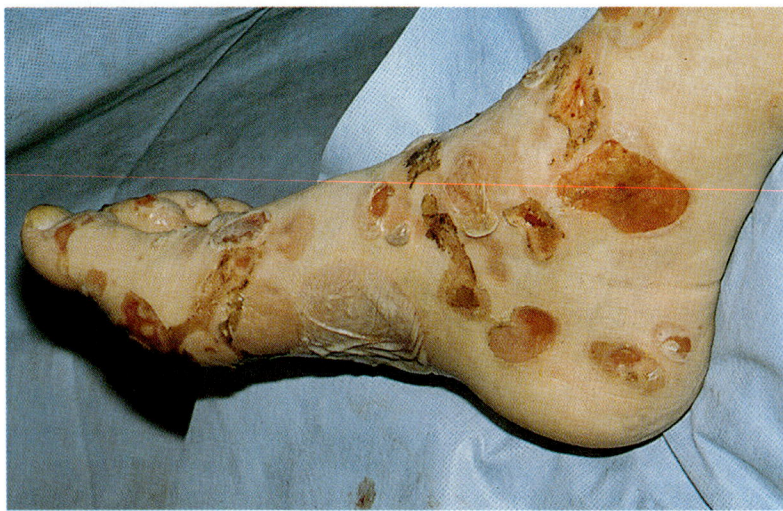

FIGURE 4-5. Eroded blisters on foot of patient with bullous pemphigoid.

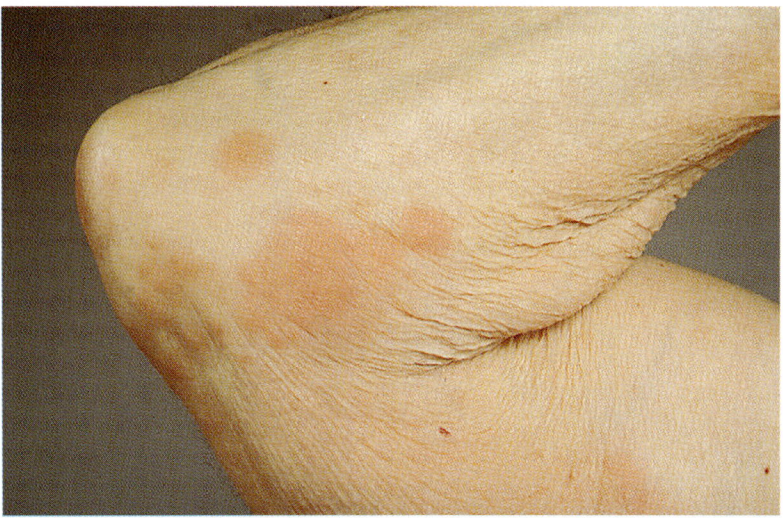

FIGURE 4-6. Urticarial papules and plaques around elbow of patient with bullous pemphigoid.

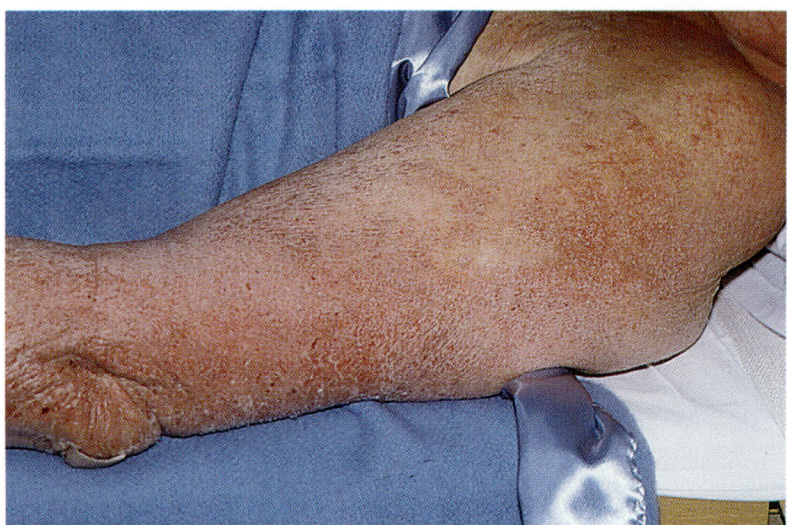

FIGURE 4-7. Confluent eczematous lesions in bullous pemphigoid on left arm and shoulder.

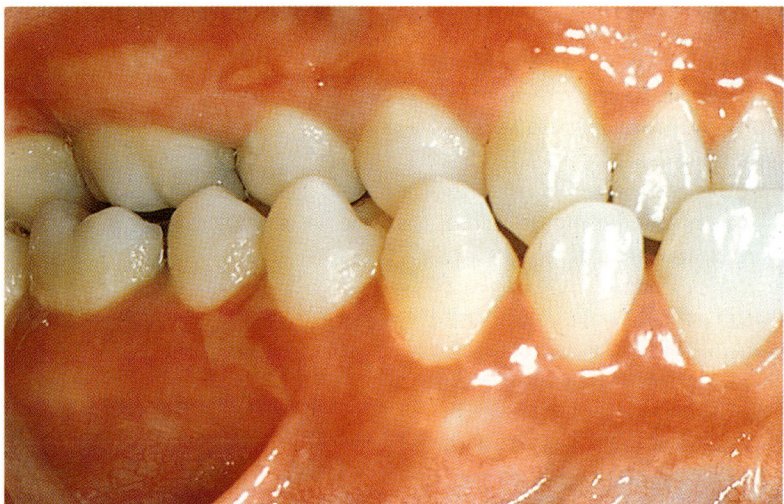

FIGURE 4-8. Desquamative gingivitis with multifocal erosive lesions of bullous pemphigoid.

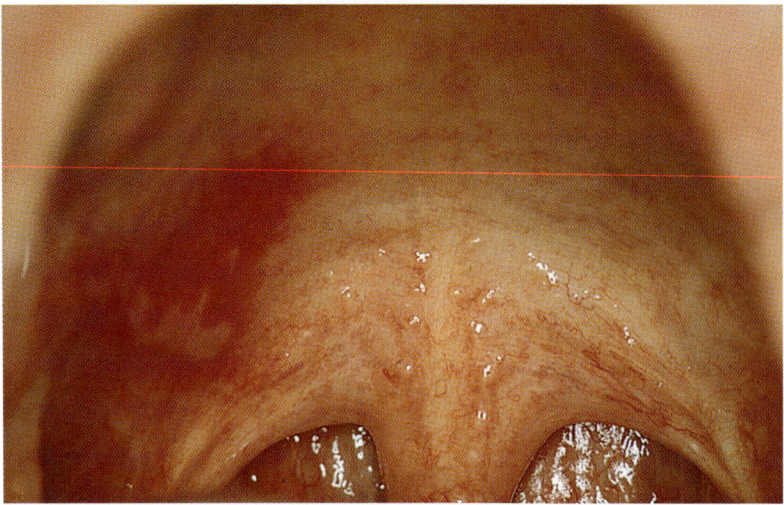

FIGURE 4-9. Oral mucosa involvement with variably-sized aphthous-like lesions on hard and soft palate of patient with bullous pemphigoid.

Clinical Variants

Several clinical presentations may be seen in bullous pemphigoid (Box 4-1). In children, the involvement of palms and soles and mucous membranes is observed with a higher frequency than in adults (Figure 4-11) and clinically resembles chronic bullous disease of childhood. Vulvar erosions and blisters may be the only manifestation in prepubescent girls. In these atypical cases, IF studies and demonstration of circulating autoantibodies reactive with the 230-kD protein have established the diagnosis of bullous pemphigoid.[10]

Although uncommon, localized forms of bullous pemphigoid develop in some patients, particularly middle-aged to elderly women, who present with lesions of the lower extremities (Figure 4-12). Localized bullous pemphigoid may also be confined to the palms and soles and resemble dyshidrotic eczema (Figure 4-13). A rare variant consists of chronic vegetating or verrucous plaques limited to the groin and axillae that tend to become secondarily infected; this clinical picture is reminiscent of pemphigus vegetans but with the immunopathologic features of bullous pemphigoid.

As in classic bullous pemphigoid, linear deposition of IgG and C3 at the BMZ is found by direct IF of perilesional skin from patients with localized disease. The same target antigens are recognized by serum antibodies in immunoblotting or immunoprecipitation studies.[8] Localized bullous pemphigoid is often chronic and refractory to treatment.[1] Lesions may persist in a localized distribution or may evolve into generalized disease.

Other variants of bullous pemphigoid have been described. Pemphigoid nodularis (Figure 4-14) mimics the clinical and histopathologic features of prurigo nodularis

BOX 4-1. CLINICAL FEATURES OF BULLOUS PEMPHIGOID

CLASSIC PRESENTATION
Elderly patients
Pruritus
Tense bullae on urticarial or erythematous bases in flexural areas

ATYPICAL NONBULLOUS PRESENTATIONS
Generalized pruritus with excoriations
Exfoliative erythroderma
Eczematous lesions

VARIANT PRESENTATIONS
Localized, lower extremities
Vegetating plaques, groin and axillae
Vulva, in prepubertal children
Herpetiform, vesicles
Dyshidrosiform, palmar and plantar lesions resembling dyshidrotic eczema
Pemphigoid nodularis, prurigo nodularis-like lesions on extremities

but has subepidermal bullae and the typical IF findings of bullous pemphigoid. Lesions of bullous pemphigoid may appear as small, tense grouped blisters that resemble dermatitis herpetiformis; this presentation is classified as vesicular pemphigoid. Bullous pemphigoid may also rarely present as a exfoliative erythroderma (Figure 4-15).[8] Keeping bullous pemphigoid in the differential diagnosis of patients with a variety of bullous and nonbullous lesions can prompt the clinician to perform IF testing.

Chapter 4 *Bullous Pemphigoid* 51

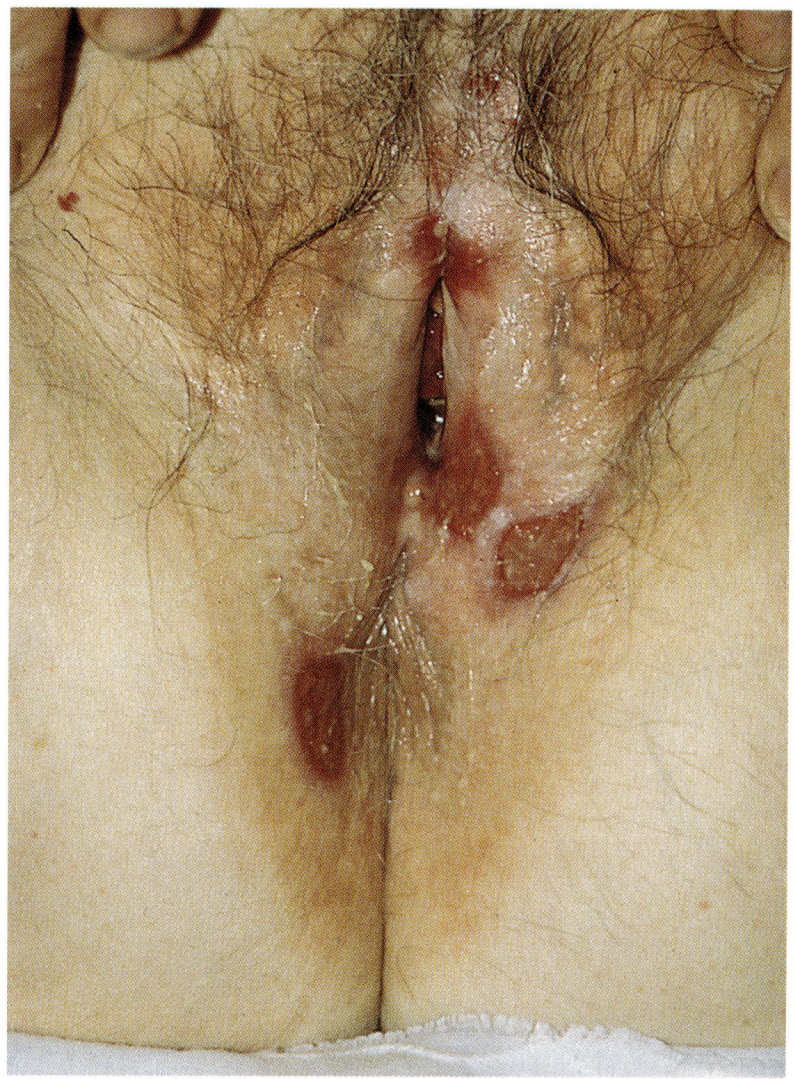

FIGURE 4-10. Erosive/ulcerative lesions of bullous pemphigoid involving vulvar and perianal areas.

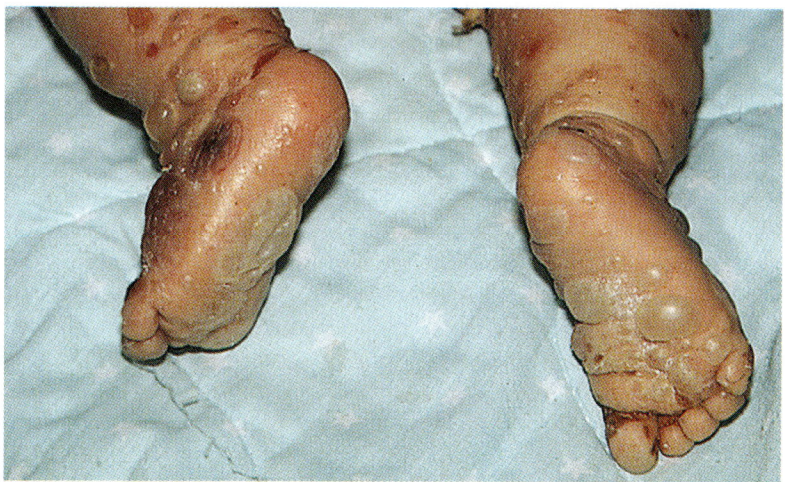

FIGURE 4-11. An infant with coalescing tense blisters of legs and feet, including plantar aspects.

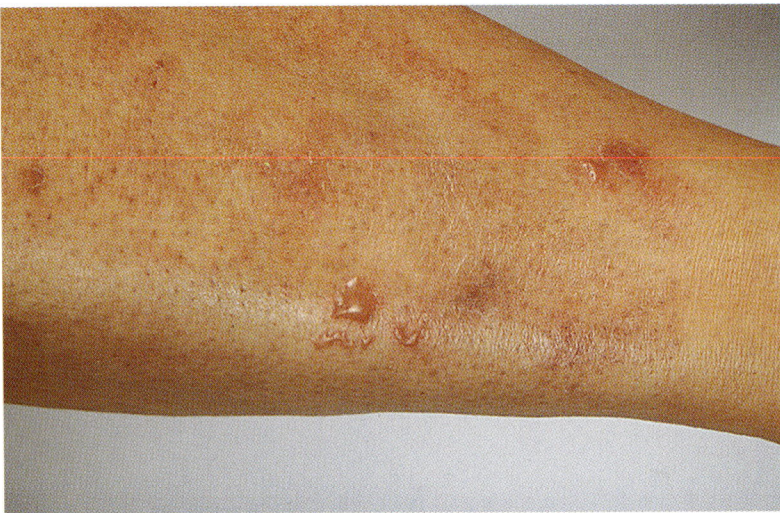

FIGURE 4-12. Left lower leg showing localized papulovesicular lesions; lower extremities were the only affected areas in this patient with bullous pemphigoid.

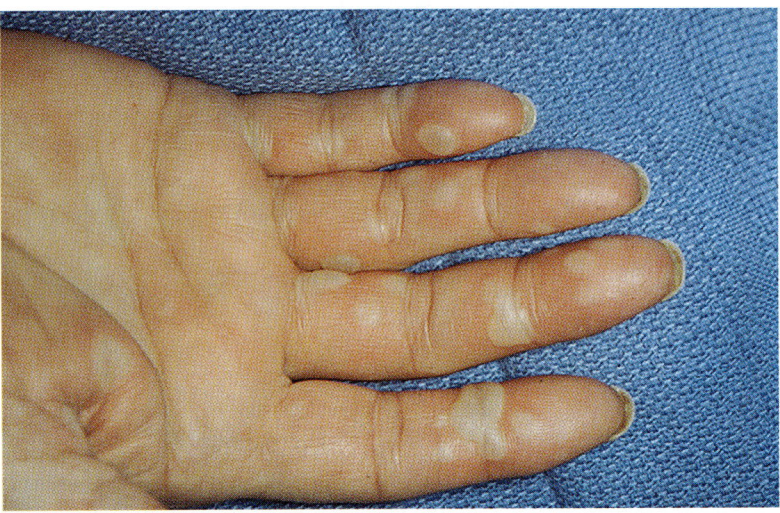

FIGURE 4-13. Vesicular lesions of bullous pemphigoid on palms may resemble dyshidrotic eczema.

Associated Diseases

Bullous pemphigoid has been reported in association with other autoimmune disorders, such as systemic lupus erythematosus (SLE), rheumatoid arthritis, multiple sclerosis, and vitiligo; metabolic diseases, such as diabetes mellitus, and other cutaneous conditions, including psoriasis and lichen planus. Because some of these associations were described before IF studies were available as diagnostic tools or have been noted in small numbers of patients, a reported relationship between bullous pemphigoid and the disorder must be interpreted with caution. However, recent comparisons with matched control patient groups demonstrate a statistically increased association between bullous pemphigoid and diabetes mellitus and between bullous pemphigoid and psoriasis than cannot be explained by the serendipitous coexistence of the diseases.[1,8]

Lichen planus in association with bullous pemphigoid has been termed *lichen planus pemphigoides*. In contrast to bullous lichen planus in which bullae develop on preexisting lichenoid papules and direct IF studies do not show linear C3 or IgG BMZ deposition, blisters occur either on preexisting lichenoid lesions or on normal-appearing skin. The histopathologic findings show subepidermal clefting and a mainly lymphocytic infiltrate, but immunopathology reveals the presence of immunoreactants at the dermal-epidermal junction as in bullous pemphigoid. Whether the same BMZ antigens are recognized in lichen planus pemphigoides as in bullous pemphigoid is still undetermined. Limited immunoprecipitation or immunoblotting studies have been performed, and the results are not definitive.

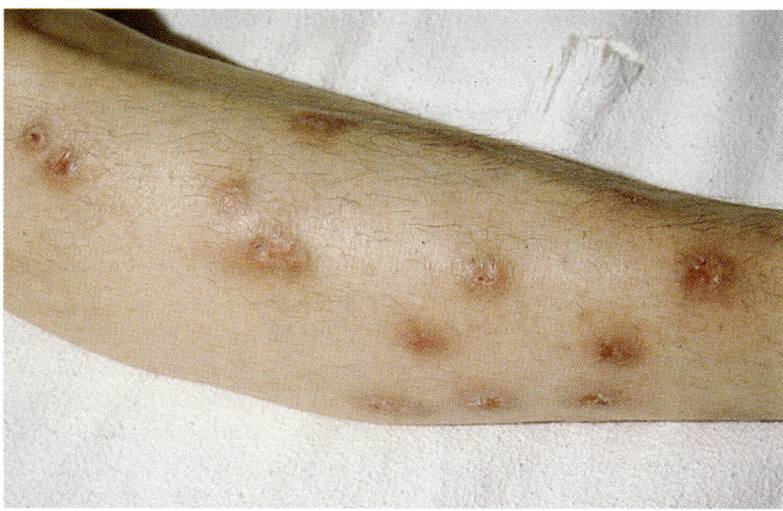

FIGURE 4-14. Prurigo nodularis-like appearance of bullous pemphigoid on anterior lower extremity.

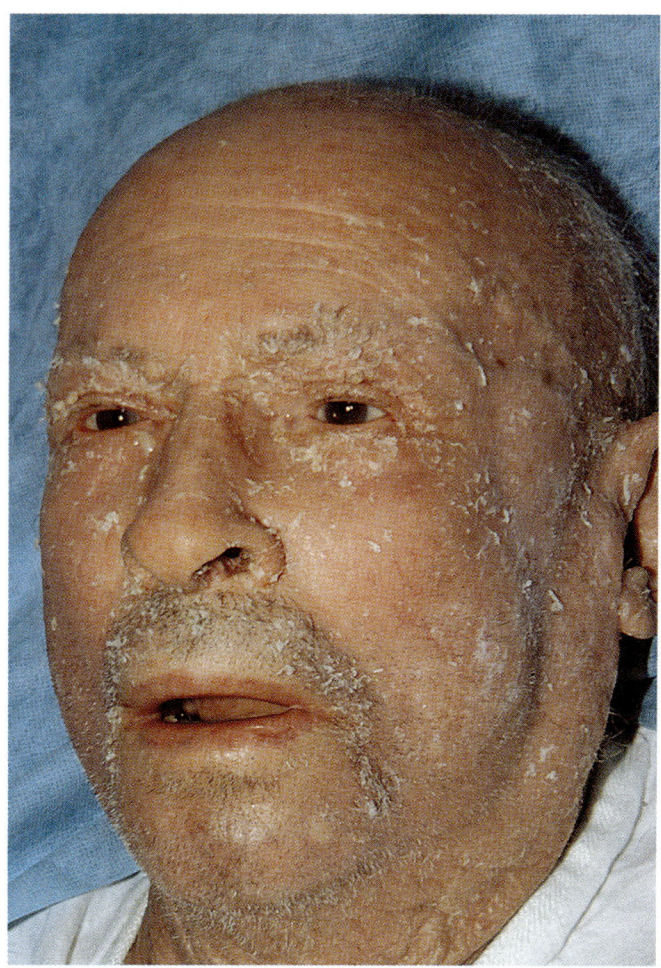

FIGURE 4-15. Exfoliative erythroderma in a patient in whom typical immunopathologic findings of bullous pemphigoid were identified by both direct and indirect IF.

Bullous pemphigoid has been reported in patients with lymphoreticular malignancies and solid tumors. However, a consistent correlation of bullous pemphigoid with neoplasias has not been found. Large retrospective studies comparing patients with bullous pemphigoid and controls with other dermatoses matched for age and gender have been performed, and the results have not shown an increased incidence of malignancies in bullous pemphigoid patients.[1,8]

Bullous Pemphigoid Induced by Drugs or Other Treatment Modalities

Although direct evidence of causality between drug intake and development of bullous pemphigoid has not been available in most cases in which a relationship was suspected, rechallenge studies demonstrated that furosemide and phenacetin are two drugs implicated in the induction of bullous pemphigoid. Other implicated medications include penicillins, ibuprofen, and IL-2.[11]

Rarely, bullous pemphigoid has apparently been induced by other agents, including electron beam treatment, radiotherapy, ultraviolet light, therapy with psoralens and ultraviolet light A (PUVA), and topical 5-fluorouracil.

Pathology

Histopathologic Features

Bullous pemphigoid is characterized by an inflammatory subepidermal bulla. However, the histopathologic findings vary, depending on the age and type of the clinical lesion. Typical features are more commonly observed in biopsy specimens taken from lesions on erythematous bases, urticarial-type lesions, or early blisters. Diffuse interstitial mixed inflammatory cell infiltration is observed in earlier erythematous or urticarial-type lesions. Eosinophils are characteristically prominent in bullous and urticarial lesions.[7,12] Eosinophils commonly localize along

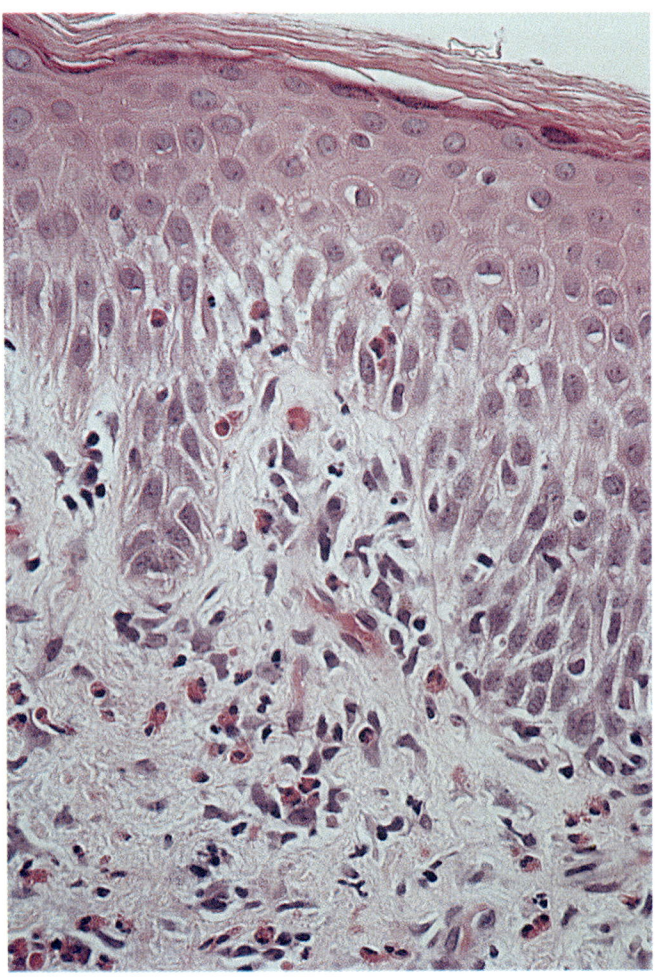

FIGURE 4-16. Mixed inflammatory cell infiltrate, including eosinophils, along the BMZ and within the epidermis (eosinophilic spongiosis) and superficial dermal edema. (H&E stain, original magnification ×400.)

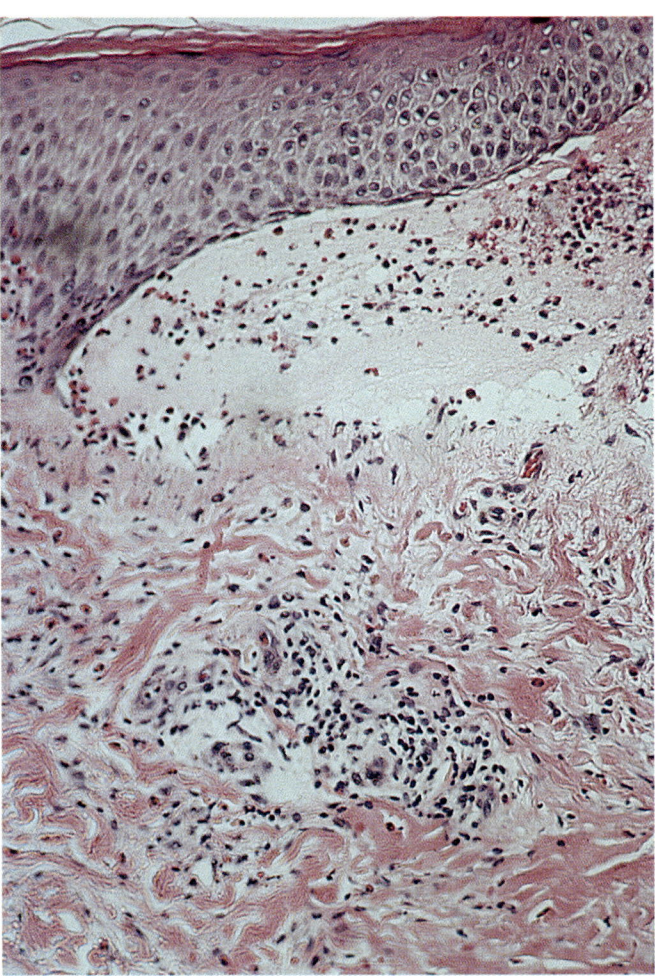

FIGURE 4-17. Subepidermal bulla containing eosinophils and fibrin with eosinophilic spongiosis at the margin as typically found in bullous pemphigoid. (H&E stain, original magnification ×200.)

the BMZ and may migrate into the epidermis, the so-called eosinophilic spongiosis (Figure 4-16).

Eosinophilic spongiosis represents an important diagnostic clue for immunobullous disease. Although initially recognized in lesions of pemphigus, eosinophilic spongiosis is most commonly seen in bullous pemphigoid,[13] and it may be seen in other subepidermal bullous diseases such as herpes gestationis. Early lesions of bullous pemphigoid may exhibit eosinophilic spongiosis without subepidermal bullae, and eosinophilic spongiosis may be seen at the margin of an inflammatory subepidermal bulla. In addition, eosinophils are usually present in the perivascular areas of the upper dermis, beneath and adjacent to a developing blister. Although eosinophils are usually most conspicuous, the infiltrate may also contain neutrophils, lymphocytes, and histiocytes. In biopsy specimens from blisters on erythematous or urticarial bases, unilocular subepidermal separation typically is observed and eosinophils are found in blister cavities (Figure 4-17) along with prominent dermal inflammation. In contrast, biopsy specimens from bullous lesions arising on normal-appearing skin often show sparse inflammatory cell infiltration. Biopsy specimens from older lesions may reveal an intraepidermal blister (Figure 4-18), instead of the typical subepidermal separation, as a result of epithelial regeneration.

Histopathologic findings in the variants of bullous pemphigoid show some of the characteristic features of bullous pemphigoid along with features of the variant type. For example, in pemphigoid vegetans and pemphigoid nodularis, acanthosis is usually prominent, reflecting the epidermal reaction observed in these lesions. In vesicular pemphigoid, subepidermal bullae tend to be small. In lichen planus pemphigoides, the features of lichen planus, including hypergranulosis and a superficial bandlike lymphocytic infiltrate, are combined with subepidermal clefting or bullae and eosinophils (Figure 4-19). In patients presenting with gener-

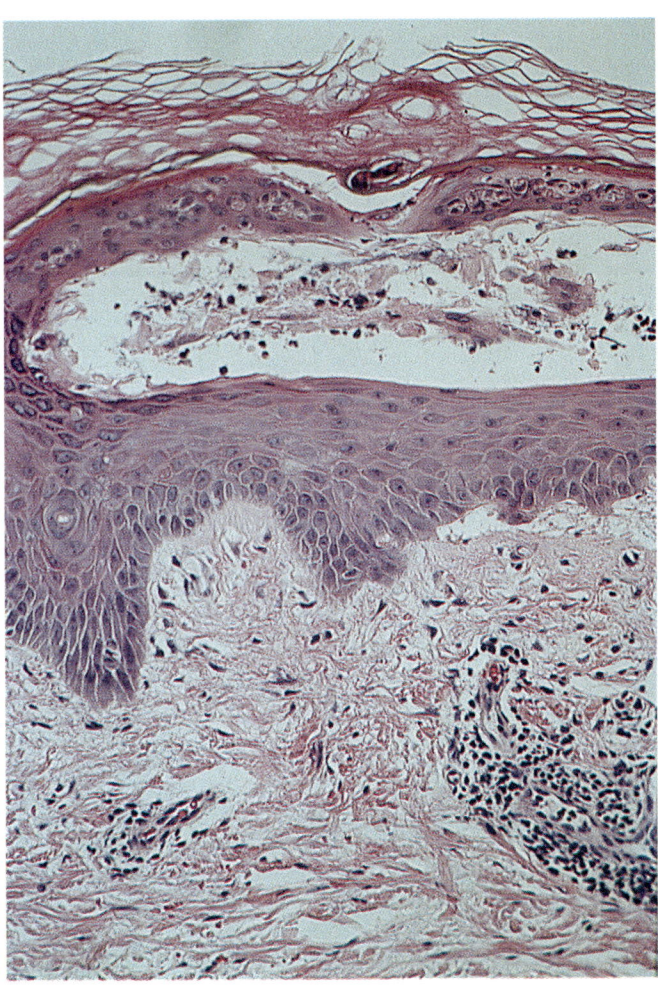

FIGURE 4-18. Intraepithelial bulla as a result of epithelial regeneration in an old lesion of bullous pemphigoid. (H&E stain, original magnification ×160.)

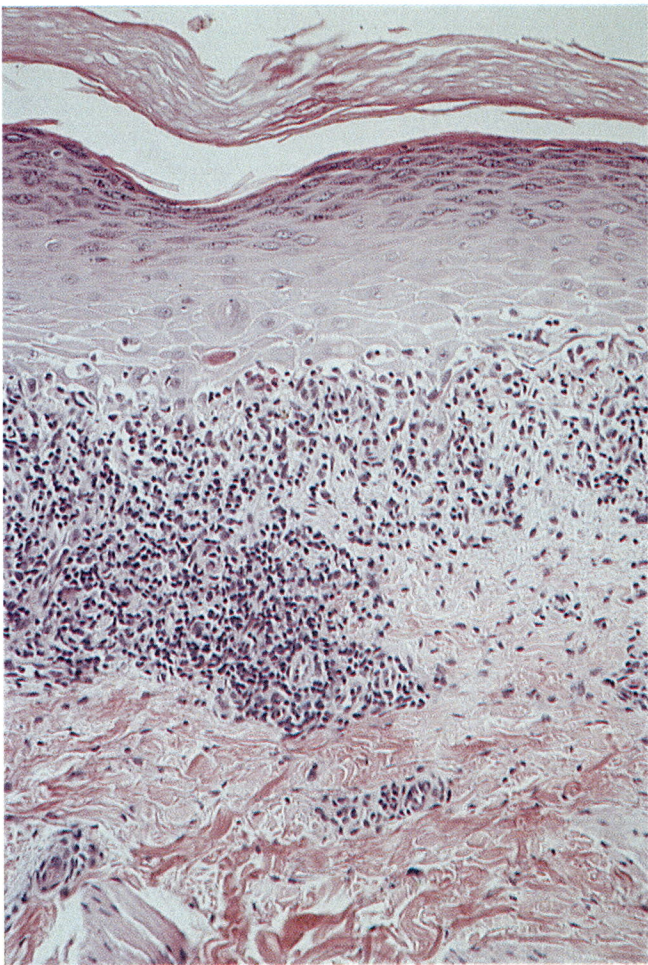

FIGURE 4-19. Lichen planus pemphigoides shows the typical histologic features of lichen planus with a bandlike inflammatory infiltrate; direct IF (not shown) revealed linear IgG and C3 at the BMZ. (H&E stain, original magnification ×200.)

Table 4-2. *Bullous Pemphigoid: Clinical and Histopathologic Differential Diagnosis*

DISEASE	TYPICAL AGE AT PRESENTATION	CLINICAL FINDINGS	HISTOPATHOLOGIC FINDINGS
Bullous pemphigoid	Elderly	Tense bullae of flexural areas, mucosal involvement limited	Subepidermal bulla with prominent infiltration of eosinophils
Epidermolysis bullosa acquisita	Middle age	Classic form with bullae, milia, and scarring on extensor surfaces of extremities; inflammatory type with widespread lesions and without scarring and milia	Subepidermal bulla with mixed inflammatory cell infiltrate or "cell-poor"
Cicatricial pemphigoid	Elderly	Prominent oral and ocular mucosal lesions with scarring sequelae; extramucosal cutaneous lesions in 20%	Subepidermal bulla with variable/limited cellular infiltrate
Antiepiligrin cicatricial pemphigoid	Middle age	Prominent oral and ocular mucosal lesions with scarring sequelae	Subepidermal bulla with variable/limited cellular infiltrate
Herpes gestationis	Young woman	Tense bullae of flexural areas, particularly abdomen; occurs in pregnancy, puerperium, or with hormonal changes, including exogenous hormones	Subepidermal bulla with eosinophils
Linear IgA bullous dermatosis, chronic bullous disease of childhood	Middle age, elderly, or childhood	May resemble bullous pemphigoid or dermatitis herpetiformis; higher frequency of oral mucosal involvement than in bullous pemphigoid	Subepidermal bulla with neutrophils or mixed inflammation with eosinophils
Bullous LE	Young adults	Blisters on head and neck areas and other sun-exposed sites	Subepidermal bulla or vesicle with neutrophils
Dermatitis herpetiformis	Young adults or middle age	Vesicles in symmetric distribution on extensor surfaces	Subepidermal vesicle with neutrophils

LE, Lupus erythematosus.

alized pruritus and in whom physical examination reveals only excoriations, histopathologic examination usually shows nonspecific findings and therefore appropriate IF examinations are essential.

Associated Diseases

Inflammatory subepidermal immunobullous diseases may be impossible to distinguish by clinical and histologic features (Table 4-2). The histopathology of herpes gestationis resembles that of bullous pemphigoid except for occasional basal keratinocyte necrosis in herpes gestationis, but the clinical presentation of herpes gestationis is distinctive. The histologic differential diagnosis of eosinophilic spongiosis includes not only other immunobullous diseases but also a variety of usually nonbullous inflammatory diseases with eosinophilia such as arthropod bite reactions and Well's syndrome. Subepidermal blisters with mixed inflammatory cell infiltration of eosinophils and neutrophils may be seen in other immunobullous disorders such as cicatricial pemphigoid, dermatitis herpetiformis, and linear IgA bullous dermatosis.[1] Bullous LE may also be considered in the differential diagnosis, although the neutrophil-rich lesions typical of bullous LE more closely resemble dermatitis herpetiformis than bullous pemphigoid. Moreover, bullous LE rarely demonstrates eosinophils.

Bullous pemphigoid lesions with subepidermal bullae and sparse or absent inflammatory cell infiltration are histologically indistinguishable from epidermolysis bullosa acquisita, cicatricial pemphigoid, and porphyria cutanea tarda. Erythema multiforme may be included in the clinical differential diagnosis of a patient with bullous pemphigoid and histopathologically may exhibit a subepidermal bulla. However, erythema multiforme is further characterized histologically by epidermal necrosis affecting multiple keratinocytes or large areas of necrotic epidermis overlying the bulla, as in toxic epidermal necrolysis.

Diagnosis

The diagnosis of bullous pemphigoid is made on the combined basis of clinical presentation, histopathologic

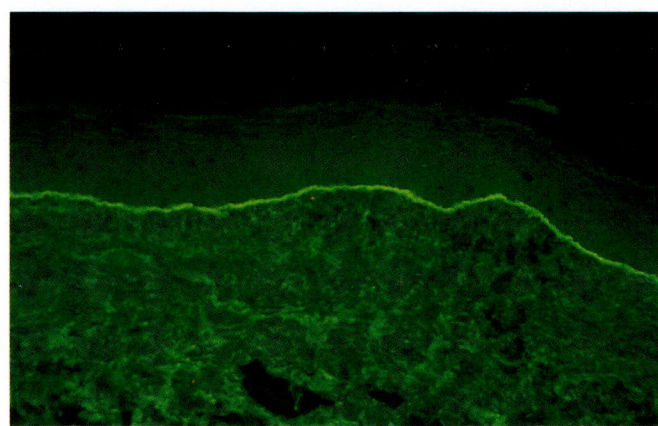

FIGURE 4-20. Direct IF of skin biopsy specimen showing linear IgG deposition at the BMZ; C3 was also present in this case. (Original magnification ×200.)

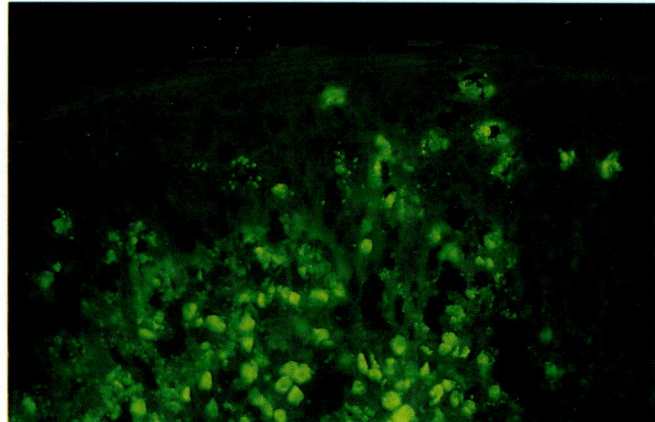

FIGURE 4-21. Direct IF of skin biopsy specimen showing eosinophilic spongiosis based on the nonspecific staining of eosinophils with fluorescein conjugates. (Anti-IgA stain, original magnification ×400.)

features, and distinctive immunopathologic findings. IF studies are essential for establishing the diagnosis in patients with characteristic clinical features and in patients with atypical clinical presentations.

Direct Immunofluorescence

The characteristic IF pattern in tissue from patients with bullous pemphigoid consists of continuous thin linear deposition of IgG and C3 along the BMZ. Approximately 90% of specimens show linear deposition of IgG (Figure 4-20) and nearly all specimens show C3 deposition. In addition to IgG and C3, linear deposition of IgM or IgA has been found at the BMZ but in less than 30% of specimens.[1] Although not specific for the diagnosis of bullous pemphigoid, prominent eosinophil infiltration is often present in the dermal papillae, along the BMZ or within the epidermis. This infiltrate is readily seen because of the nonspecific staining of eosinophils with any fluorescein-labeled protein (Figure 4-21). Eosinophil infiltration and degranulation may also be observed by immunohistologic staining with specific antibodies to eosinophil granule proteins.[7]

The optimal site for obtaining biopsy specimens for direct IF examination is perilesional skin or early urticarial-type lesions located in flexural areas. Regional differences exist in the expression of bullous pemphigoid antigens detected by direct IF, presumably because Ig deposition in the disease is most detectable where the antigens are most densely expressed. These differences correlate with the predominant sites of lesional development. Therefore scalp, face, and extensor areas are less likely to yield diagnostic IF results than flexural sites. In addition, direct IF examination of biopsy specimens from lower extremities for evidence of pemphigoid may show false-negative results.[14] Furthermore, biopsy specimens taken from involved tissue, especially blisters of several days' duration are unlikely to show characteristic staining by direct IF because immunoreactants may have been eliminated in the inflammatory process.

Direct IF staining of tissues from patients with bullous pemphigoid typically shows linear C3 or linear IgG and C3 deposition at the BMZ. Although distinctive, this staining pattern alone does not confirm the diagnosis of bullous pemphigoid because the same pattern may be seen in cicatricial pemphigoid, herpes gestationis, epidermolysis bullosa acquisita, and bullous SLE (Table 4-3). Furthermore, approximately 10% to 15% of bullous pemphigoid tissues show both linear IgG and IgA BMZ deposition, and in these cases, linear IgA bullous dematosis is also a diagnostic possibility (Table 4-3).

Indirect Immunofluorescence

Indirect IF is an important technique for detecting autoantibodies to BMZ antigens circulating in a patient's serum. Indirect IF of serum in combination with direct IF of tissue is necessary for establishing a diagnosis of bullous pemphigoid. Serum from patients suspected of having bullous pemphigoid is reacted with a BMZ-containing substrate. Normal human skin (flexural sites are preferred) and monkey esophagus substrates are commonly used for routine clinical testing. Exposing human skin to a 1 M NaCl solution for 48 to 72 hours at 4° C induces splitting at the level of the lamina lucida in the BMZ; incubation of patient serum with this salt-split human skin substrate allows identification of autoantibodies that bind to either epidermal or dermal antigens. The distal third of rhesus monkey esophagus is useful for determining whether circulating antibodies are

Table 4-3. *Bullous Pemphigoid: Immunopathologic Differential Diagnosis*

	Tissue	Serum		
Disease	Direct IF	Indirect IF on Human Salt-Split Skin	Indirect IF on Monkey Esophagus	Immunoprecipitation and/or Immunoblotting
Bullous pemphigoid	Linear BMZ deposition of IgG (90%), C3 (>90%), and other Ig (<30%)	Epidermal pattern	IgG BMZ antibodies (>70%)	230-kD (>90%) and 180-kD (30%) proteins
Cicatricial pemphigoid	Indistinguishable from bullous pemphigoid	Epidermal pattern	Low titer of IgG BMZ antibodies (15%)	180-kD and/or 230-kD proteins
Anti-epiligrin cicatricial pemphigoid	Indistinguishable from bullous pemphigoid	Dermal pattern	Low titer of IgG BMZ antibodies	175-, 145-, 125-, 117?-kD proteins
Epidermolysis bullosa acquisita	Broad linear BMZ deposition of IgG, C3, and other Ig	Dermal pattern	IgG BMZ antibodies (50%)	290-kD and/or 145-kD proteins (collagen VII)
Herpes gestationis	Linear BMZ deposition of C3 (IgG also present in approximately 40%)	Epidermal pattern	Herpes gestationis factor (90%-100%)	180-kD (230-kD?) protein
Linear IgA bullous dermatosis (epidermal type)	Linear BMZ deposition of IgA with or without C3	Epidermal pattern	Low titer of IgA BMZ antibodies (20%)	97-kD protein
Linear IgA bullous dermatosis (dermal type)	Linear BMZ deposition of IgA with or without C3	Dermal pattern	Low titer of IgA BMZ antibodies	290-kD and/or 145-kD proteins (collagen VII)
Bullous LE	Linear or granular BMZ deposition of Ig or C3	Dermal pattern*	Low titer of BMZ antibodies (50%)	290-kD and/or 145-kD proteins (collagen VII)
Dermatitis herpetiformis	Stippled IgA deposition in dermal papillae	NA	IgA endomysial antibodies (70%)	?

IF, Immunofluorescence, *BMZ*, basement membrane zone; *Ig*, immunoglobulins; *SLE*, systemic lupus erythematosus; *NA*, not applicable.
*Combined patterns and rare epidermal patterns have been reported.

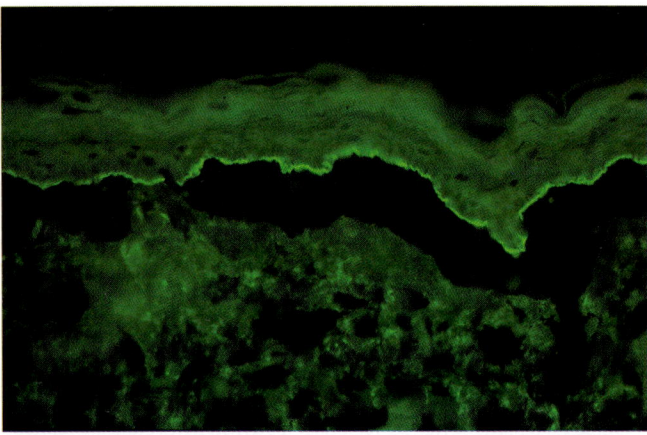

FIGURE 4-22. Indirect IF with bullous pemphigoid serum on human salt-split skin substrate showing an "epidermal pattern" of IgG staining. (Original magnification ×200.)

present and the titers of such antibodies. With monkey esophagus substrate, circulating autoantibodies directed against pemphigoid antigens located in the BMZ (Figure 4-22) can be differentiated from circulating autoantibodies to pemphigus antigens located on epithelial cell surfaces.

Other disorders (see Table 4-3) with circulating IgG autoantibodies that show a "dermal pattern" of BMZ staining include bullous SLE and a newly recognized immunobullous disease with the clinical features of cicatricial pemphigoid in which autoantibodies develop to epiligrin (laminin-5). However, distinguishing bullous pemphigoid from cicatricial pemphigoid may be difficult because most cicatricial pemphigoid sera show an "epidermal pattern" by indirect IF on human salt-split skin. Using anti-IgA as the secondary antibody, the subtype of linear IgA bullous dermatosis in which antibodies develop to collagen VII shows a dermal pattern on human salt-split skin substrate. In contrast to pemphigus in which titers of circulating epithelial antibodies are useful for monitoring disease activity and response to therapy, the presence or titer of circulating BMZ antibodies has not been shown to reflect disease activity or extent in bullous pemphigoid.

Differential Diagnosis

In the prodromal stage of the disease, before the development of vesiculobullous lesions, urticarial and eczematous reactions are diagnostic considerations. Pruritus is a common feature in all of these conditions, and while lesions of urticaria usually are evanescent, the urticarial type of lesions observed in bullous pemphigoid tend to last more than 24 hours. Histologic findings in the urticarial and eczematous lesions of bullous pemphigoid may be nonspecific and similar to other urticarial and eczematoid dermatoses. Thus IF examination of tissue and serum is required for an early diagnosis.

Scabies should be considered in the differential diagnosis of patients presenting with generalized pruritus in whom excoriations are the only finding on physical examination. However, bullous pemphigoid may present in elderly patients as unexplained persistent generalized pruritus. Again, IF studies are important to diagnose this occult form of the disease.

When the patient presents with vesicular or bullous lesions, other immunobullous diseases are included in the differential diagnosis (see Table 4-2). These diagnoses include cicatricial pemphigoid, epidermolysis bullosa acquisition, herpes gestationis, linear IgA bullous disease, dermatitis herpetiformis, and bullous SLE. Histopathologic features and IF findings that differentiate these diseases are listed in Tables 4-2 and 4-3.

Treatment

If left untreated, bullous pemphigoid follows a chronic course characterized by periodic remissions and exacerbations over a period of time, usually lasting less than 5 years. Spontaneous remission eventually occurs, and thereafter the disease remains inactive. A therapeutic plan is established on the basis of the dermatologic evaluation and general health of the patient.[15] Before glucocorticoids were available for treatment, mortality was estimated to occur in about 25% of patients with bullous pemphigoid.[2,15] This prognosis was better than that observed in patients with pemphigus in whom a fatal outcome occurred in more than half of the patients.[2] Although with modern therapies, especially glucocorticoids, the prognosis of the disease has improved, 10% mortality is still found in patients with bullous pemphigoid. This mortality may result because the elderly are more commonly affected, and adverse effects from treatment, as well as coexistent illnesses, increase with age.

The extent of disease has been classified in three gradations according to the number of cutaneous blisters and the number of mucosal lesions.[15] Therefore mild bullous pemphigoid is present in patients with fewer than 20 blisters or one to five lesions of mucosae; moderate disease is based on 20 to 40 skin blisters or five to ten lesions on mucosal surfaces; and bullous pemphigoid is severe if patients have more than 40 skin blisters or more than ten mucosal lesions or extensive erosions. Although treatment must be individualized for every patient, this classification may provide a helpful guide to establish the type and dosage of therapeutic agent(s).[15]

Since bullous pemphigoid is a chronic disease, treatment is directed at accomplishing the following goals:

1. Control of the disease by inhibiting or reducing the development of new vesiculobullous lesions and control of pruritus
2. Maintenance of disease remission without new lesion formation
3. Use of the lowest possible doses of drugs to maintain remission.

Withdrawal of therapy often is possible after a period of time and should be attempted gradually.

Most patients with bullous pemphigoid require systemic therapy with glucocorticoids. Other immunosuppressive agents may be added for therapeutic benefit or glucocorticoid-sparing activity. In milder cases or with localized disease, topical glucocorticoids may be a therapeutic option. This general therapeutic approach has been proven to be successful in childhood, as well as adult, disease (Table 4-4); however, the use of immunosuppressive drugs should be used more cautiously in children.[10] Cases of drug-induced bullous pemphigoid may respond to discontinuation of the implicated drug, but in most cases systemic therapy is also necessary to achieve more effective control of the disease.[11]

Systemic glucocorticoids are the drugs of choice to induce remission in bullous pemphigoid. Therapeutic benefit is likely the result of the known antiinflammatory properties of glucocorticoids rather than their immunosuppressive effects.[8] Doses of prednisone from 40 to 80 mg daily (equivalent to 0.75 to 1.25 mg/kg/day) control the disease in most patients, although exceptional patients may require higher doses. Improvement is usually noted within days to weeks. Glucocorticoids should be tapered promptly as the disease improves and when possible, administered every other day to limit the adverse effects that contribute to the high incidence of

Table 4-4. *Bullous Pemphigoid Therapy*

Drug	Dose	Main adverse effects
Prednisone	40-80 mg/day	Glucose intolerance, hypertension, diabetes mellitus, osteoporosis, increased susceptibility to infection
Azathioprine	100-150 mg/day	Bone marrow depression, idiopathic hepatitis, infection susceptibility, teratogenicity, malignancy risk; **excessive myelosuppression if thiopurine methyltransferase deficient**
Cyclophosphamide	100 mg/day	Nausea, vomiting, bone marrow depression, hemorrhagic cystitis, sterility, alopecia, teratogenicity, malignancy risk
Chlorambucil	5-10 mg/day	Bone marrow suppression, thrombocytopenia, hematologic malignancy risk
Cyclosporine	5-8 mg/day	Nephrotoxicity, hypertension, hepatotoxicity, malignancy risk
Dapsone	50-150 mg/day	Hemolysis, methemoglobinemia, exfoliative dermatitis, peripheral neuropathy, hepatotoxicity; **enhanced hemolysis if glucose-6-phosphate dehydrogenase deficient**
Antibiotics and niacinamide	Tetracycline 2 g/day or minocycline 200 mg/day with niacinamide 1.5-2.5 g/day	Gastrointestinal intolerance, photosensitivity
Topical glucocorticoids	Clobetasol propionate, 0.05%/12 hr or triamcinolone acetonide 0.1%/tid-qid	Atrophy and increased fragility of skin with long-term use

morbidity and mortality. "Pulse therapy" with intravenous glucocorticoids has been successfully used in resistant cases; most commonly, methylprednisolone (1 g in 5% dextrose or normal saline) is infused over 60 to 90 minutes on 3 to 5 consecutive days and then followed by oral glucocorticoid maintenance therapy. Rapid clinical responses have been observed with this regimen, but fatal complications have occurred in the elderly.[15] Topical therapy with glucocorticoids may be used in mild or localized bullous pemphigoid and is also very useful as an adjuvant to systemic glucocorticoid therapy in more severe cases. The most potent topical glucocorticoids are preferred, such as clobetasol propionate, 0.05%, applied twice daily. Lesions may heal within 2 weeks of treatment, or long-term therapy may be needed. To avoid adverse effects and for prolonged maintenance therapy (2 months to 1 year), less potent topical glucocorticoids are recommended. Intralesional triamcinolone acetonide 3-10 mg/ml has also been tried for resistant lesions.

Other therapeutic agents that minimize the systemic glucocorticoid dose are often used concomitantly with glucocorticoids in bullous pemphigoid. These alternate therapies may be the only treatment needed for milder cases or may be a desirable therapeutic option for patients in whom the use of glucocorticoids may exacerbate an underlying disease such as diabetes mellitus, tuberculosis, or hypertension.[1]

Azathioprine is one of the commonly prescribed nonsteroidal immunosuppressive agents for treatment of bullous pemphigoid. It has been used in combination with glucocorticoids for steroid-sparing effect, for maintenance after steroid withdrawal, or as a solitary treatment for mild disease. However, before initiating therapy, thiopurine methyltransferase (TPMT) levels must be obtained to detect individuals with low levels who will have excessive myelosuppression when taking azathioprine. If TPMT levels are normal, a usual starting dose of azathioprine for severe disease is 100 to 150 mg/day (equivalent to 2 to 2.5 mg/kg/day). Side effects from azathioprine include bone marrow depression, idiopathic hepatitis, increased susceptibility to infection, teratogenicity, and increased risk of malignancies. Baseline laboratory studies before starting therapy should include (in addition to a TPMT level) a complete blood count, serum and urine electrolyte panel, and renal and liver function tests. Blood counts should be repeated weekly during the first 2 months or as long as the dose is being increased. Thereafter blood counts should be checked every month along with renal and liver function studies. Monitoring should be performed throughout treatment. Because azathioprine has a delayed onset of therapeutic action, approximately 4 to 8 weeks, it should be started concurrently with glucocorticoid administration. In general, the therapeutic strategy for bullous pemphigoid is to rapidly control disease activity with glucocorticoids and to minimize glucocorticoid side effects and maintain disease control with nonsteroidal immunosuppressives.

Cyclophosphamide has also been used as an effective steroid-sparing agent in the treatment of bullous pemphigoid. An average daily dose of cyclophosphamide is 100 mg/kg, doses equivalent to 1 to 3 mg/kg/day are recommended, and it has also been used intravenously in a pulse-therapy regimen in combination with glucocorticoids. Side effects include nausea and vomiting, bone marrow depression, hemorrhagic cystitis, sterility, alopecia, teratogenicity, and an increased incidence of internal malignancy. Monitoring is similar to azathioprine, but urinalysis also must be done weekly during the first 2 to 3 months of therapy and twice a month thereafter to monitor for hemorrhagic cystitis. The toxicity of cylcophosphamide is greater than that of azathioprine and is usually not considered a first-line therapy for bullous pemphigoid. It is more often used to treat cicatricial pemphigoid, which tends to be more refractory to therapy and has scarring sequelae.

Chlorambucil used at a starting dose of 0.1 mg/kg/day and reduced over 6 weeks to a daily maintenance dose of 2 mg has proven beneficial in combination with prednisolone 40-60 mg/day. Hematologic toxicity with bone marrow suppression and reversible thrombocytopenia is a common side effect. With the dosages of chlorambucil over a 5-month treatment time as stated, reversible thrombocytopenia has been observed in 30% of patients. Monitoring must be performed with baseline and weekly blood counts. Occurrence of acute myeloid leukemia has been reported and appears to be related to cumulative doses of more than 1g. The potential risk of inducing hematologic malignancies discourages use of chlorambucil in clinical practice.

Cyclosporine, at doses of 5 to 8 mg/kg/day, is therapeutically beneficial when combined with glucocorticoids in some patients with bullous pemphigoid; however, its benefit as a monotherapeutic agent has not been demonstrated. Because of potential nephrotoxicity and expense, it is probably best considered an adjunctive therapy for selected unresponsive cases. Side effects include hypertension, renal dysfunction, increased serum lipid levels, hypertricosis, gingival hyperplasia, hepatotoxicity, and increased risk of malignancy. Assessment before treatment should include blood pressure, blood counts, renal and liver function tests, fasting lipids, 24-hour urinary protein level, and urinalysis. These tests should be repeated every 1 to 2 weeks during the first 3 months of treatment and monthly thereafter. Creatinine clearance should be checked periodically as indicated by the patient's age and test results.

Methotrexate has been tried in a limited number of patients with bullous pemphigoid but seems to be less therapeutically effective than other immunosuppressive agents. For this reason, its use has not been widely accepted in bullous pemphigoid.[15]

Dapsone doses of 50 to 150 mg/day in combination with topical steroids have been reported to be beneficial in treating bullous pemphigoid. Improvement in some patients has been rapid, within 2 weeks of initiating treatment. Interestingly, histopathologic studies in the responsive cases have revealed a predominantly neutrophilic infiltrate instead of the eosinophil predominance more commonly observed in patients with bullous pemphigoid. Up to 15% of bullous pemphigoid patients may respond to this treatment modality, and in milder cases it may be the only therapy needed to maintain disease remission. Some patients with bullous pemphigoid, presenting with generalized pruritus without evidence of bulla or other typical features of the disease (forme fruste), may successfully be treated with sulfones with good control of the pruritus. Sulfones may also be tried as an alternative treatment in patients in whom glucocorticoids and other immunosuppressives are either contraindicated or not tolerated. Adverse effects from dapsone include hemolysis and methemoglobinemia, exfoliative dermatitis, peripheral neuropathy, anorexia, nausea and vomiting, hepatotoxicity, and neuropsychiatric disturbances. Before starting treatment, a glucose-6-phosphate dehydrogenase (G-6-PD) level should be obtained to exclude a deficiency, which will result in acute or enhanced hemolysis with sulfone administration. Necessary baseline and weekly laboratory investigations include complete blood counts with reticulocyte count, electrolyte panel, and renal and liver function tests. During therapy, detection of methemoglobinemia may be assessed clinically and confirmed by laboratory tests.[1,15]

Antibiotics and niacinamide have been used in combination for the treatment of bullous pemphigoid. Tetracycline 2 g/day and niacinamide 1.5 to 2.5 g/day have been shown to be as effective as prednisone 20 mg/day in some clinical trials. Minocycline 200 mg/day has been used as an alternative to tetracycline for patients in whom gastrointestinal side effects have been a problem, and erythromycin alone has been beneficial in some cases. The effectiveness of these treatments may be related to antiinflammatory properties of the drugs. Side effects include gastrointestinal symptoms, renal disturbances, drug exanthems, photosensitivity, hyperpigmentation (minocycline), and those effects related to the use of broad-spectrum antibiotics such as candidiasis and pseudomembranous colitis.[1,15] Topical antibiotics may be beneficial for treating secondarily infected blisters.

Other modalities have been tried in the treatment of bullous pemphigoid. Plasmapheresis, in combination with glucocorticoids, has steroid-sparing effects and reduces the rate of relapses compared to treatment with glucocorticoids alone. However, this procedure is not simple to administer; cardiac monitoring is required and treatments must be given in special transfusion/blood bank units. Ig therapy has been used in bullous pemphigoid patients but has only temporary effects with relapses observed within 2 weeks of administration.

Localized mucosal lesions in patients with bullous pemphigoid do not usually represent a therapeutic problem because they are often transient, in sharp contrast to patients with cicatricial pemphigoid in whom treatment must be started promptly and vigorously to avoid scarring sequelae. Oral bullous pemphigoid, including desquamative gingivitis, usually responds to topical glucocorticoids. Clobetasol propionate 0.05% or betamethasone valerate 0.1% may be applied twice daily, and the ointment should contact the affected surface for at least 30 minutes. Triamcinolone in an adhesive base, such as Orabase, has also been used effectively. Aerosol or intralesional glucocorticoids are usually not needed for the treatment of oral bullous pemphigoid. Anecdotally, topical cyclosporine has been beneficial. Oral hygiene with antiseptic mouthwashes several times a day may contribute to a better therapeutic response from topical therapies used in the mouth.[15]

References

1. Anhalt GJ, Morrison L: Pemphigoid: bullous, gestational, and cicatricial. In Provost TT, Weston WL, eds: *Bullous diseases,* St. Louis, 1993, Mosby.
2. Lever WF: Pemphigus, *Medicine* 32:1-123, 1953.
3. Jordon RE, Beutner EH, Witebsky E, et al: Basement membrane zone antibodies in bullous pemphigoid, *JAMA* 200:91-96, 1967.
4. Stanley JR: Cell adhesion molecules as targets of autoantibodies in pemphigus and pemphigoid, bullous diseases due to defective epidermal cell adhesion, *Adv Immunol* 53:291-325, 1993.
5. Giudice GJ, Liu Z, Diaz LA: An animal model of bullous pemphigoid: what can it teach us? *Proc Assoc Amer Phys* 107:237-241, 1995.
6. Dahl MV: The bullous diseases: Pemphigus, pemphigoid, dermatitis herpetiformis, and others. In Dahl MV, ed: *Clinical immunodermatology,* ed 3, St. Louis, 1996, Mosby.
7. Borrego L, Maynard B, Peterson EA, et al: Deposition of eosinophil granule proteins precedes blister formation in bullous pemphigoid: Comparison with neutrophil and mast cell granule proteins, *Am J Pathol* 148:897-909, 1996.
8. Korman NJ: Bullous pemphigoid. *Dermatol Clin* 11:483-498, 1993.
9. Asbrink E, Hovmark A: Clinical variations in bullous pemphigoid with respect to early symptoms, *Acta Derm Venereol* (Stockh) 61:417-421, 1981.
10. Rico MJ: Autoimmune blistering diseases in children, *Semin Dermatol* 14:54-59, 1995.
11. Fellner MJ: Drug-induced bullous pemphigoid, *Clin Dermatol* 11:515-520,1993.
12. Weedon D: The vesiculobullous reaction pattern. In Weedon D, ed: *The skin,* ed 3, New York, 1992 Churchill Livingstone.
13. Crotty C, Pittelkow M, Muller SA: Eosinophilic spongiosis: a clinicopathologic review of seventy-one cases, *J Am Acad Dermatol* 8:337-343, 1983.
14. Weigand DA: Effect of anatomic region on immunofluorescence diagnosis of bullous pemphigoid, *J Am Acad Dermatol* 12:274-278, 1985.
15. Huilgol SC, Black MM: Management of the immunobullous disorders. I. Pemphigoid, *Clin Exp Dermatol* 20:189-201, 1995.

Cicatricial Pemphigoid

Neil J. Korman
Kevin D. Cooper

Cicatricial pemphigoid is a disease phenotype consisting of a group of subepithelial blistering diseases that involve primarily mucosal surfaces and occasionally the skin. Recent studies, utilizing sophisticated immunopathologic and immunochemical techniques, revealed that the entity known as cicatricial pemphigoid, benign mucous membrane pemphigoid, and ocular pemphigoid is best understood when it is divided into several groups.[1]

The first group includes patients with anti-epiligrin cicatricial pemphigoid.[2] These patients are immunochemically distinct in that they have circulating immunoglobulin G (IgG) autoantibodies that bind to the dermal side of salt-split skin and recognize epiligrin, now known as laminin-5 and occasionally laminin-6,[3] but they lack distinguishing clinical features that separate them from other cicatricial pemphigoid variants. The other three major groups that form the cicatricial pemphigoid spectrum have been delineated in a large study of 123 patients with immune-mediated subepithelial blistering diseases who were categorized on the basis of clinical and immunopathologic features.[1] The first distinct group of patients have pure ocular disease in the absence of skin, oral, or other mucous membrane disease and are characterized as having pure ocular pemphigoid. In this study, the investigators found that these patients rarely had circulating IgG antibodies and had negative serologic reactivity to bullous pemphigoid antigens or other defined basement membrane zone (BMZ) antigens. Recently, another group demonstrated that many patients with pure ocular pemphigoid have IgG antibodies directed against the β4 integrin,[4] whereas other patients have been found to have circulating IgA antibodies that react with an uncharacterized 45-kD antigen.[5]

The next group of patients defined in this large study are those who have mucosal disease along with skin lesions and circulating IgG antibodies and serologic reactivity to bullous pemphigoid antigens that occur at the same frequency as patients with bullous pemphigoid. These patients have been classified as having anti-bullous pemphigoid antigen mucosal pemphigoid. The last group is a heterogeneous one that includes patients who have oral mucosal disease (along with ocular and other mucous membrane lesions) in the absence of any skin lesions, as well as patients with oral disease alone; these patients' disease is sometimes referred to as *oral mucosal pemphigoid*. Whether any of these variants within the cicatricial pemphigoid phenotype may eventually prove to be distinct pathomechanistically remains the subject for future study.

Etiology

The etiology and pathogenesis of cicatricial pemphigoid are not well understood. A reasonable explanation for the pathogenesis is that an abnormal immune response occurs in the mucosal-associated lymphoid tissue. Because cicatricial pemphigoid often has similar immunopathologic findings as bullous pemphigoid, it may be logical to assume that these conditions share a similar pathogenesis. In bullous pemphigoid, circulating bullous pemphigoid autoantibodies bind to bullous pemphigoid antigens and activate the complement cascade that produces the anaphylatoxins C3a and C5a. Mast cell activation occurs secondary to anaphylatoxin release. After activation, mast cells degranulate and release many proinflammatory mediators. As a consequence of the many released mast cell products and probably also a result of the chemotactic properties of C5a, neutrophils and eosinophils are recruited to the epidermal BMZ. Complement factors previously fixed at the BMZ may facilitate immune adherence of neutrophils and eosinophils. These activated neutrophils and eosinophils release their own inflammatory mediators, including lysosomal proteolytic enzymes. Mononuclear macrophages and lymphocytes also participate in the inflammatory process. Dermal-epidermal junction separation occurs either due to direct cytotoxic action or proteolytic enzymes; the end result is subepidermal blister formation. Mucosal scarring may result from activated fibrotic repair mechanisms

CICATRICIAL PEMPHIGOID SUMMARY

ETIOLOGY

Cicatricial pemphigoid is an autoimmune mucocutaneous blistering disease. The etiology and pathogenesis of cicatricial pemphigoid are not well understood. Cicatricial pemphigoid is best understood when it is divided into several groups. Patients in different subgroups may have circulating antibodies directed against different BMZ molecules, including both bullous pemphigoid antigens, laminin-5, and the β4 integrin.

CLINICAL FEATURES

Subepithelial blisters involve primarily mucosal surfaces and occasionally the skin.

PATHOLOGY

Histologic examination of skin or mucosal lesions reveals a subepithelial vesicle with an inflammatory infiltrate with lymphocytes, neutrophils, eosinophils, or plasma cells.

DIAGNOSIS

Clinical presentation and characteristic histopathologic and immunopathologic features.

DIFFERENTIAL DIAGNOSIS

Bullous pemphigoid, epidermolysis bullosa acquisita, linear IgA bullous disease, paraneoplastic pemphigus, and pseudopemphigoid are considered.

TREATMENT

Patients with involvement limited to the nasopharynx or oropharynx are treated with topical or intralesional steroids, short bursts of oral corticosteroids, or dapsone. If the eyes, esophagus, or larynx become involved, then aggressive therapy with systemic corticosteroids and immunosuppressive agents is warranted.

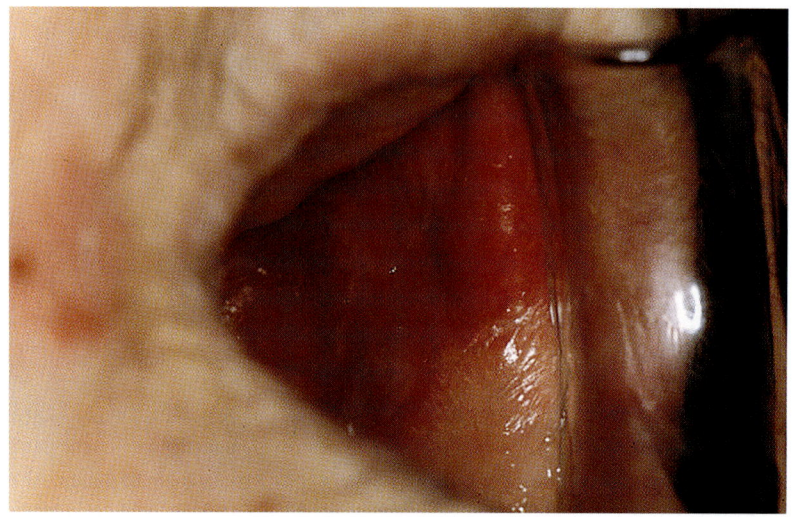

FIGURE 5-1. Confluent erythema of the buccal mucosa in a patient with cicatricial pemphigoid.

induced by mast cell products and activated leukocytes, resulting in fibrosis and adhesions.

In the eye, the scarring process may induce loss of cellular elements critical for the oil and mucous layers of tear formation. The result is a tear that does not spread uniformly and evaporates quickly, causing corneal dryness and eventual corneal keratinization leading finally to corneal opacity. Patients with pure ocular cicatricial pemphigoid seem to have an immunogenetic predisposition to develop this disease because of a markedly increased occurrence of the HLA-DQB1*0301 allele.[6]

Clinical Features

Cicatricial pemphigoid involves primarily mucosal surfaces, including (in decreasing order of frequency) the oropharynx, conjunctiva, nasopharynx, larynx, genitalia, and esophagus.[7-9] Morbidity and mortality are caused by the scarring that results from recurrent lesions. In the past, clinical criteria were used to differentiate cicatricial pemphigoid from bullous pemphigoid. Patients with cicatricial pemphigoid usually have prominent scarring and mucosal predominant disease, whereas patients with bullous pemphigoid usually have nonscarring skin lesions.

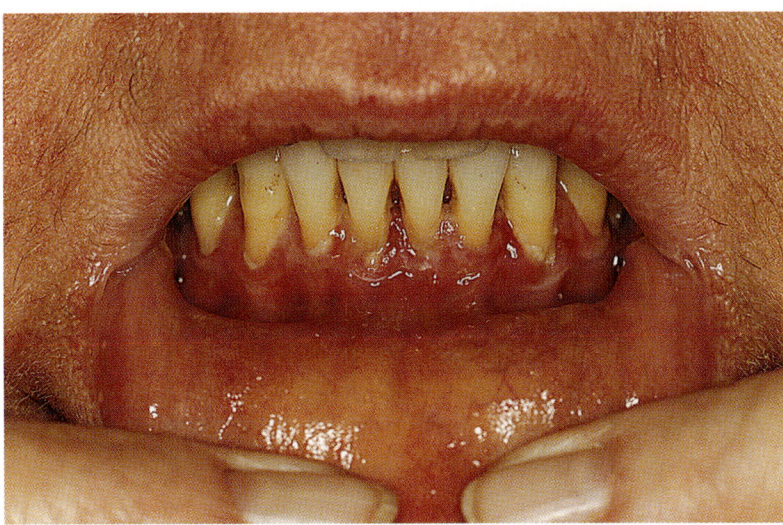

FIGURE 5-2. Desquamative gingivitis seen in a patient with significant oral mucosal involvement.

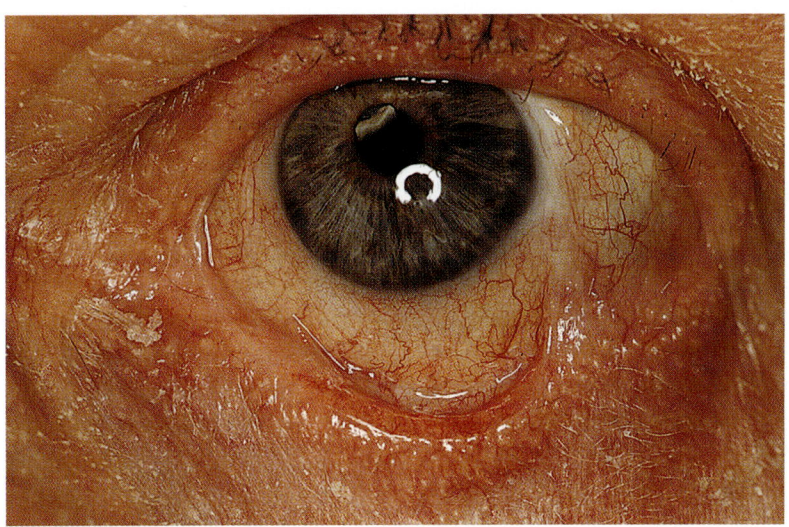

FIGURE 5-3. Early ocular inflammation in a patient with cicatricial pemphigoid showing conjunctival injection, early symblepharon, and forniceal shortening.

More recent studies suggest that these patients should be classified by their immunopathologic and immunochemical profiles to determine whether patients have bullous pemphigoid with ocular or oral involvement, as opposed to cicatricial pemphigoid or oral mucosal pemphigoid with skin involvement.

The oral mucosa is most frequently involved in cicatricial pemphigoid. Although ulcers and erosions are often seen in the oral mucosa (Figure 5-1), the most typical presentation is desquamative gingivitis, which is characterized by gingival erythema and edema (Figure 5-2). While the cicatricial pemphigoid spectrum of disease is the most common etiology for desquamative gin-

givitis, patients with pemphigus vulgaris, lichen planus, epidermolysis bullosa acquisita, and linear IgA bullous disease may also develop desquamative gingivitis.

Ocular manifestations of cicatricial pemphigoid include unilateral or bilateral conjunctival irritation presenting as dryness or a burning or foreign body sensation, which some patients describe as "grittiness."[7,8] Bullae formation is rarely seen in the conjunctiva, and physical findings may include loss of the normally deep architecture of the inferior or superior fornices. With progression of disease, scarring becomes more evident with focal vertical fusions of the bulbar and palpebral conjunctivae, which are known as *symblepharon* (Figure 5-3). Similarly, hori-

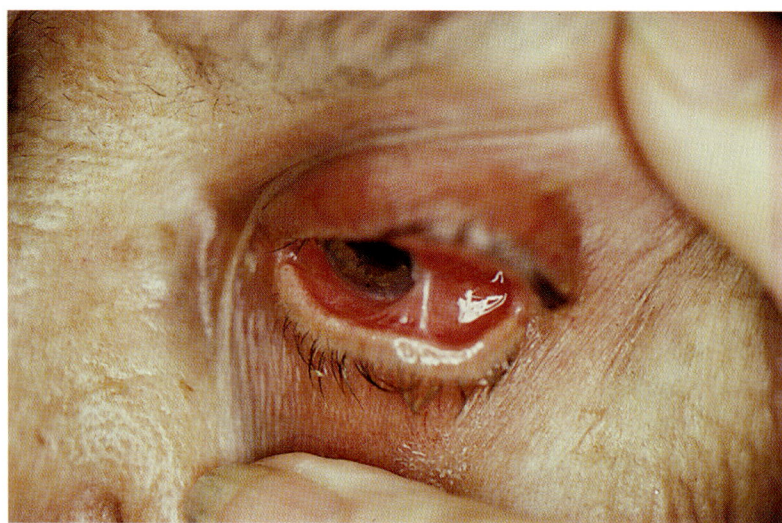

FIGURE 5-4. Late ocular disease in a patient with cicatricial pemphigoid showing much more pronounced symblepharon formation along with ankyloblepharon.

zontal fibrosis may occur, leading to progressive fusion of the superior and inferior palpebral conjunctivae known as *ankyloblepharon* and visible as a shortening of the inferior fornix (Figure 5-4). This can be quantitated as millimeters of depth of fornix or as percent shortening relative to the depth of normal fornix. With extensive fibrosis, the conjunctiva contracts and the eyelids become inverted. This inversion, known as *entropion,* causes the process, *trichiasis,* in which the eyelashes scrape the corneal surface. Corneal damage occurs and leads to corneal neovascularization and corneal ulceration, as well as improper tear coverage and keratinization. These processes, if left untreated, can result in blindness.

Esophageal lesions occur infrequently in patients with cicatricial pemphigoid. Symptoms include heartburn and dysphagia and an inability to swallow large pieces of food, which is a sign of potential esophageal stenosis. This stenosis is a result of the scarring from recurrent blister formation and can be serious. Definitive diagnosis is by barium-swallow studies followed with endoscopy and biopsies for histology and immunofluorescence (IF). Laryngotracheal disease is quite rare but can be life-threatening because of a compromised airway. Other sites of involvement include the genital and rectal areas with blisters, leading to scarring and loss of function in these areas.

Skin lesions in cicatricial pemphigoid may occur in a generalized distribution as seen in bullous pemphigoid, although it has been reported that the lesions in cicatricial pemphigoid tend to be relatively transient in nature, whereas the skin lesions in bullous pemphigoid last for longer periods of time. Classification based on antigen specificity of the circulating autoantibodies may be required to determine whether such patients have bullous pemphigoid with mucosal involvement, as opposed to cicatricial pemphigoid or oral mucosal pemphigoid with skin involvement.

The other type of skin lesion that occurs in patients with cicatricial pemphigoid is localized blisters that heal with scarring. Lesions may occur in skin adjacent to the involved mucous membranes or may be localized to the head and neck region in patients who lack any mucous membrane involvement. This condition, *Brunsting-Perry pemphigoid,* is characterized by the development of one to several circumscribed erythematous patches on top of which appear crops of recurrent blisters (Figure 5-5) that heal with atrophic scarring.[10] This condition is often marked by significant pruritus and may last for many years. The nosology of Brunsting-Perry pemphigoid is not completely clear since it has some features that favor a diagnosis of bullous pemphigoid (the presence of skin lesions only) and other features that favor a diagnosis of cicatricial pemphigoid (the presence of scarring). Some of these patients may have epidermolysis bullosa acquisita or other related entities. One patient with Brunsting-Perry pemphigoid had typical clinical features, as well as circulating IgA antibodies (unpublished data). Since circulating IgA antibodies are more commonly seen in cicatricial pemphigoid, this observation supports the concept that Brunsting-Perry pemphigoid is more likely to be a variant of cicatricial pemphigoid rather than bullous pemphigoid.

Cicatricial pemphigoid is generally a disease of older patients. The typical patient is over age 60. The natural history of the disease demonstrates a very low spontaneous remission rate.

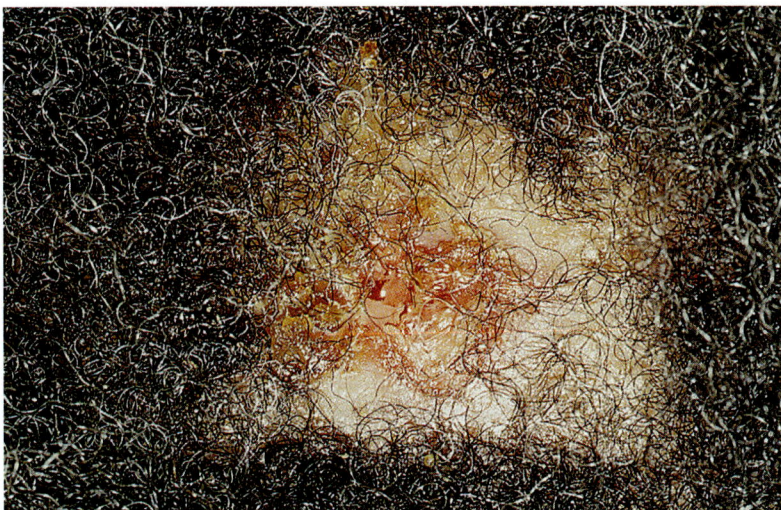
FIGURE 5-5. Scalp lesion in a patient with Brunsting-Perry pemphigoid revealing alopecia and an old blister.

Pathology

Histology

Histologic examination of skin or mucosal lesions reveals a subepithelial vesicle with an inflammatory infiltrate that may include lymphocytes, neutrophils, eosinophils, or plasma cells. Mucosal lesions tend to show a greater predominance of plasma cells. Although by no means diagnostic, some studies suggest that in bullous pemphigoid there is a higher frequency of eosinophils, whereas in cicatricial pemphigoid, there is a higher frequency of neutrophils.

Immunopathology

Direct IF studies in patients with presumed cicatricial pemphigoid are positive in most cases. The major immune reactants observed are IgG and C3 and IgA to a lesser degree. The immune reactants are deposited in a linear pattern along the epithelial BMZ (Figure 5-6). The presence of linear IgA deposits at the epithelial BMZ along with IgG and C3 is more commonly seen in cicatricial pemphigoid than in bullous pemphigoid and can occasionally be a helpful clue to distinguishing these two entities. Linear deposits of fibrin at the epidermal BMZ may also be prominent in cicatricial pemphigoid. The best results for direct IF examination are obtained from perilesional mucosal specimens, but occasionally perilesional skin specimens may also yield positive findings. Technical difficulties, however, can sometimes lead to a loss of mucosal epithelium rendering these studies difficult to interpret. Buccal mucosal biopsy for direct IF, even in the absence of oral disease, has a higher rate of positivity than a skin biopsy in patients with pure ocular disease and helps to avoid the morbidity of obtaining a conjunctival biopsy. Early indirect IF studies in patients with presumed cicatricial pemphigoid revealed low titer IgG anti-BMZ antibodies in low percentages of patients. More recent studies revealed that higher percentages of patients with cicatricial pemphigoid have circulating IgG antibodies when salt-split skin is used as a substrate (Figure 5-7).[11] Some patients with cicatricial pemphigoid have circulating IgA antibodies along with circulating IgG antibodies directed against the BMZ. Circulating IgA anti-BMZ antibodies in the absence of circulating IgG anti-BMZ antibodies have been found in occasional patients with cicatricial pemphigoid. The demonstration of circulating IgA anti-BMZ antibodies may therefore serve as another clue to aid in differentiating cicatricial pemphigoid from bullous pemphigoid. Although most patients with cicatricial pemphigoid have circulating antibodies that bind to the epidermal side of salt-split skin, there is a recently recognized variant of cicatricial pemphigoid, *anti-laminin-5 cicatricial pemphigoid*, in which patients have circulating IgG antibodies that bind to the dermal side of salt-split skin.[2] When multiple different substrates are used to screen a given patient's serum, up to 88% of cases may be positive for circulating IgG anti-BMZ antibodies. Recently, a very high frequency of circulating IgG and IgA antibodies were demonstrated in patients with cicatricial pemphigoid when assayed utilizing nondiluted patient sera.[12] Following up on this observation, another study demonstrated that the use of a simple concentrated serum assay allowed for the detection of very low titer circulating IgG and/or IgA antibodies in some patients.[13] This concentrated serum indirect IF assay may therefore be a

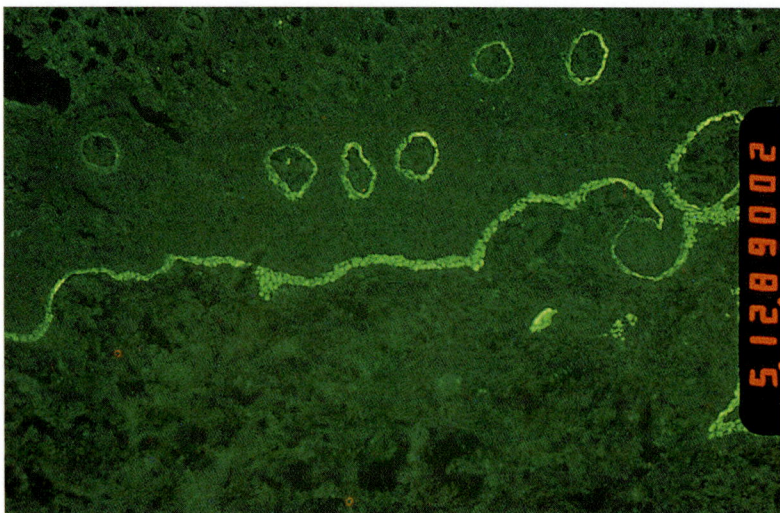

FIGURE 5-6. Direct IF perilesional mucosa from a patient with cicatricial pemphigoid revealing linear deposits of IgG at the epithelial submucosal BMZ.

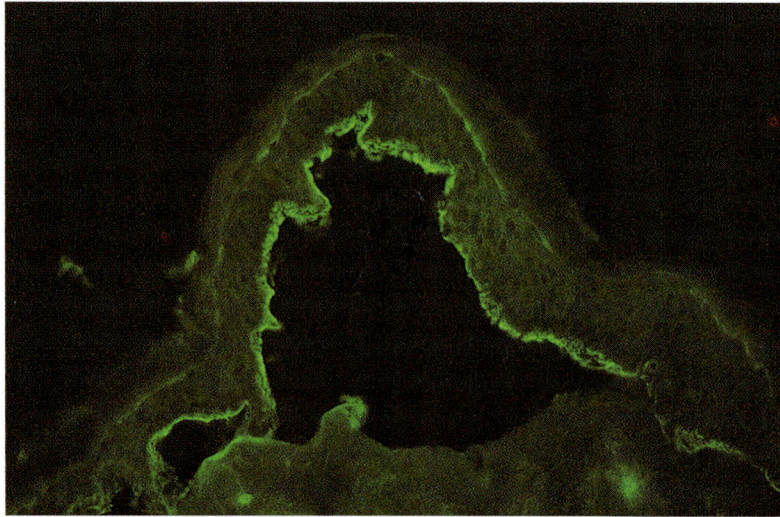

FIGURE 5-7. Indirect IF of serum from a patient with cicatricial pemphigoid assayed on 1.0 M NaCl-split human epidermis reveals the presence of a circulating IgG antibody that binds to the epidermal side of the blister cavity.

valuable tool in improving the diagnostic evaluation of patients with cicatricial pemphigoid.

Immunoelectron Microscopy

Both direct and indirect immunoelectron microscopy studies reveal the deposition of IgG immune reactants within the lower portions of the lamina lucida or in the lamina densa in most patients.

Immunochemistry

The use of sophisticated immunochemical techniques, including immunoblotting and immunoprecipitation, in the evaluation of patients with cicatricial pemphigoid has helped considerably in understanding the nosology of this condition. The original studies demonstrated that patients with cicatricial pemphigoid had circulating IgG antibodies that recognized either one or both of the 230- and 180-kD bullous pemphigoid antigens.[7] This point is still controversial, since recent studies evaluating large numbers of patients reveal that patients with cicatricial pemphigoid with bullous pemphigoid antibodies tend to have skin lesions and are best classified as a variant of bullous pemphigoid.[1] Recent studies demonstrated that some patients with cicatricial pemphigoid have IgG antibodies directed against laminin-5 and laminin-6.[2,3] Patients with pure ocular disease may have IgG antibodies directed against the β4 integrin, and other patients may have IgA antibodies directed against an incompletely characterized 45-kD protein.[4,5] These immunochemical studies demonstrate that there are several distinct variants within the cicatricial pemphigoid phenotype and that further work is necessary to ascertain all of the different subtypes within this disease spectrum.

Diagnosis

Diagnosis of cicatricial pemphigoid is based on the presence of the appropriate clinical, histologic, immunopathologic and immunochemical features. When a patient presents with the onset of a blistering disease of the mucous membranes, appropriate evaluation includes careful examination, biopsies for histology and direct IF, and serum studies for indirect IF. The diagnosis of cicatricial pemphigoid should be suspected in patients with erosions or blisters of the mucous membranes, particularly if there is scarring present. The appropriate evaluation depends on the areas of involvement. Diagnostic evaluation of patients with suspected cicatricial pemphigoid is presented here and in Box 5-1.

Patients with skin disease should have a biopsy of lesional skin for histology, a perilesional skin biopsy for direct IF, and serum studies for indirect IF performed on salt-split skin. Patients with oral mucous membrane involvement should have lesional mucosa, preferably an

---

BOX 5-1. DIAGNOSTIC EVALUATION OF PATIENTS WITH SUSPECTED CICATRICIAL PEMPHIGOID

1. Skin disease
   A. Lesional skin biopsy for histology
   B. Perilesional skin biopsy for direct IF
   C. Serum for indirect IF using salt-split skin
2. Oral mucous membrane disease
   A. Early lesional mucosal biopsy for histology
   B. Perilesional of uninvolved mucosa or skin biopsy for direct IF
   C. Serum for indirect IF using salt-split skin
3. Ocular disease
   A. Uninvolved buccal mucosal biopsy for direct IF
   B. Serum for indirect IF using salt-split skin
   C. If both the direct IF and indirect IF are negative, perform indirect IF on concentrated sera
   D. If the indirect IF on concentrated sera is negative, perform another uninvolved buccal mucosal biopsy or a skin biopsy and salt-split this biopsy before performing direct IF
   E. If all studies continue to be negative, have an ophthalmologist perform conjunctival biopsy for histology and direct IF

---

early lesion such as an intact blister or a new erythematous patch, examined for histology. For direct IF examination, either uninvolved buccal mucosa, uninvolved perilesional mucosa, or uninvolved skin can be utilized. Occasionally, patients with cicatricial pemphigoid have such fragile mucosa that the epithelium is lost whenever any type of biopsy is obtained. To circumvent this problem a technique has been developed whereby the epithelium is obtained by rolling over the uninvolved mucosa to dislodge a piece of epithelium.[14] Direct IF is then performed on this piece of epithelium. Additionally, indirect IF on salt-split skin should be performed.

Patients with ocular disease often present the greatest diagnostic challenge. In an attempt to avoid ocular biopsies (unless they are absolutely necessary), a buccal mucosal biopsy for direct IF is recommended. If this biopsy is positive for linear BMZ deposits of IgG and C3, then proceed to indirect IF studies on salt-split skin in order to further characterize the particular subgroup of cicatricial pemphigoid to which the patient belongs. If the buccal mucosal direct IF biopsy is negative, routine salt-split skin indirect IF studies should be performed. If necessary, concentrated serum salt-split skin studies should also be done. If neither of these tests can confirm the presence of an autoimmune blistering disease as suspected, another biopsy of buccal mucosa or facial skin near the eye should be taken. This biopsy should be incubated with 1.0 M NaCl for 3 days. A direct IF study should be performed on this salt-split perilesional skin. Only after extensive attempts to document the presence of tissue bound or serum antibodies have failed, should conjunctival biopsies be performed. An ophthalmologist should obtain lesional tissue for histology and uninvolved conjunctiva for direct IF.

Differential Diagnosis

Subepithelial blisters of the mucous membranes may occur in numerous conditions besides cicatricial pemphigoid, including bullous pemphigoid, epidermolysis bullosa acquisita, linear IgA bullous dermatosis, the bullous eruption of systemic lupus erythematosus (SLE), and anti-p105 pemphigoid. Paraneoplastic pemphigus and pseudopemphigoid should also be discussed, although they do not typically demonstrate subepithelial blisters of the mucous membranes.

Bullous Pemphigoid

Bullous pemphigoid is an acquired subepidermal blistering disease that occurs most commonly in the elderly.[15] Patients develop IgG antibodies that are directed against molecules found in the epidermal BMZ and are thought to mediate cell-to-matrix adhesion. The primary lesions of bullous pemphigoid are tense blisters that occur on normal-appearing skin or on an erythematous base and are most commonly seen on the flexor surfaces of the arms and legs, axilla, groin, and abdomen.

Histologic examination of a lesion of bullous pemphigoid reveals a subepidermal blister with a predominance of eosinophils in the inflammatory infiltrate. Direct IF studies demonstrate the presence of linear deposits of IgG and C3 at the epidermal BMZ. Circulating IgG autoantibodies that bind to the epidermal BMZ are found in at least 70% of patients with bullous pemphigoid. When assayed on 1.0 M NaCl-split human skin, antibodies from bullous pemphigoid patients bind to the epidermal side of the split. The antigens recognized by these circulating antibodies are the hemidesmosomal 230-kD and 180-kD molecular weight bullous pemphigoid antigens, BPAG1 and BPAG2, respectively.

Bullous pemphigoid is a comparatively benign disease with a self-limited course that may vary from several months up to 10 years and with a mortality rate of 5% to 10% in untreated patients. Systemic glucocorticosteroids are the mainstay of therapy. Patients with mild disease that is localized can often be controlled with topical corticosteroids, but patients with more significant disease often require treatment with systemic glucocorticosteroids, sometimes with immunosuppressive agents.

Epidermolysis Bullosa Acquisita

Epidermolysis bullosa acquisita is an acquired autoimmune blistering disease, which most commonly occurs in middle age and is characterized by the presence of circulating autoantibodies directed against type VII collagen.[16] Patients with epidermyolysis bullous acquisita may have mechanobullous noninflammatory trauma-induced blisters similar to those in inherited epidermolysis bullosa, but patients may also present with inflammatory blisters of the skin and mucous membrane involvement clinically indistinguishable from bullous or cicatricial pemphigoid. The extent of mucous membrane involvement varies from minor oral disease to severe mucous membrane disease, including scarring ocular and esophageal lesions.

Histology reveals a subepidermal blister with few inflammatory cells when mechanobullous lesions are sampled or a neutrophil-rich leukocyte infiltrate when inflammatory blisters are sampled. Direct IF studies reveal linear deposits of IgG and occasionally the third component of complement at the epidermal BMZ. Circulating IgG autoantibodies that bind to the epidermal BMZ are found in about 50% of patients with epidermyolysis bullousa acquisita. When assayed on 1.0 M NaCl-split human skin, antibodies from patients with epidermyolysis bullousa acquisita bind to the dermal side of the split. The antigen recognized by these circulating antibodies is a 290-kD protein, which is a part of the carboxy terminal domain of type VII collagen.

The course of the disease is chronic and is very difficult to treat. Patients with noninflammatory lesions are largely resistant to therapy. Patients with inflammatory lesions are also difficult to treat but will respond to systemic glucocorticosteroids alone or with other agents such as dapsone or an immunosuppressive agent (such as cyclophosphamide, azathioprine, or particularly, cyclosporine). Recent success has been anecdotally reported with the use of extracorporeal photopheresis.

Linear IgA Bullous Dermatosis

Linear IgA bullous dermatosis is a subepidermal blistering disease that until recently was considered a variant type of dermatitis herpetiformis.[17] Clinical lesions consist of papulovesicles or blisters along with urticarial plaques; sometimes the patients may have an arcuate pattern with a "cluster of jewels" grouping of blisters. Lesions of the oral mucous membranes are frequently seen. Rarely, ocular involvement with subsequent scarring may occur that is similar to the scarring in cicatricial pemphigoid. Linear IgA bullous disease may occur with increased frequency in patients over 60 years of age but may be seen at any age throughout adulthood. A blistering disease found in children, known as chronic bullous disease of childhood, appears to be the childhood counterpart of linear IgA bullous disease.

The histology of linear IgA bullous disease reveals a subepidermal blister with an infiltrate of neutrophils. Direct IF studies reveal linear BMZ deposits of IgA. Indirect IF studies performed on salt-split skin often reveal a low-titer circulating IgA antibody, which usually binds to the epidermal side. The majority of patients with linear IgA disease respond to dapsone. Occasional patients may require the addition of systemic glucocorticosteroids to control their disease; α-interferon has been helpful in the treatment of some patients with linear IgA disease. Rare patients with ocular disease must be treated aggressively with systemic glucocorticosteroids and cyclophosphamide to control the disease and prevent ocular scarring.

Bullous Lupus Erythematosus

Bullous lupus erythematosus (LE) is characterized by the presence of blisters occurring in a patient with systemic LE (SLE). It occurs in a small percentage of patients with SLE, usually during a flare of their disease. Tense vesicles, urticarial papules, and plaques that may resemble either bullous pemphigoid or dermatitis herpetiformis may be present.[18] The lesions have a predilection for the upper body, including the face, neck, arms, and shoulders and can also involve the oral mucous membranes. The histology of these lesions reveals dermal papillary microabscesses of neutrophils. Routine direct IF testing reveals the presence of linear or granular deposits of IgG, IgA, IgM, and C3 at the dermal-epidermal junction. Indirect IF studies reveal the presence of circulating IgG antibodies that bind to the dermal side of salt-split skin in a pattern indistinguishable from epidermolysis bullosa acquisita antibodies. The antigen recognized by these circulating antibodies appears to be identical to the 290-kD type VII collagen recognized by circulating antibodies in epidermolysis bullosa acquisita. Bullous LE is usually treated with dapsone with good results.

Paraneoplastic Pemphigus

Paraneoplastic pemphigus is a recently recognized autoimmune syndrome that occurs in patients with an underlying malignancy, usually lymphoreticular in origin.[19] The disease is characterized by ocular and oral blisters and erosions along with generalized skin lesions that may resemble toxic epidermal necrolysis, lichen planus, bullous pemphigoid, or erythema multiforme. It is a rapidly progressive condition leading to death in most patients who have an associated malignant neoplasm (such as lymphoma). Paraneoplastic pemphigus may resolve in patients who have an associated benign neoplasm (such as thymoma) that has been surgically removed. Histologic features of both pemphigus vulgaris and erythema multiforme may be present, and rarely the histology may show features of pemphigoid. IF studies of paraneoplastic pemphigus show the presence of circulating and tissue bound IgG antibodies that bind to the cell surface of stratified squamous epithelia in a pattern indistinguishable from pemphigus. These circulating IgG antibodies also recognize the cell surface of simple epithelia, such as liver and heart, and transitional epithelia, such as bladder. Pemphigus IgG antibodies, however, only recognize the cell surface of stratified squamous epithelia. The circulating antibodies in paraneoplastic pemphigus recognize a complex of epidermal proteins that include a 250-kD protein (desmoplakin I), the 230-kD bullous pemphigoid antigen, a 210-kD protein (envoplakin), and the uncharacterized 190- and 170-kD proteins. While the etiology of this disease is poorly understood, it may result from the combination of both a cellular and humoral immune response to tumor antigens, which also have overlapping reactivity with normal components of skin and other epithelia.

Anti-p105 Pemphigoid

Recently, a new clinical entity has been described in a patient presenting with a nonscarring dermatosis characterized by the sudden onset of severe bullae and erosions of the skin and oral mucous membranes. Histology revealed subepidermal blister formation along with a neutrophilic dermal papillary infiltrate and linear deposits of IgG and C3 along the epidermal basement membrane by direct IF.[20] More extensive immunochemical investigation of this patient revealed circulating IgG antibodies directed against a novel component of the epidermal BMZ, a 105-kD molecule. This patient's disease may represent a new entity called anti-p105 pemphigoid.

Pseudopemphigoid

Pseudopemphigoid is a clinical entity known to ophthalmologists as a scarring ocular disease that is difficult to distinguish from cicatricial pemphigoid.[7] Patients develop this condition, which only involves the eyes and most commonly only one eye, as an unusual complication of long-term use of topical eyedrops for glaucoma treatment. The most commonly implicated agents include pilocarpine, guanethidine, idoxuridine, phosphochiline, and ephedrine. Although the histology of this lesion may sometimes reveal a subepithelial blister, immunopathology is almost always negative.

Treatment

Treatment of patients with cicatricial pemphigoid is predicated on the extent and severity of disease with careful consideration given to the involved tissues. In patients with mild disease, characterized by the presence of small numbers of blisters or erosions of the oral mucous membranes, treatment with topical or intralesional steroids seems to be the most prudent measure, particularly when combined with appropriate oral hygiene methods to prevent further oral trauma. These methods should include making sure that if the patient is wearing dentures or other oral appliances that they fit well. Other helpful measures include the use of topical viscous lidocaine to diminish the pain of oral erosions and the use of half-strength hydrogen peroxide rinses after meals and before bed to minimize the incidence of secondary infections. Use of topical steroids in the oral cavity can be difficult; the use of an acrylic mold to ensure adequate delivery of drug to the involved gingivae has been helpful in many patients. Another viable therapy for patients with oral mucous membrane disease is topical cyclosporine. Those patients who have more significant oral disease are often treated with dapsone in doses up to 150 mg daily as tolerated.[21] As the extent and severity of the disease worsens, the tendency to use more aggressive therapy increases. Those patients who have the worst oral disease with severe gingivitis and with loosening of the teeth should be treated with systemic therapy that may include dapsone, as well as oral corticosteroids, to suppress the immune reaction and prevent major dental problems, which may include loss of numerous teeth.

A major morbidity in cicatricial pemphigoid is ocular involvement. These patients often are referred from and managed with an ophthalmologist. The most worrisome physical signs are a rapidly progressive conjunctival inflammation and significant scarring. These patients require aggressive therapy to prevent the destruction of the Meibomian glands and mucous glands that play an important role in ocular lubrication. Often, if these glands are destroyed, it is extremely difficult to preserve adequate ocular function. All patients with ocular disease require systemic therapy, although disagreement exists regarding the specifics of therapy. Some experts believe that prednisone with dapsone is a reasonable first-line therapy for patients with moderate ocular disease, with progression to oral corticosteroids combined with azathioprine in those patients who have progressive disease, and finally to cyclophosphamide for those with the worst disease. Others insist that all patients with ocular disease be treated at onset with the combination of prednisone and cyclophosphamide. Significant experience with this regimen demonstrates that approximately 75% of these patients may experience a prolonged remission after 18 to 24 months of treatment.[22] However, there are significant risks with this therapy, including hemorrhagic cystitis, bone marrow suppression, increased risk of infections, and most worrisome of all a significantly increased risk of developing bladder carcinomas and lymphomas. Recently, the use of pulse cyclophosphamide with glucocorticosteroids has been reported to also be a successful treatment in a small number of patients with ocular cicatricial pemphigoid.[23] Whether this form of therapy will prove to be as efficacious and perhaps less toxic than oral cyclophosphamide is not known at this time.

Patients who have involvement of the skin or genitalia may be managed with either topical or occasionally in the more severe cases, systemic steroids. Other major morbidities in cicatricial pemphigoid occur when patients have esophageal or laryngotracheal involvement, and the consensus is that these patients should be treated aggressively with a combination of prednisone and cyclophosphamide to prevent the potentially life-threatening complications of asphyxiation and esophageal stenosis. In patients with severe esophageal stenosis, esophageal dilation may be required.

Patients with cicatricial pemphigoid may develop severe scarring that requires surgical intervention. It is crucial that this surgical intervention not occur until the disease is under control because there may be more inflammation created with further scarring if surgery is performed while the disease is still clinically active. If surgical procedures that injure mucosal epithelium become necessary, such as lysing conjunctival adhesions, dilating the esophagus, or resecting laryngeal stenosis, it is prudent to increase the level of immunosuppression for a period of 2 weeks after the procedure.

REFERENCES

1. Chan LS, Yancey KB, Hammerberg C, et al: Immune-mediated subepithelial blistering diseases of mucous membranes, *Arch Dermatol* 129:448-455, 1993.
2. Domloge-Hultsch N, Anhalt GJ, Gammon WR, et al: Anti-epiligrin cicatricial pemphigoid. A subepithelial bullous disorder, *Arch Dermatol* 130:1521-1529, 1994.
3. Chan LS, Majmudar AA, Tran HH, et al: Laminin-6 and Laminin-5 are recognized by autoantibodies in a subset of cicatricial pemphigoid, *J Invest Dermatol* 108:848-53, 1997.
4. Tyagi et al: Ocular cicatricial pemphigoid antigen: Partial sequence and biochemical characterization, *Proc Nat Acad Sci* 93: 14714-9, 1996.
5. Smith EP, Taylor TB, Meyer LJ, et al: Identification of a basement membrane zone antigen reactive with circulating IgA antibody in ocular cicatricial pemphigoid, *J Invest Dermatol* 101:619-623, 1993.
6. Chan LS, Hammerberg C, Cooper KD: Significantly increased occurrence of HLA-DQB1*0301 allele in patients with ocular cicatricial pemphigoid, *J Invest Dermatol* 108:129-132, 1997.
7. Mutasim DF, Pelc NJ, Anhalt GJ: Cicatricial pemphigoid, *Dermatol Clin* 11:499-510, 1993.
8. Ahmed AR, Hombal SM: Cicatricial pemphigoid, *Int J Dermatol* 25:90-96, 1986.
9. Hardy KM, Perry JO, Pingree GC, et al: Benign mucous membrane pemphigoid, *Arch Dermatol* 104:467-475, 1971.
10. Brunsting LA, Perry HO: Benign Pemphigoid? A report of seven cases with chronic, scarring, herpetiform plaques about the head and neck, *Arch Dermatol* 75:489-501, 1957.
11. Kelly SE, Wojnarowska F: The use of chemically split tissue in the detection of circulating anti-basement membrane zone antibodies in bullous pemphigoid and cicatricial pemphigoid, *Br J Dermatol* 118:31-40, 1988.
12. Sarret Y, Hall R, Cobo LM, et al: Salt-split human skin substrate for the immunofluorescent screening of serum from patients with cicatricial pemphigoid and a new method of immunoprecipitation with IgA antibodies, *J Am Acad Dermatol* 24:952-58, 1991.
13. Korman NJ, Watson RD: Immune-mediated subepithelial blistering diseases of the mucous membranes: Improving the detection of circulating autoantibodies by the use of concentrated sera, *Arch Dermatol* 132:1194-1198, 1996.
14. Siegel MA, Anhalt GJ: Direct immunofluorescence of detached gingival epithelium for diagnosis of cicatricial pemphigoid, *Oral Surg Oral Med Oral Path* 75:296-302, 1993.
15. Korman NJ: Bullous pemphigoid, *Dermatol Clin* 11:483-498, 1993.

16. Gammon WR, Briggaman RA, Woodley DT, et al: Epidermolysis bullosa acquisita-a pemphigoid-like disease, *J Am Acad Dermatol* 11:820-832, 1984.
17. Leonard JN, Wright P, Williams DM, et al: The relationship between linear IgA disease and benign mucous membrane pemphigoid, *Br J Dermatol* 110:307-314, 1984.
18. Gammon WR, Briggaman RA: Bullous SLE: A phenotypically distinctive but immunologically heterogenous bullous disorder, *J Invest Dermatol* 100:28S-34S, 1993.
19. Korman NJ: Paraneoplastic pemphigus: A distinctive autoimmune syndrome, *Med Surg Derm* 2:3-6, 1995.
20. Chan LS, Fine JD, Briggaman RA, et al: Identification and partial characterization of a novel 105 kd lower lamina lucia autoantigen associated with a novel immune-mediated subepidermal blistering disease, *J Invest Dermatol* 101:262-267, 1993.
21. Rogers RS, Seehafer JR, Perry HO: Treatment of cicatricial pemphigoid with dapsone, *J Am Acad Dermatol* 6:215-223, 1982.
22. Foster CS: Cicatricial pemphigoid, *Trans Am Ophthalmol Soc* 84:527-660, 1986.
23. Pandya AG, Warren KJ, Bergstresser PR: Cicatricial pemphigoid successfully treated with pulse intravenous cyclophosphamide, *Arch Dermatol* 133:245-247, 1997.

6

Pemphigoid (Herpes) Gestationis

Rachel E. Jenkins
Martin M. Black

Etiology

Pemphigoid gestationis is a rare autoimmune bullous disease occurring during pregnancy and the puerperium, occasionally associated with trophoblastic tumors, hydatidiform mole, and choriocarcinoma.[1] Historically it has been called a variety of names with Milton first applying the name *herpes gestationis* in 1872 (Box 6-1). Clinically and immunopathologically, pemphigoid gestationis is closely related to the pemphigoid group of bullous disorders; therefore the term *pemphigoid gestationis* is preferable to *herpes gestationis*, which may otherwise encourage confusion with viral-mediated disease. Despite clinical resemblances to herpetic lesions, viral studies in pemphigoid gestationis have been consistently negative.

Pemphigoid gestationis has been previously shown to be associated with the HLA antigens, DR3 and DR4. Approximately 61% to 80% of patients express DR3, 52% to 53% express DR4, and 43% to 50% express both compared with 3% of normal controls.[2] Advances in molecular analytical techniques, such as restriction fragment length polymorphism (RFLP) and sequence-specific oligonucleotide probing, now allow the identification of HLA alleles previously difficult to define by serologic assays. HLA DRB1*0301 (DR3) and DRB1* 0401/040X (DR4; the "X" denoting the combined subtypes of DR4 other than 0401) have recently been shown to be associated with pemphigoid gestationis.[3] There is no obvious relationship between HLA type and clinical severity, onset, duration, or recurrence nor is there any relationship between HLA type and the presence or absence of immunoglobulin G (IgG) along the basement membrane zone (BMZ) by direct immunofluorescence (IF). A significant increase in the frequency of paternal HLA DR2 antigens also led to the conclusion that both paternal HLA type and maternal HLA antibodies are important in the development of pemphigoid gestationis. The MHC class II genes, DR, DP, and DQ, are located immediately adjacent to the class III genes that encode the complement components C4 with the isomers C4A and C4B, factor B and C2. There are in fact 13 alleles of C4A and 22 of C4B. A recent study has demonstrated the universal presence of nonfunctioning, so-called C4 null allele in patients with pemphigoid gestationis.[4] In particular, a C4A rather than C4B null allele was identified and this may be important with regards to impaired immune complex degradation. However, because the C4 locus is adjacent to the DR locus on chromosome 6, with strong linkage disequilibrium, it makes it extremely difficult to determine what is the primary genetic marker in pemphigoid gestationis, whether it is DRB1* 0301, DRB1*0401/040X, or a C4 null allele.

BOX 6-1. HISTORICAL TERMINOLOGY OF PEMPHIGOID GESTATIONIS

NAME AND REFERENCE
Pemphigus gravidarum, von Martius, 1829
Pemphigus pruriginosus, Chausit, 1852
Herpes circinatus bullosus, Wilson, 1867
Pemphigus hystericus, Hebra, 1868
Herpes gestationis, Milton, 1872
Dermatitis multiformis gestationis, Allen, 1889
Pemphigoid gestationis, Holmes and Black, 1982

Clinical Features

Pemphigoid gestationis is estimated to complicate 1 in 40,000 to 60,000 pregnancies.[1] The disease has no particular racial predisposition, although there is evidence that the incidence may vary according to the incidence of HLA-DR3 and DR4 in different populations.

Onset of Disease

Pemphigoid gestationis may develop at any time from 9 weeks' gestation to 1 week postpartum but usually presents during the second and third trimesters. First trimester onset has been reported but this is exceptional

PEMPHIGOID GESTATIONIS SUMMARY

ETIOLOGY
Pemphigoid gestationis is a rare autoimmune bullous disease occurring during pregnancy and the puerperium. It is associated with HLA DR3 AND DR4, especially the subtypes DRB1*0301 and DRB1*0401/040X. The etiology is unknown.

CLINICAL FEATURES
Onset of disease is characteristically in the second and third trimester of pregnancy and often flares immediately postpartum. Early lesions consist of erythematous, annular, urticated plaques on which vesicles develop; periumbilical involvement is common. Bullae and rings of vesicles may later develop especially on limbs, palms, and soles.

PATHOLOGY
Subepidermal bullae develop with prominent eosinophils within blister fluid and edematous upper dermis. There is a mixed, perivascular lymphohistiocytic infiltrate admixed with eosinophils. Direct IF shows linear deposition of complement, with or without IgG, along BMZ of perilesional skin and placenta. Indirect IF demonstrates circulating anti-BMZ IgG in 25% of patients.

DIAGNOSIS
Typical clinical findings supported by characteristic laboratory techniques of direct (on skin) and indirect (on serum) IF.

DIFFERENTIAL DIAGNOSIS
Polymorphic eruption of pregnancy, bullous pemphigoid, dermatitis herpetiformis, linear IgA bullous dermatosis, erythema multiforme, contact dermatitis, urticaria, bullous drug eruption.

TREATMENT
Topical corticosteriods, systemic antihistamines, and systemic corticosteriods are the mainstay and occasionally other immunosuppressive agents are used after delivery.

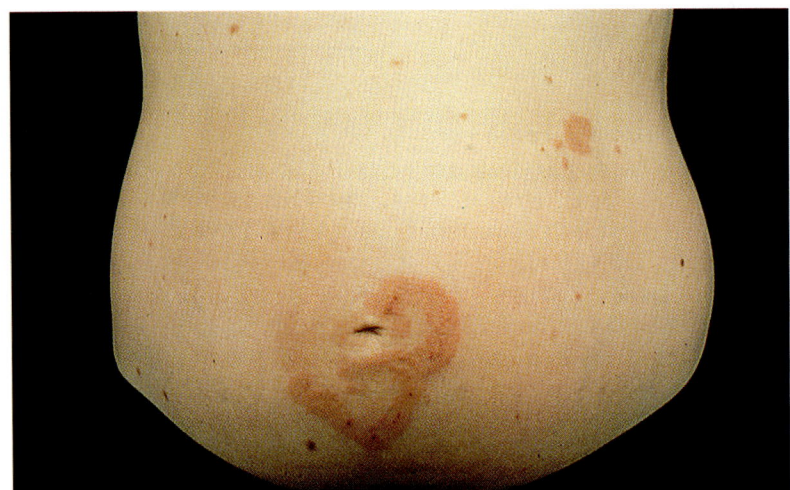

FIGURE 6-1. Periumbilical plaque in pemphigoid gestationis.

even with recurrent disease. The disease may present in the first pregnancy or later and is likely to recur, usually with an earlier onset and more florid expression. When pemphigoid gestationis develops during the middle trimester there is often a period of relative remission in the last few weeks of pregnancy, but this is frequently followed by abrupt relapse postpartum.[1] Initial presentation postpartum may be "explosive" and occurs in approximately 20% of women, but onset more than 3 days' postpartum makes pemphigoid gestationis unlikely as the diagnosis.

Occasionally, subsequent pregnancies are unaffected. Such *skip pregnancies* have an incidence of approximately 5% but remain unpredictable on a prospective basis using available data. What is clear, however, is that recurrence is not universal. Previous reports have suggested that such pregnancies may be more likely after a change in partner or when the mother and fetus are fully compatible at the HLA-D locus but this is certainly not always the case.[1]

Rash of Pemphigoid Gestationis

Typical early lesions consist of pruritic, erythematous, urticated papules, and plaques (Figure 6-1) that may become targetlike, develop into annular wheals (Figure 6-2), or become polycyclic. After a variable period, ranging from a few days to a month, vesicles develop (Figure 6-3). Bullae and rings of vesicles develop at the margins of edematous, erythematous plaques. Bullae may appear *de novo* on otherwise clinically uninvolved skin. Blisters are usually tense and contain serous fluid; however, pustules may be seen, albeit rarely. In 90% of patients the eruption is initially confined to the periumbilical area with later spread to the abdomen (Figure 6-4), thighs (Figure 6-5), palms, and soles (Figure 6-6).[1] The condition often becomes widespread, but the face (Figure 6-7) and oral mucosa are usually spared. The blisters tend to resolve first with the plaques of erythema persisting longer. In the absence of secondary infection, resolution usually occurs without scarring.

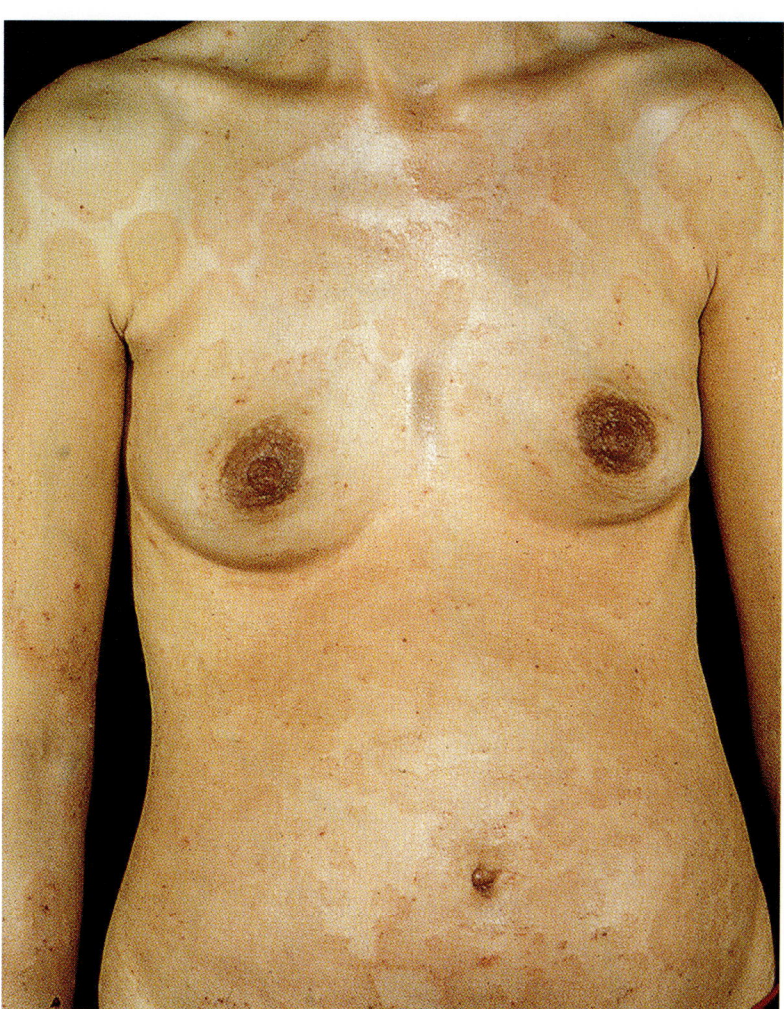

FIGURE 6-2. Widespread annular erythema in pemphigoid gestationis.

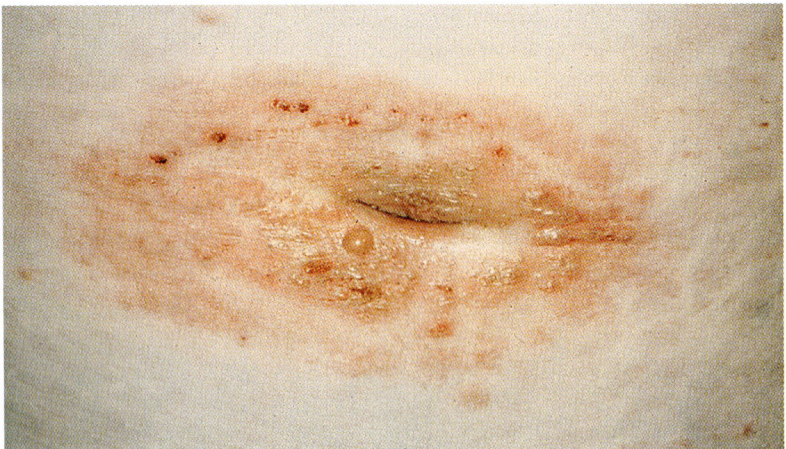

FIGURE 6-3. Peri-umbilical annular plaque with early vesiculation in pemphigoid gestationis.

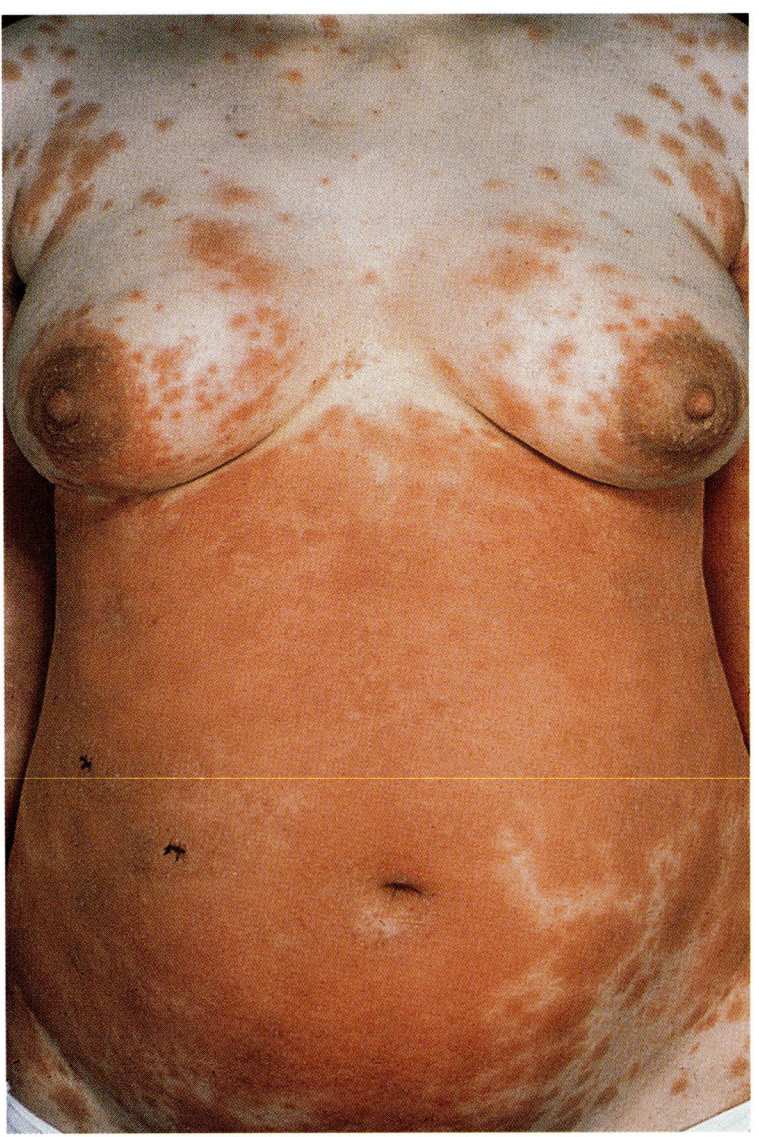

FIGURE 6-4. Widespread erythema on trunk in pemphigoid gestationis.

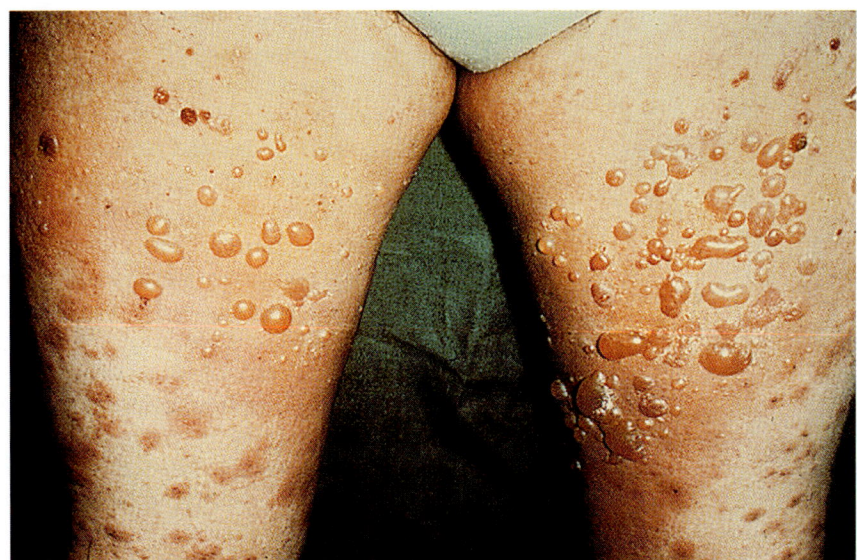

FIGURE 6-5. Bullous lesions on anterior thighs in pemphigoid gestationis.

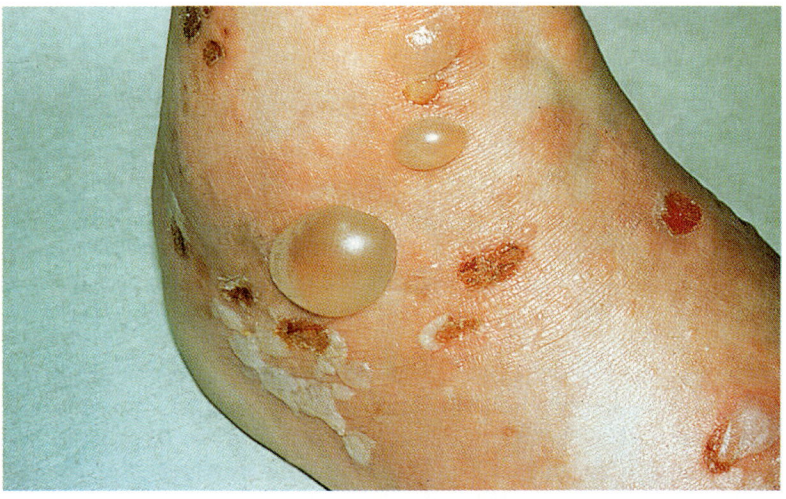

FIGURE 6-6. Tense bullae, erosions and urticarial lesions on ankle in pemphigoid gestationis.

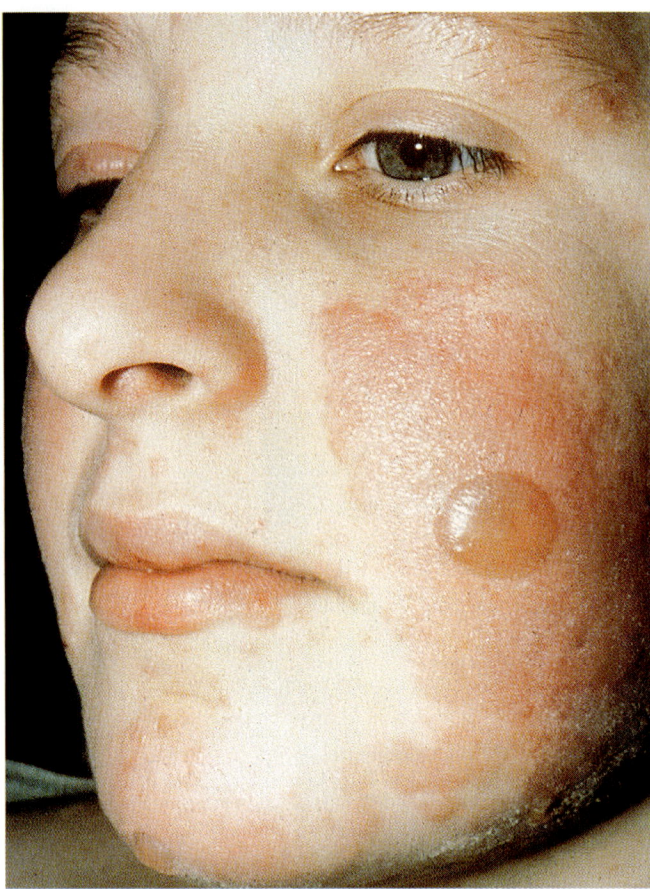

FIGURE 6-7. Blisters and urticarial lesions on face in pemphigoid gestationis.

Natural History

Occasionally there is spontaneous clearing of the disease during the latter part of pregnancy. Exacerbation with delivery is the rule, however, even in those with a previous history of spontaneous resolution. Such exacerbation occurs in 75% to 80% of cases. Postpartum flares of disease are seen in 50% to 75%, typically beginning within 24 to 48 hours of delivery. The duration of postpartum flares is variable but usually ranges from weeks to several months of involvement.

The duration of continued disease activity beyond delivery is variable, and there is no correlation between disease activity and serum antibody titers. The bullous lesions tend to resolve within a month of delivery, but pruritic, urticated plaques may persist for several months or even years with premenstrual exacerbations. Some patients have been described with disease activity for as long as 11 to 12 years.[5] Minor flares during menstruation for weeks or months postpartum are common and often is the only time when symptoms occur. Some women (20% to 50%) with a history of pemphigoid gestationis develop recurrences if treated with oral contraceptives (oestrogens or progestogens).

Hydatidiform Mole and Choriocarinoma

Rarely, pemphigoid gestationis is associated with trophoblastic tumors such as hydatidiform mole and choriocarcinoma.[1] Hydatidiform mole and choriocarcinoma are entirely derived from the sexual consorts in that the 46 chromosomes of the hydatidiform mole consist of a pair of identical paternal chromosomes with no maternal contribution.[6] Since pemphigoid gestationis occurs in both pregnancy and trophoblastic tumors, it is possible that paternally-derived antigens reside on the trophoblastic cells or cells of the chorioamniotic membranes. If any of these cross-react with antigens in the BMZ of skin, then immune responses to the trophoblast could result in autoimmune response to the skin.

Interestingly, there are no reports of a disease in men similar to pemphigoid gestationis with choriocarcinoma. This malignancy is relatively common and biochemically similar to normal pregnancy. Cytogenetic studies have demonstrated that the chromosomes in choriocarcinoma in men are also entirely of paternal origin.[6] It would therefore appear that placental tissue is required for the initial development of disease not simply the presence of germinal tissue nor actual presence of fetus. The allogeneic state of pregnancy is therefore required to develop PG.

Fetal/Neonatal Disease

Cutaneous lesions occur in 5% to 10% of infants born to mothers with pemphigoid gestationis.[1] They are generally mild and may be present at birth or appear at any time up to the third day postpartum. The lesions are often not frankly bullous but take the form of an erythematous or urticarial papular rash that regresses spontaneously around 3 weeks. Very rarely, large (3 to 4 cm diameter) bullae develop and may persist for about a month. Neonatal cutaneous disease is usually mild and transient, resolving untreated over days to weeks presumably as transferred maternal antibodies are catabolized. Long-term sequelae of disease have not been reported in children born to affected mothers nor has an increase in other autoimmune diseases.

Neonatal pemphigoid gestationis results from the passive transfer across the placenta of maternal IgG anti-BMZ autoantibodies. These antibodies may be demonstrated in cord blood and in neonatal skin. Some reports have shown complement deposition in skin specimens even in the absence of clinical disease. By the end of the first month of life, direct IF of these infants' skin biopsy specimens is normal, and circulating IgG anti-BMZ autoantibodies can no longer be detected.

The risks to the fetus or neonate in pemphigoid gestationis have historically been controversial with few studies large enough to provide a definitive answer. In 1969 Kolodny remarked that there was no evidence of an increased incidence of stillbirth or spontaneous abortion associated with pemphigoid gestationis.[7] Lawley

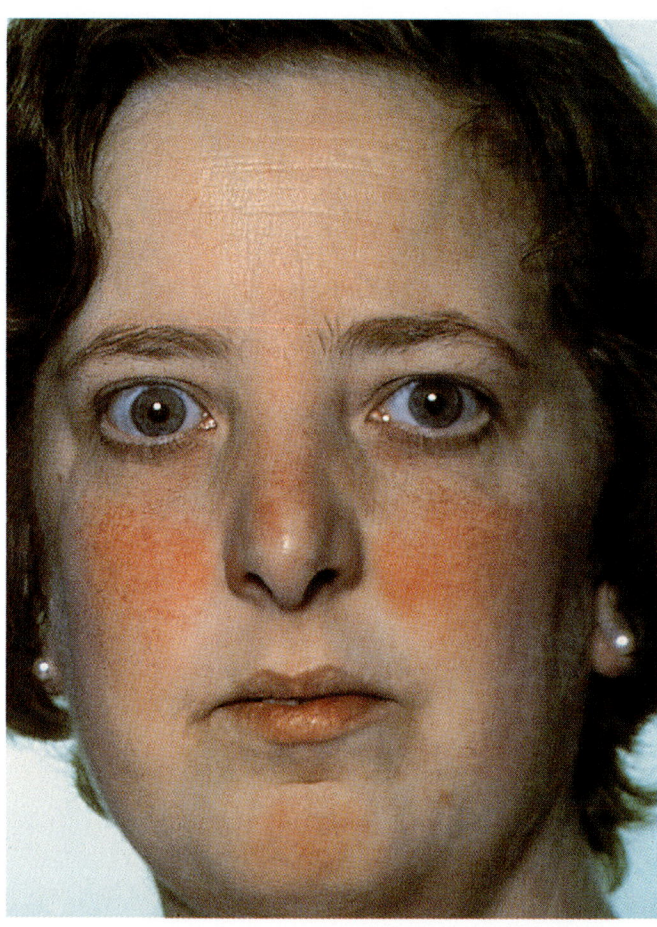

FIGURE 6-8. Thyrotoxicosis, which developed 10 years after the onset of severe pemphigoid gestationis in same patient as Figure 6-7.

et al reviewed 41 cases of immunologically confirmed pemphigoid gestationis and by contrast, reported increased fetal morbidity and mortality.[8] This study, however, relied on published cases that may have overestimated complications after selective reporting. A study of 50 pregnancies affected by pemphigoid gestationis demonstrated a significant increase in the frequency of infants that had small-for-gestation dates.[9] Because such infants have increased mortality and morbidity, these authors concluded that the fetal prognosis in pemphigoid gestationis was impaired. A more recent large study found no evidence of an increased rate of spontaneous abortion or significant mortality but did demonstrate an increased incidence of both prematurity and small-for-dates babies with pemphigoid gestationis.[10] These observations would be consistent with low-grade placental dysfunction.

Associated Autoimmune Diseases

There have been a few anecdotal case reports of pemphigoid gestationis occurring in association with other immunologically mediated disease, e.g., alopecia areata or Crohn's disease, but this is unusual. However, a study of 75 patients with pemphigoid gestationis reported 11% also had Graves' disease (Figure 6-8).[11] Graves' disease is known to be associated with DR3 with a 0.4% female prevalence. This study also documented a slight increase in other autoantibodies in patients with pemphigoid gestationis, including antithyroid antibodies and gastric parietal cell antibodies. In addition, there was a 25% incidence of autoimmune diseases in the relatives of those with pemphigoid gestationis, particularly Graves' disease, Hashimoto's thyroiditis, and pernicious anemia. The secondary association of other autoimmune disease with pemphigoid gestationis is important and suggests that these patients should be assessed at regular intervals for the rest of their lives.

Pathology

Histopathology

The histopathologic features of pemphigoid gestationis are distinctive for a rash occurring in pregnancy with a spectrum of appearances running parallel to the clinical manifestations. The histopathology of pemphigoid gestationis classically shows subepidermal blistering, eosinophils within the blister fluid and an edematous upper dermis that contains a mixed, perivascular lymphohistiocytic infiltrate admixed with eosinophils (although these characteristic findings are seen only in the minority of cases). More common findings include spongiotic vesicle formation or eosinophilic spongiosis (Figure 6-9). Spongiosis is often present along with focal necrosis of the basal cells over the tips of the dermal papillae. The necrotic basal cells can resemble the cytoid bodies of lichen planus. Liquefactive degeneration has been reported in up to 50% of cases. Eosinophils are common and may be seen singly or within spongiotic vesicles. Dermal changes that are seen in virtually all specimens include papillary dermal edema and perivascular infiltration of lymphocytes, histiocytes, and eosinophils. Inflammatory infiltrates may extend into or occasionally beyond the mid-reticular dermis. Eosinophils, neutrophils, or occasional lymphocytes may be seen to line up along the BMZ (Figure 6-10). The presence of eosinophils is the most constant feature in pemphigoid gestationis, being seen in nearly every case (Figure 6-11). The degree of edema or vesiculaton is variable. Early urticarial lesions are characterize by epidermal and marked papillary dermal edema. There is a moderately dense perivascular mixed inflammatory cell infiltrate with lymphocytes, histiocytes, and conspicuous eosinophils around the vessels of both the superficial and deep dermal plexuses.

Subepidermal separation results from basal cell necrosis leading to subepidermal bullae (Figure 6-12). The blister cavities typically contain large numbers of

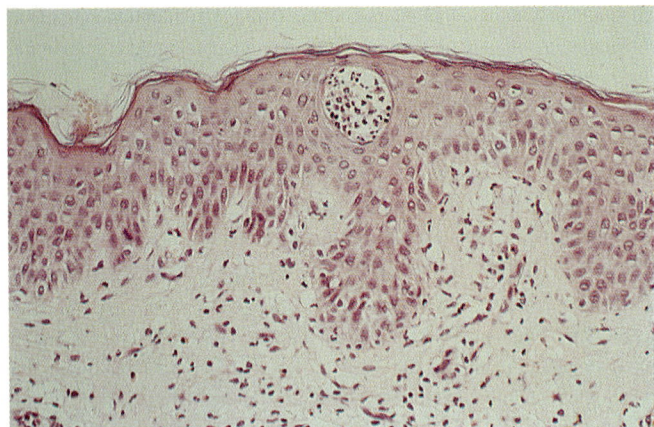

FIGURE 6-9. Vesicles containing eosinophils in epidermis (H&E; ×25) in pemphigoid gestationis.

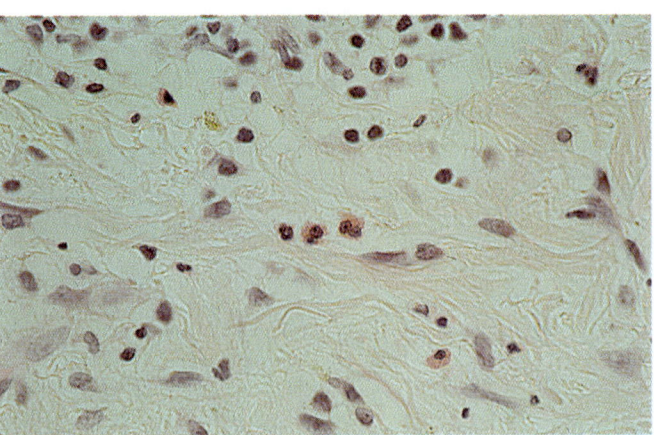

FIGURE 6-11. High magnification showing prominent eosinophils in dermal infiltrate (H&E; ×40) in pemphigoid gestationis.

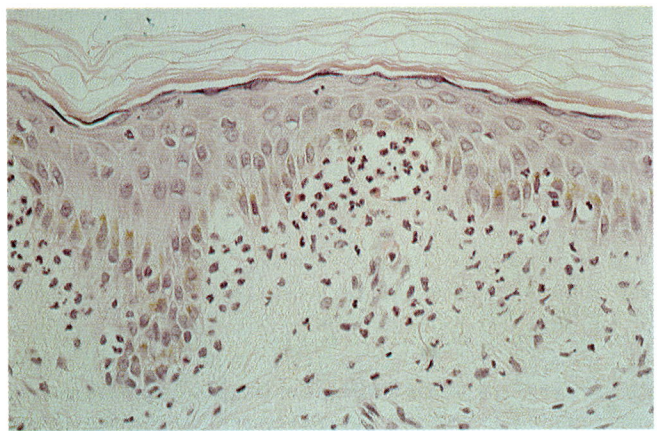

FIGURE 6-10. Early lesion showing eosinophilic spongiosis in upper dermis (H&E; ×25) in pemphigoid gestationis.

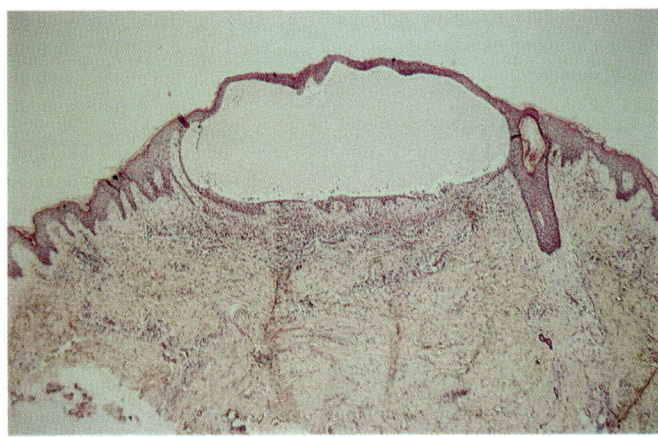

FIGURE 6-12. PG. Late lesion showing subepidermal blister (H&E; ×4) in pemphigoid gestationis.

eosinophils in addition to lymphocytes and other mononuclear cells. Severe edema of the papillary dermis can result in bulbous, tear drop-shaped dermal papillae. Sections cut to the side of these papillae can give the appearance of intraepidermal vesicles and examination of serial sections avoids misinterpretation.

Immunopathology

The most characteristic finding in pemphigoid gestationis is linear deposition of C3, with or without IgG, along the BMZ of perilesional skin. Direct IF demonstrates C3 in the BMZ of clinically uninvolved skin in all patients with pemphigoid gestationis (Figure 6-13) and linear IgG deposition in about 25% of cases. IgG deposition may be demonstrable in patients with negative routine IF with refined multi-step techniques. For example, the use of split-skin specimens, chemically separated through the lamina lucida, demonstrates IgG deposits in the lamina lucida even when conventional direct IF is negative. There appears to be no difference in disease expression in those patients who have deposition of complement alone compared with those who have IgG in addition to complement.

The *herpes gestationis factor*, now known as pemphigoid gestationis factor, is an IgG1 autoantibody directed against a normal cell surface component of cutaneous BMZ.[1] By contrast, in bullous pemphigoid the predominant autoantibody is IgG4 subclass. IgG1 avidly fixes complement by the classical pathway unlike IgG4, which activates complement deposition via the alternative pathway (Table 6-1). Circulating anti-BMZ IgG is detected in about 25% of patients using an indirect IF technique (Figure 6-14)

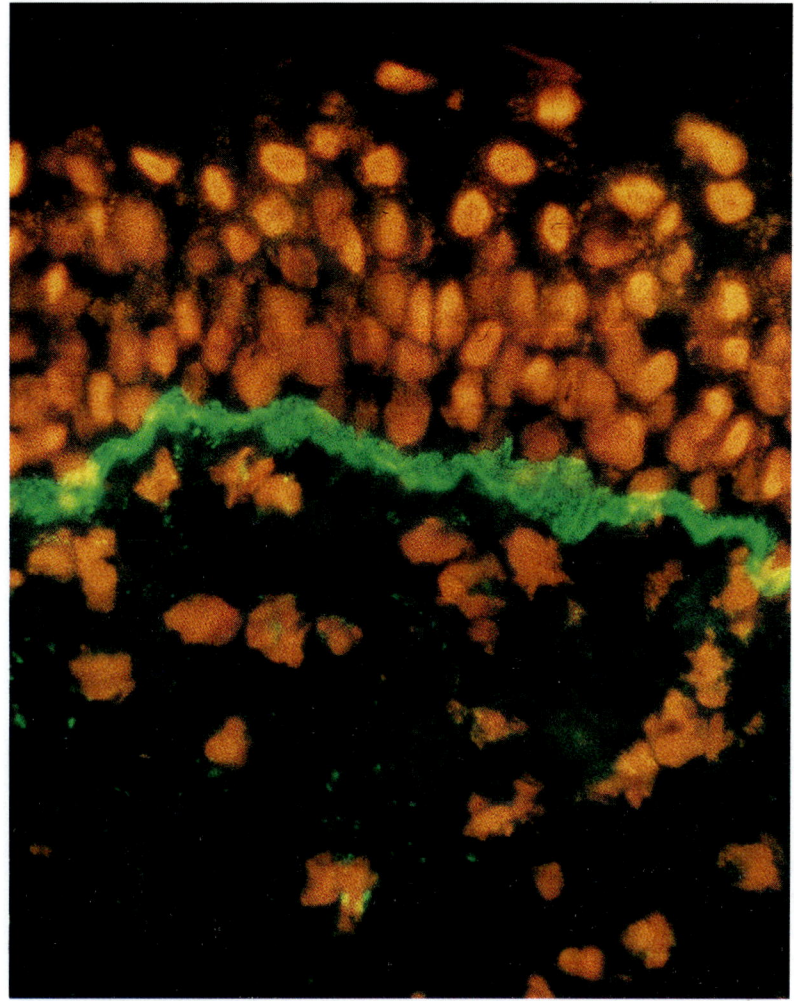

FIGURE 6-13. PG. Direct IF of perilesional skin showing linear deposition of C3 counterstained with propidium iodide.

Table 6-1. *Activation of Complement by Immunoglobulins of Different Class and Subclass*

Class	Subclass	Classical Pathway	Alternative Pathway
IgM		++++	++
IgG	IgG1	++++	++
	IgG2	+	++
	IgG3	+++	++
	IgG4	—	++
IgA		—	+++
IgE		—	++
IgD		—	++

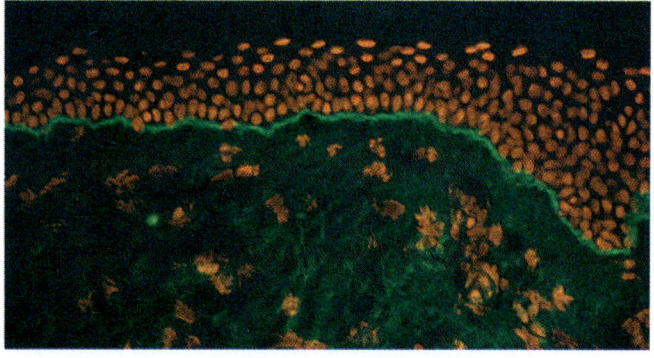

FIGURE 6-14. PG. Indirect IF showing linear IgG binding of serum to BMZ counterstained with propidium iodide.

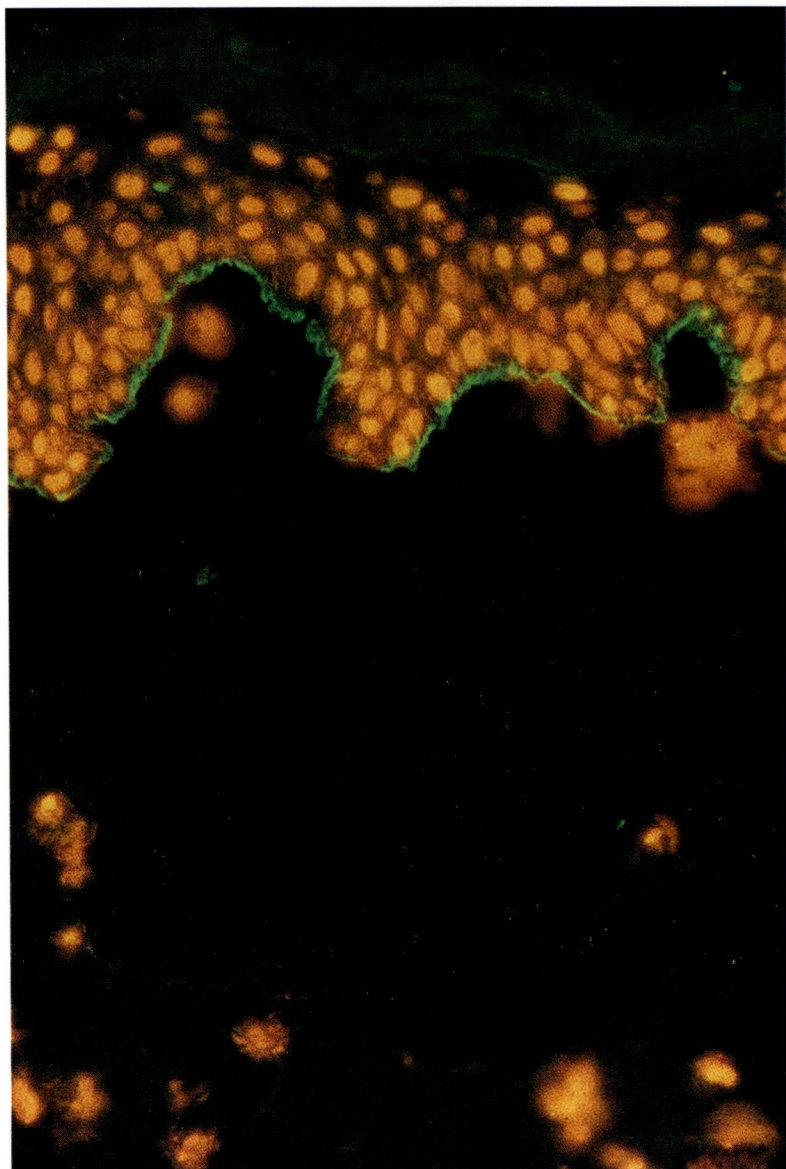

FIGURE 6-15. PG. Indirect IF showing serum binding to the epidermal aspect of salt-split skin.

and binding is to the epidermal side of NaCl-split skin (Figure 6-15). Titers do not correlate with disease severity; however, some authors have suggested that patients with high titers do have more severe and persistent disease.

There have been two reports of atypical IF staining in patients with pemphigoid gestationis, the significance of which is yet to be established. Hashimoto et al demonstrated IgG anti-keratinocyte cell surface antibodies using indirect IF in pemphigoid gestationis sera in addition to linear IgG and C3 BMZ staining.[12] Vaughan Jones et al reported a case of pemphigoid gestationis with intercellular IgG staining using direct and indirect IF in addition to linear BMZ staining with IgG and C3.[13]

Immunopathogenesis

Studies using immunoelectron microscopy (immuno-EM) demonstrated that anti-BMZ IgG is directed towards a component just below the hemidesmosome in the upper lamina lucida of the BMZ. Immunoprecipitation has previously demonstrated that the majority (>95%) of bullous pemphigoid sera react with a 230-kD epidermal polypeptide known as BPAg1[14] with about 50% also reacting with a second epidermal antigen of 180 kD, known as BPAg2.[15] The majority of pemphigoid gestationis sera recognize BPAg2 and some react to both BPAg2 and BPAg1. Cloning and sequencing have demonstrated that the 2 antigens are distinct gene products of different chromosomal locations, BPAG1 at locus

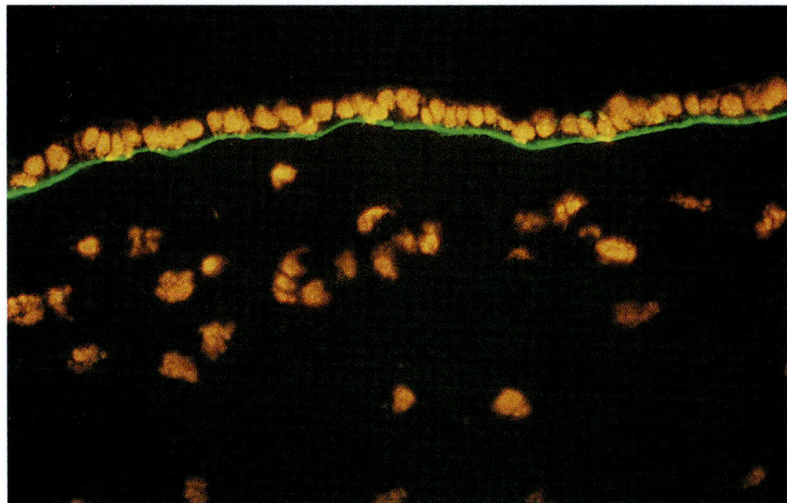

FIGURE 6-16. Direct IF showing linear BMZ staining with C3 in amniotic epithelium counterstained with propidium iodide.

6p11-12[16] and BPAG2 at locus 10q24.3.[17] BPAG2 has recently also been identified as COL171A1.[18] Pemphigoid gestationis and bullous pemphigoid therefore appear to share antigenic determinants, but in pemphigoid gestationis, antibodies directed against the 180-kD antigen are prevalent while in bullous pemphigoid antibodies to the 230-kD antigen are more frequent.

Other evidence, produced by immuno-EM using immunogold techniques, have shown that BPAg2 is a type II transmembrane constituent of the hemidesmosome with collagenous segments in its extracellular domain. For this reason, this constituent is also known as type XVII collagen. BPAg1 is an intracellular, cytoplasmic plaque component. The actual target epitope in pemphigoid gestationis has recently been localized to the NC16A region of the BPAg2 extracellular domain positioned immediately adjacent to the plasma membrane of hemidesmosomes.[19] This immunodominant epitope is recognized by more than 50% of bullous pemphigoid sera and 70% of pemphigoid gestationis. It has been further mapped to a 16 amino acid peptide.

Since BPAg1 is restricted to the intracellular compartment of the basal keratinocyte, it is not directly accessible to circulating antibodies. Anti-BPAg1 autoantibodies would be predicted to arise as a secondary event in response to an initial insult to the basal keratinocyte. In contrast, BPAg2 is a transmembrane protein and is recognized by both pemphigoid gestationis and bullous pemphigoid autoantibodies. Therefore anti-BPAg2 autoantibodies may play an initiator role in subepidermal blister formation in pemphigoid gestationis and bullous pemphigoid. Circulating autoantibodies in both diseases are likely to have access to this newly defined antigenic site on the surface of intact keratinocytes.

Pathophysiologically, pemphigoid gestationis factor fixes to the BMZ, triggering complement activation via the classical complement pathway. Immune complex formation leads to chemotactic factor elaboration and the progressive accumulation of inflammatory cells, in particular eosinophils, with the release of inflammatory mediators. The release of proteolytic enzymes from eosinophilic granules is probably responsible for the resulting separation between epidermis and dermis. Dermal-epidermal separation induces conformational changes in the pemphigoid gestationis antigen and may lead to exposure of previously cryptic antigens within the BMZ. Basal cell damage may also be produced in this manner. Such increased antigen exposure to the immune system results in increasing antibody production and immune complex formation, which perpetuates cellular damage. The fetus remains relatively protected from this immunologic onslaught in the majority of cases by the placenta, which prevents involvement of the fetal circulation.

Circulating autoantibodies, which bind to skin, cross-react with the BMZs of chorionic epithelium, and amnion and immune complexes are deposited in the placenta during the course of most cases of pemphigoid gestationis (Figure 6-16). In addition, there is an aberrant expression of MHC class II molecules, probably paternal origin, in the placenta by amniochorionic stromal cells and trophoblasts. These cells may be exposed to the maternal immune system, since it is known that in some anchoring villi there are focal deficiencies in the syncytiotrophoblast.[20] The cross-reactivity may be explained by the common origin of skin and amnion from the ectodermal germ layer. Within the villous stroma of chorionic villi, adjacent to

86 *Atlas of Bullous Disease*

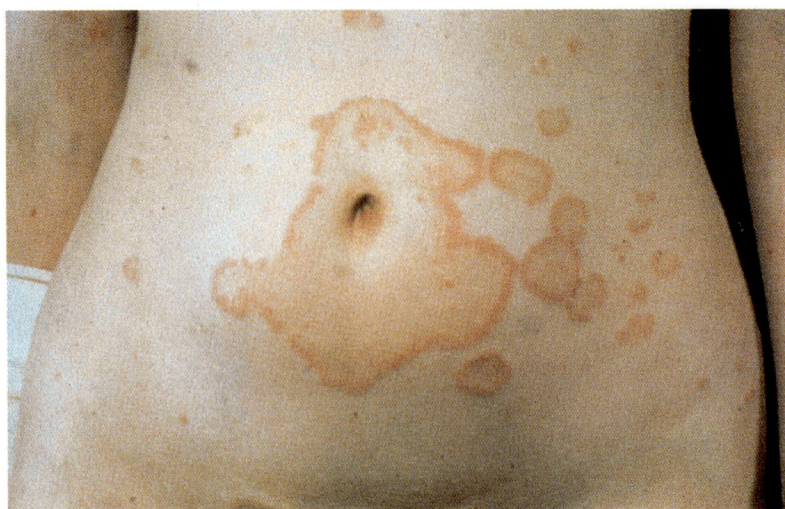

FIGURE 6-17. Pruritic, periumbilical urticarial lesions in pemphigoid gestationis.

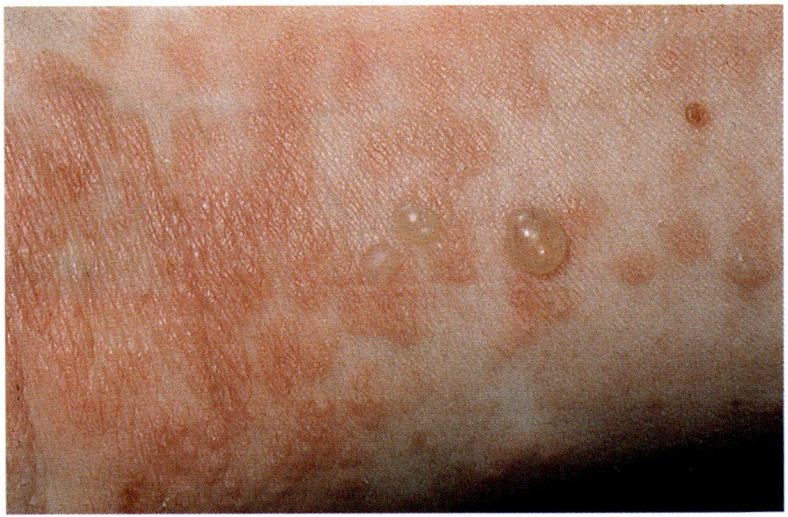

FIGURE 6-18. Bullae on urticated erythema on forearm in pemphigoid gestationis.

the maternal decidua, affected women show an abnormal expression of MHC class II antigens (-DR, -DP, -DQ), together with an increase in lymphocytes near the site of immune attack.[21] This does appear in the skin where only complement components (with or without IgG) are seen along the BMZ.

Diagnosis

Pemphigoid gestationis classically presents as a dramatic vesiculobullous disease during pregnancy, usually in the second or third trimester, or in the immediate postpartum period. It has a typically characteristic onset in which intensely pruritic, urticarial lesions on the abdomen (Figure 6-17) progress rapidly to a generalized pemphigoid-like bullous eruption (Figures 6-18 to 6-20). The disorder may spontaneously improve during late pregnancy, but even if it does improve, it usually flares at the time of delivery. The disease usually regresses spontaneously in the weeks to months after delivery, but in a few cases, the disease may remain active for many years afterwards.

Immunopathologically, pemphigoid gestationis is characterized by linear deposition of C3, with or without IgG, along the BMZ of both skin and placenta; the diagnosis of pemphigoid gestationis is confirmed on direct IF by finding a bright linear band along the cutaneous BMZ of C3 (Figures 6-21 and 6-22), with or without IgG,

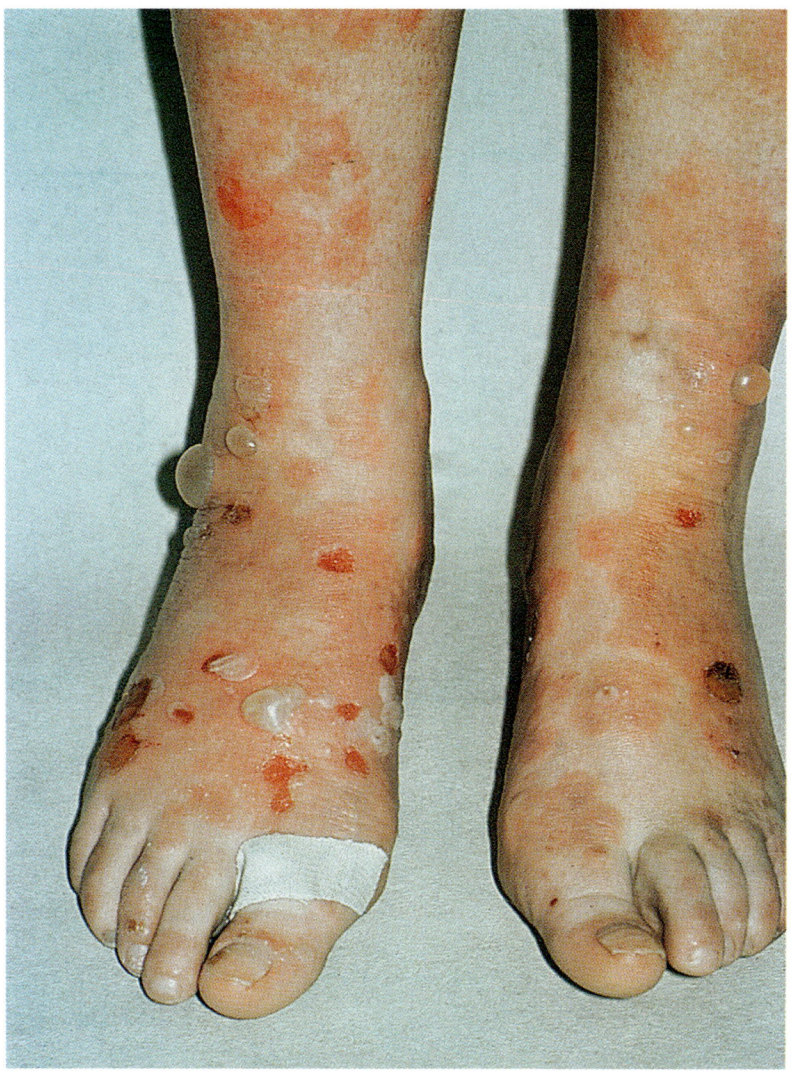

FIGURE 6-19. Blisters, erosions and urticarial lesions on legs in pemphigoid gestationis.

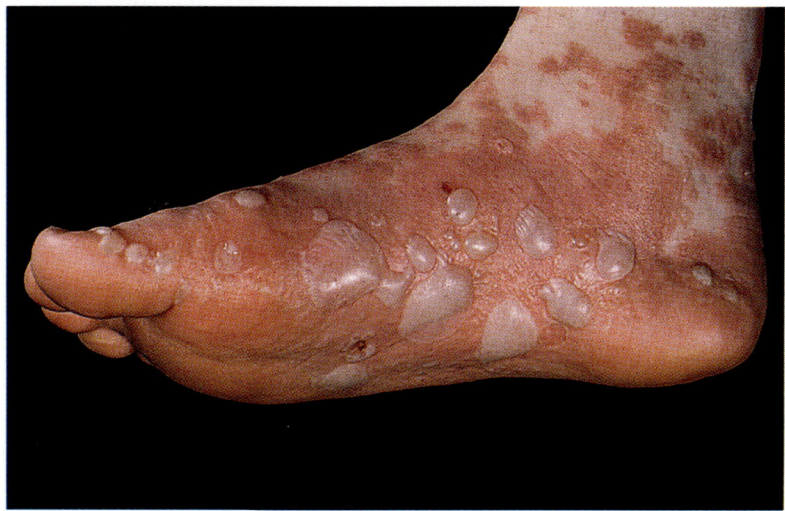

FIGURE 6-20. Tense bullous lesions on foot in pemphigoid gestationis.

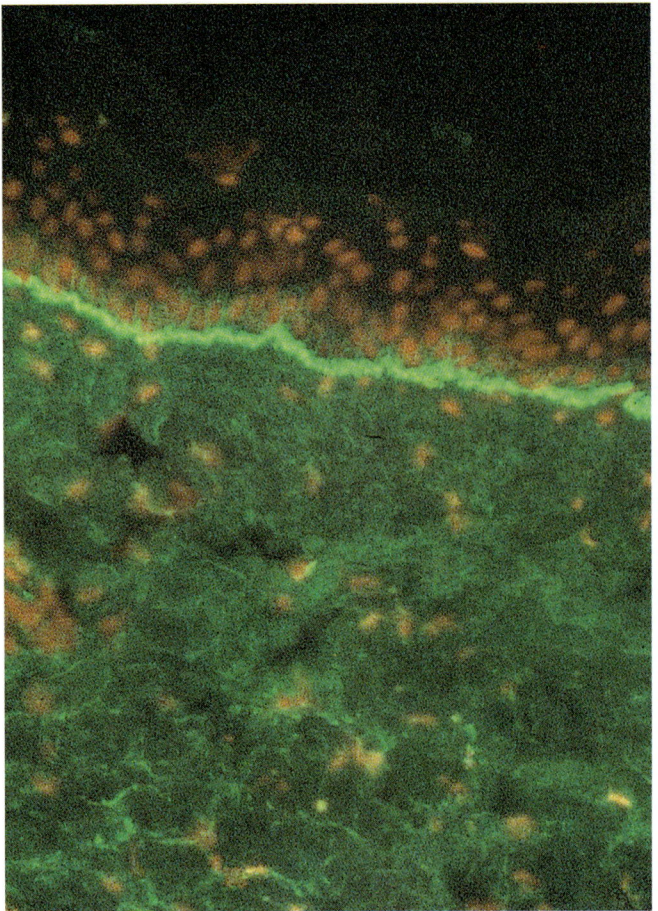

FIGURE 6-21. Direct IF of perilesional skin showing linear deposition of C3 at BMZ counterstained with propidium iodide.

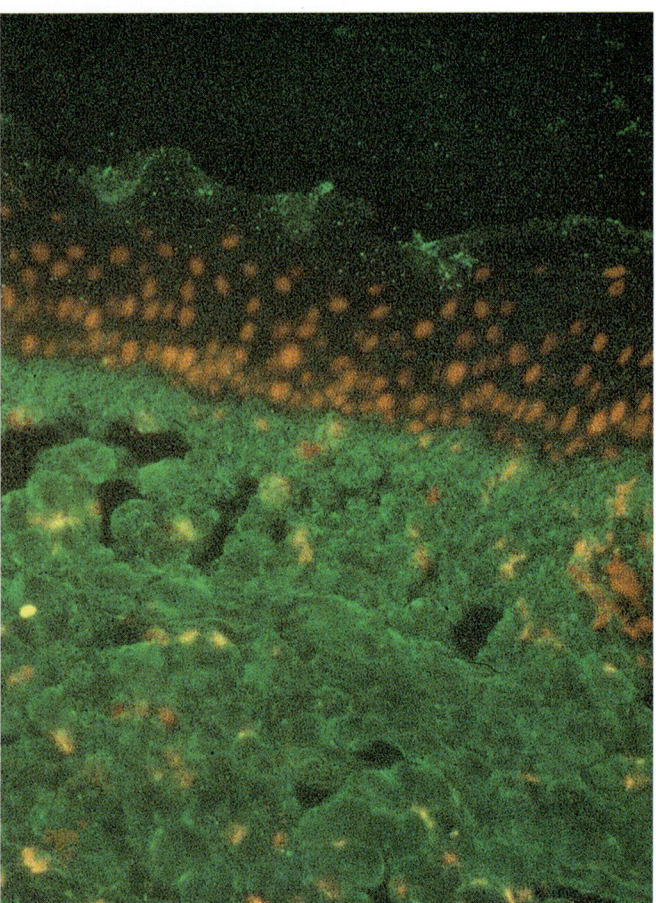

FIGURE 6-22. Negative control for direct IF.

or by the ability of serum to fix C3 to the BMZ by indirect, complement-added IF techniques (Figure 6-23).

The diagnosis of pemphigoid gestationis should not be applied to individuals with a pruritic, vesiculobullous dermatosis during pregnancy who do not demonstrate linear deposits of C3 in their epidermal BMZ. Considering that a minority of patients with pemphigoid gestationis show evidence of circulating anti-BMZ antibodies in routine indirect IF and that not all patients with pemphigoid gestationis demonstrate positive findings in complement fixation IF studies, it is apparent why it is critical to examine the patient's skin rather than the serum for the immunopathologic diagnosis of this disease.

Pemphigoid gestationis has clinical, histologic (Figure 6-24, A and B), and immunopathologic features that resemble selected aspects of bullous pemphigoid. Although many dissimilarities exist between these diseases, studies have shown that anti-BMZ antibodies in pemphigoid gestationis and bullous pemphigoid recognize related or identical antigens.

In pemphigoid gestationis there is aberrant expression of MHC class II antigens in the placenta on amniochorionic stromal cells and trophoblastic cells, which are derived from paternal genes.[21] In addition, there is a universal presence of anti-HLA antibodies that are mainly directed against class I antigens.[22] The actual role of these anti-HLA antibodies in the primary pathogenesis of pemphigoid gestationis is unknown but their presence does imply that women with pemphigoid gestationis are more able than normal women to mount an allogeneic response against their partners' antigens and this may be a clue to the etiology of the disease. Anti-HLA antibodies may develop as a consequence of a placental bleed, which may then result in the partial destruction of the placenta, exposing cryptic antigens leading to the production of IgG autoantibody.

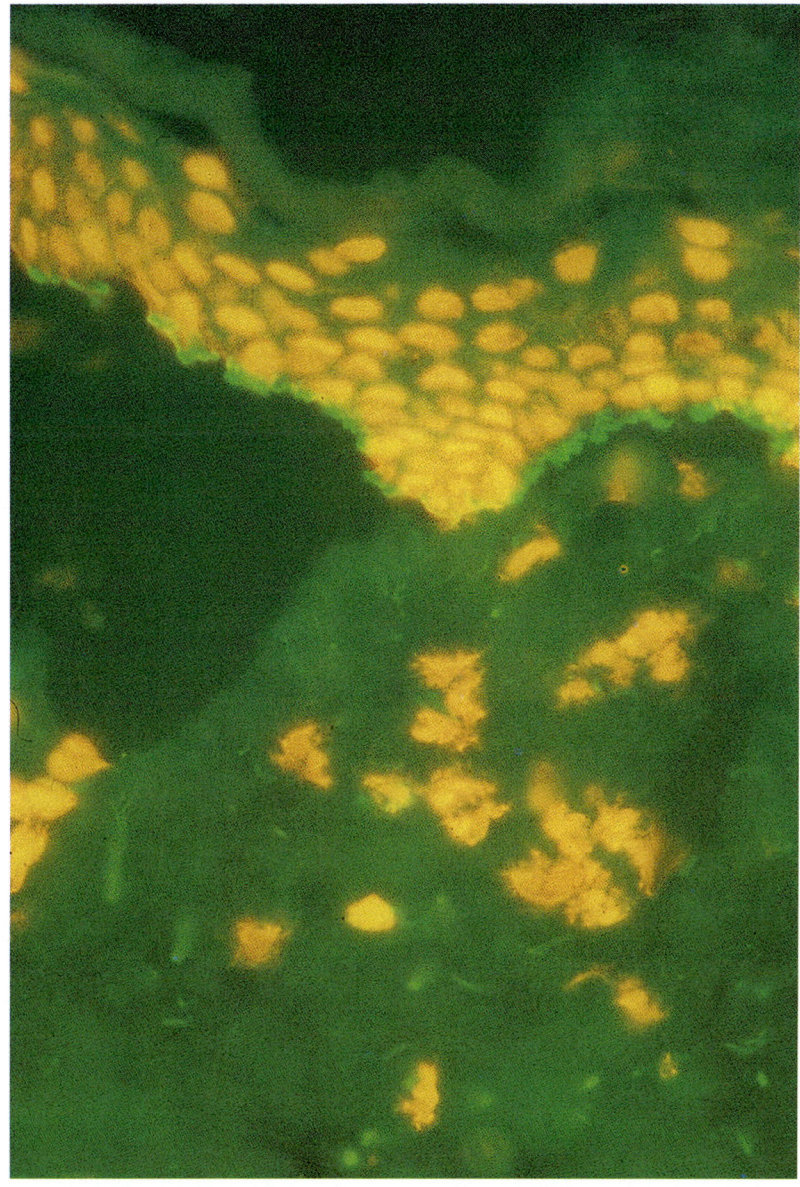

FIGURE 6-23. Indirect immunofluorescence showing serum binding to epidermal side of salt-split skin.

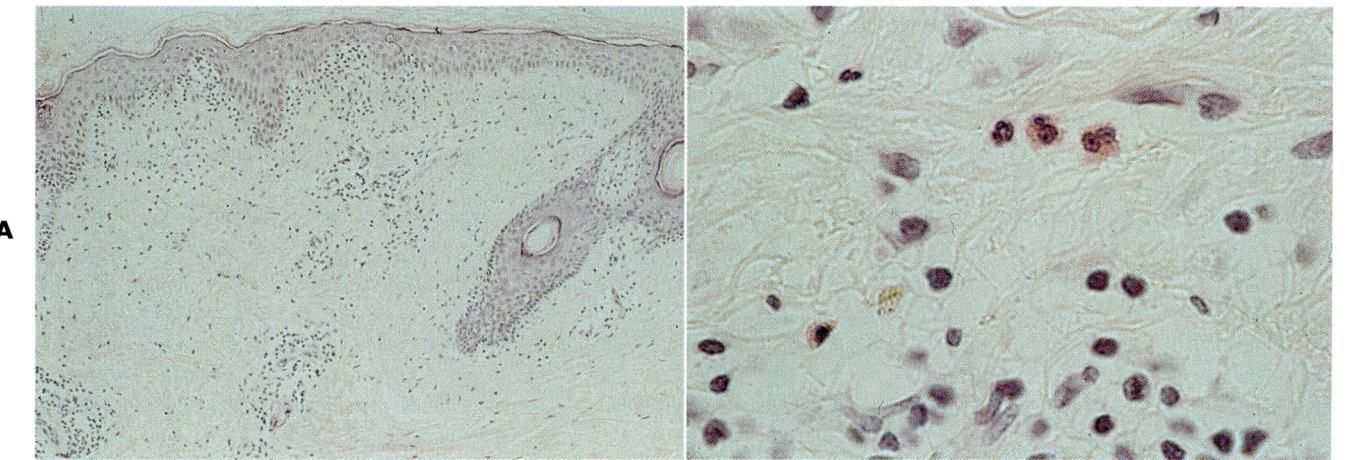

FIGURE 6-24. **A,** Eosinophilic spongiosis in epidermis and hair follicle (H&E; ×10). **B,** Prominent eosinophils in dermal infiltrate (H&E; ×40).

Table 6-2. *Differences between pemphigoid gestationis and polymorphic eruption of pregnancy*

Feature	Pemphighoid Gestationis	Polymorphic Eruption of Pregnancy
Incidence	Very rare (1:50,000)	Common (1:150)
Primiparous	50%	80%
Multiple pregnancy	−	+
Morphology		
Erythematous papules	+	+
Target lesions	+	+
Vesicles	+	+
Bullae	+	−
Prominent striae	−	+
Periumbilical lesions	+	−
Fetal prognosis	Impaired	Normal
Recurrence in subsequent pregnancies	+	−
Direct IF for C3 at BMZ	100%	−
Indirect IF for C3 at BMZ	80%	−
HLA associations	DR3, DR4	−
Associated autoimmune conditions	+	−
Etiology	Autoantibody to BMZ of skin and placenta	Unknown

IF, Immunofluorescence; *C3*, third component of complement; *BMZ*, basement membrane zone; *HLA*, human leukocyte antigen.

Table 6-3. *Comparison of Pemphigoid Gestationis and Bullous Pemphigoid*

	Pemphigoid Gestationis	Bullous Pemphigoid
DIFFERENCES		
Sex	Female	Male/female (1:1)
Age	15 to 45 years	Over 60 years
Etiologic associations	Pregnancy, hydatidiform mole, choriocarcinoma	Unknown
Predilection for umbilicus	Yes	No
Hormonal modulation	Yes	No
HLA associations	DR3, DR4	?
SIMILARITIES		
Clinical	Widespread pruritic bullous eruption	
Histopathology	Subepidermal bullae containing numerous eosinophils	
Direct IF	Deposition of C3 and IgG at the BMZ	
Indirect IF	Circulating complement fixing IgG1 autoantibody	
Immunogold EM	Deposition of the reaction product immediately below hemidesmosome at NC16A domain of BPAg2 (180 kD)	
Treatment	Invariable response to systemic corticosteriods	

IF, Immunofluorescence; *C3*, third component of complement; *BMZ*, basement membrane zone; *HLA*, human leukocyte antigen; *EM*, electron microscopy.

Differential Diagnosis

Differentiating pemphigoid gestationis from other cutaneous bullous eruptions is usually not difficult especially once blisters begin to develop. The vesicles and bullae found only in pemphigoid gestationis distinguish it from other pregnancy-related dermatoses such as papular dermatitis of pregnancy and prurigo of pregnancy. Nonclassical presentations could, however, easily be confused with polymorphic eruption of pregnancy (Table 6-2) and other autoimmune bullous diseases, e.g., bullous pemphigoid (Table 6-3), dermatitis herpetiformis, or linear IgA disease. Bullous lupus erythematosus (LE) also needs to be considered. Bullous pemphigoid is unusual in child-bearing age group. Dermatitis herpetiformis and linear IgA disease can be differentiated by routine histology or IF. In most clinical settings the most important differential diagnosis is between prebullous pemphigoid gestationis and polymorphic eruption of pregnancy. Although eosinophils are more commonly seen in pemphigoid gestationis, they may also be present in polymorphic eruption of pregnancy and the real key to differentiating the two diseases is IF. Other diseases to be considered in the differential diagnosis include erythema multiforme, contact dermatitis and bullous drug eruptions.

Polymorphic Eruption of Pregnancy

Polymorphic eruption of pregnancy (also termed late-onset prurigo of pregnancy, pruritic urticarial papules and plaques of pregnancy, and toxic erythema of pregnancy) is the most common gestational dermatosis, affecting 1 in 160 pregnancies. Presentation is usually in the last weeks of the third trimester and is mainly a disorder of first but not subsequent pregnancies. However, a recent study of 15 patients with polymorphic eruption of pregnancy (PEP) reported that only 53% of the patients

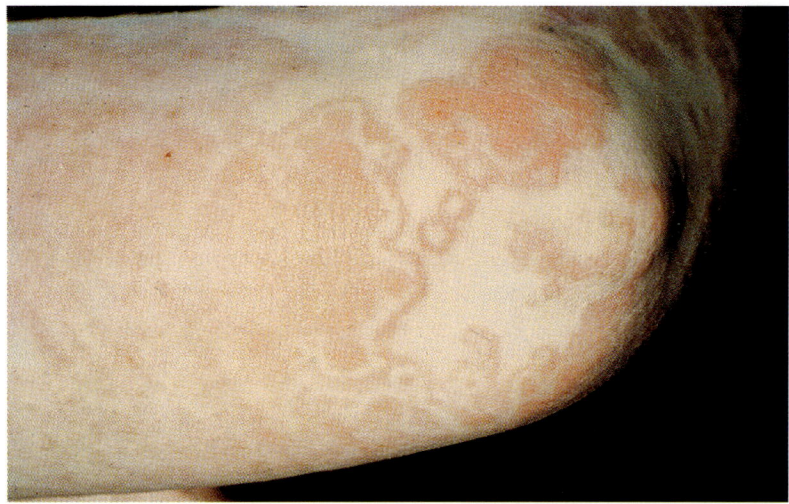

FIGURE 6-25. Targetlike and annular polycyclic lesions on elbow in PEP.

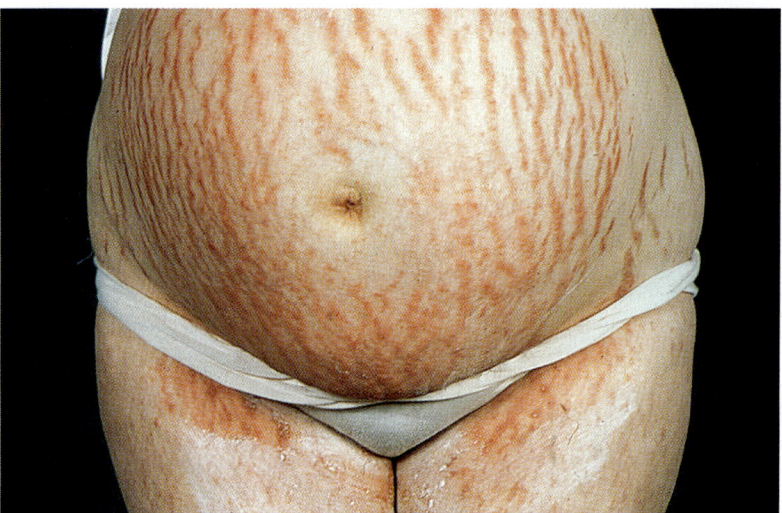

FIGURE 6-26. Urticated papules on lower abdomen in association with prominent striae distensa in PEP.

were primiparous.[23] The condition may develop in twins or multiple pregnancies for the first time. Manifestations are variable with a range that includes urticarial papules, plaques, polycyclic wheals (Figure 6-25), and vesiculation. Bullae are rare and when they do appear are unlikely to be >2 mm in diameter. Lesions typically develop over abdominal striae (Figure 6-26), with periumbilical sparing being characteristic. Bullous lesions of >5 mm diameter are not a feature of PEP; therefore it is only in the pre-bullous stage of pemphigoid gestationis that clinical distinction from PEP is a problem. The presence of periumbilical involvement and florid target lesions in pemphigoid gestationis and the presence of prominent striae in PEP are important clinical distinctions. However, histologic appearances of PEP may be similar to pemphigoid gestationis with a variable dermal perivascular lymphohistiocytic and eosinophilic infiltrate. Direct and indirect IF are negative in the majority of cases of PEP, although there have been occasional reports of equivocal direct IF findings, e.g., weak linear C3 deposition along the BMZ, perivascular C3 and fibrin in the dermis, and one report of circulating IgM anti-BMZ antibodies. Immuno-EM is negative. The etiology of PEP is unknown, although it may be due to damage to connective tissue in striae. The distribution of HLA haplotypes in affected women with PEP is comparable to controls. The disease usually

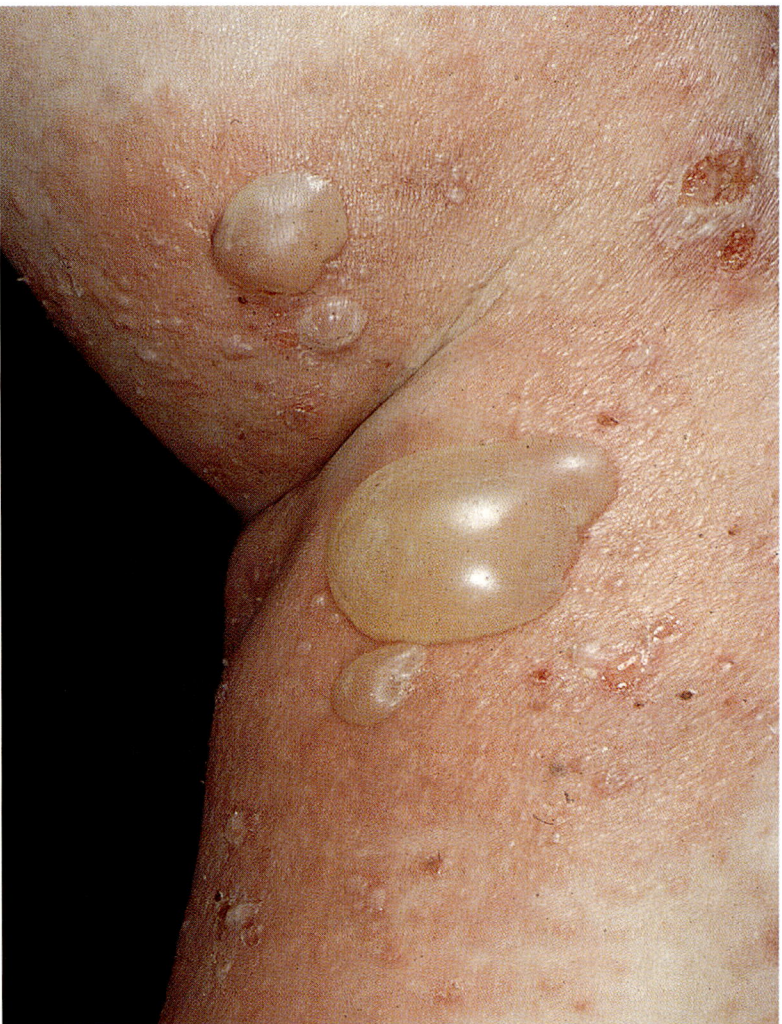

FIGURE 6-27. Blisters and erythema on posterior leg in bullous pemphigoid.

resolves spontaneously within a few weeks of parturition. In contrast to pemphigoid gestationis, there is almost no evidence to suggest that PEP is an autoimmune disease and has no defined hormonal influence.

Fetal prognosis in PEP is probably normal. There has been one report of PEP where the infant may have had a similar rash to the mother, however, the available description was nonspecific, with 1 to 2 mm-sized erythematous papules distributed on the arms, trunk, and buttocks with equivocal histology. There is little information regarding recurrence of PEP, although the risk appears low.

Bullous Pemphigoid

Bullous pemphigoid shows marked clinical, histologic and immunologic similarities to pemphigoid gestationis, but there are no reports of bullous pemphigoid complicating pregnancy. Both conditions are characterized by widespread pruritic, urticarial, and bullous eruptions that usually respond to systemic steroids. Pemphigoid gestationis appears to have a greater predilection for periumbilical skin, whereas in bullous pemphigoid the lesion distribution is mainly on the thighs (Figure 6-27) and lower abdomen. The age of onset of bullous pemphigoid is strikingly different, being usually over age 50 years.

The histopathology, with subepidermal bullae associated with marked papillary dermal edema and spongiosis and a predominantly perivascular dermal infiltrate frequently containing numerous eosinophils, can be indistinguishable. IF and immuno-EM demonstrate deposition of C3 and IgG in the lamina lucida of the BMZ. There is no evidence that bullous pemphigoid is hormonally-mediated, and there is no identified association with HLA antigens. It has been shown that the major antigen in bullous pemphigoid has a molecular weight of 230 kD, which is larger than the 180 kD in pemphigoid gestationis, although shared pathogenic

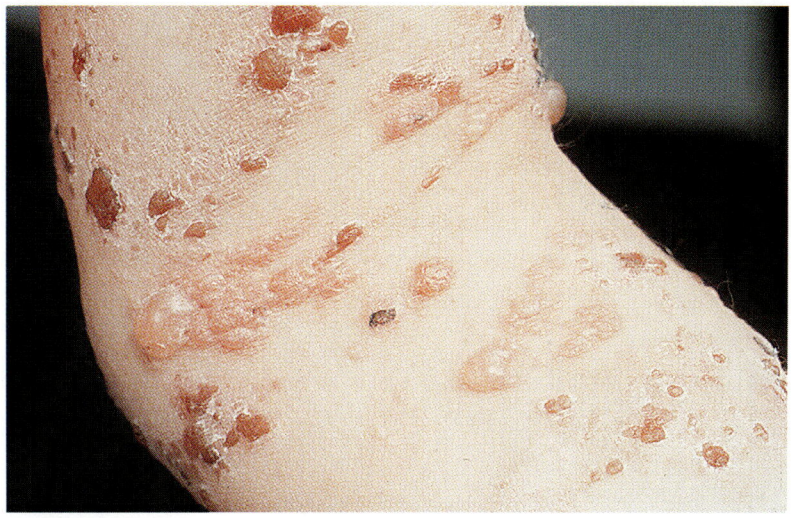

FIGURE 6-28. Blisters on arm in linear IgA disease of adults.

mechanisms appear at play. However, the actual primary target antigen in bullous pemphigoid is unknown.

Further Differential Diagnosis

Other bullous eruptions occurring during pregnancy include dermatitis herpetiformis, linear IgA disease (Figure 6-28), erythema multiforme (Figure 6-29), urticaria (Figure 6-30), contact dermatitis (Figure 6-31), and bullous drug eruptions (Figure 6-32). Dermatitis herpetiformis is characterized by grouped vesicles and papules symmetrically distributed on the extensor aspects of the elbows, knees, buttocks, shoulders, and scalp and are intensely pruritic. Mucosal involvement is usually minor and asymptomatic. There is usually histologic or symptomatic evidence of gluten-sensitive enteropathy. Biopsy of intact blister and surrounding urticarial skin shows subepidermal blister and papillary microabscesses at the tips of the dermal papillae that are full of neutrophils. The characteristic direct IF feature of normal, uninvolved skin is the presence of granular deposits of IgA in the upper papillary dermis. There are no circulating antibodies to the BMZ or dermal papillae. However, 80% have endomysial antibodies, which is a specific marker for the presence of underlying gluten-sensitive enteropathy.

Linear IgA disease is a rare, acquired subepidermal blistering disease that has been defined on the basis of its unique immunopathologic finding of linear deposits of IgA along the BMZ. It encompasses a clinically heterogeneous group of patients divided into two main forms, linear IgA of adults and chronic bullous disease of childhood. Linear IgA disease clinically resembles dermatitis herpetiformis, but some lesions develop on the trunk and limbs similar to pemphigoid gestationis. Mucosal involvement can be prominent and associated with

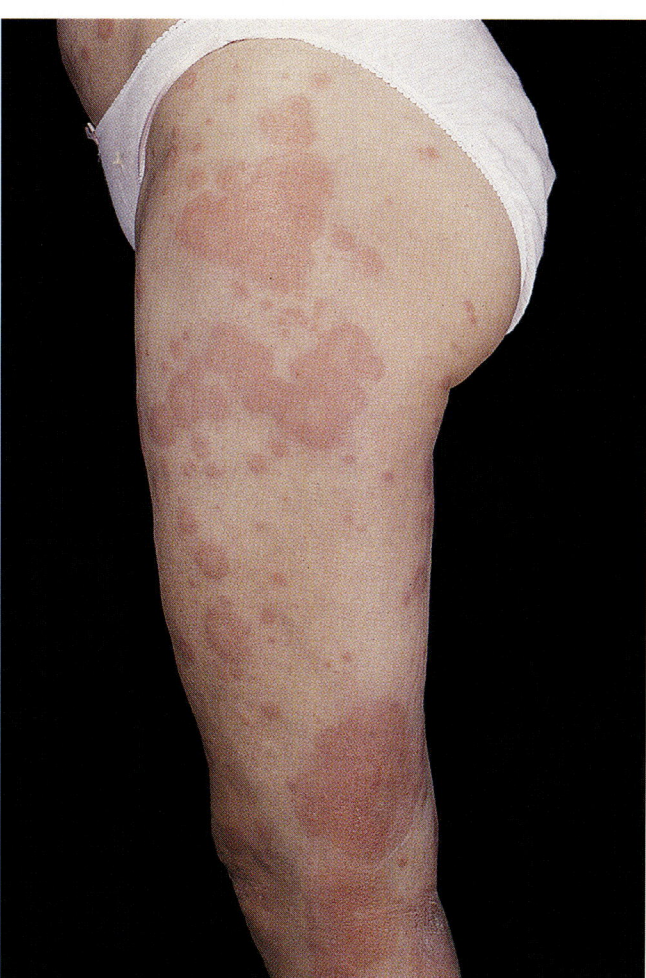

FIGURE 6-29. Well-circumscribed erythematous lesions on legs in erythema multiforme.

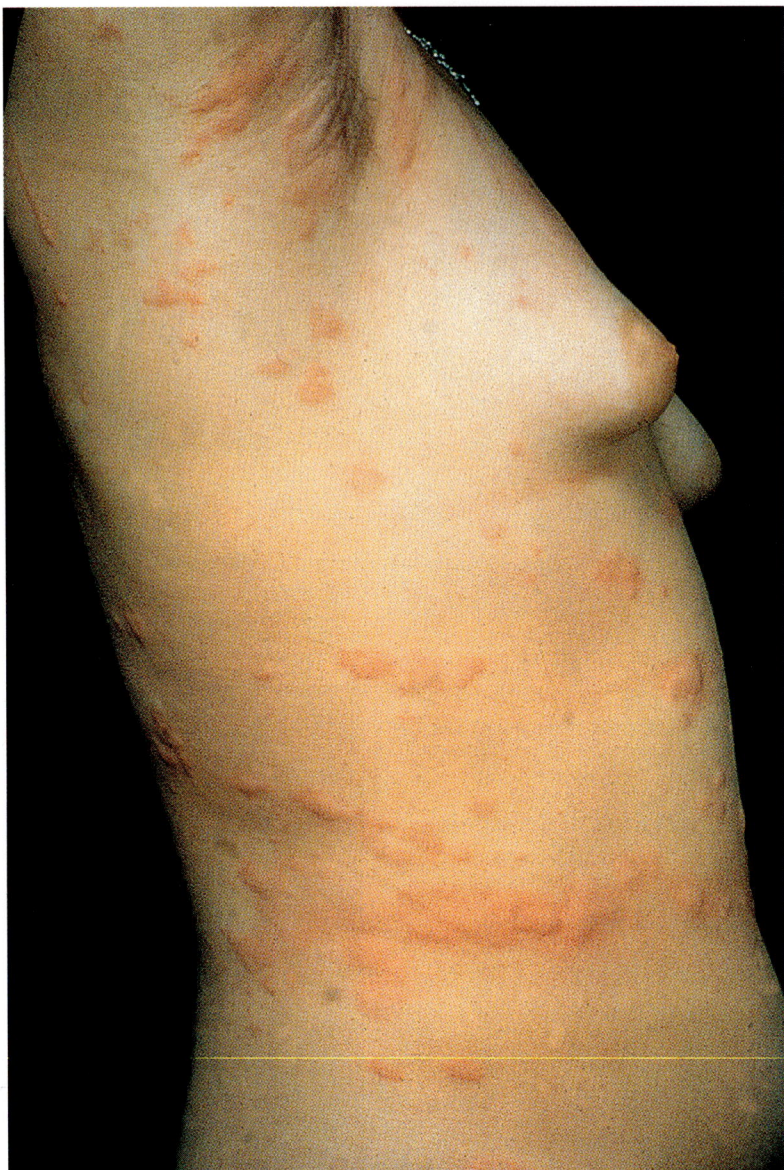

FIGURE 6-30. Chronic urticaria on trunk.

scarring. Histology shows a subepidermal blister with eosinophils and neutrophils. Direct IF shows linear IgA deposition at the BMZ. Approximately 20% of patients with linear IgA disease have circulating autoantibodies compared with 75% of patients with chronic bullous disease of childhood. Unlike dermatitis herpetiformis, there is no associated gluten-sensitive enteropathy.

Bullous LE is a rare specific manifestation of SLE. It is defined by its clinical, pathologic, and immunopathologic features, which include a diagnosis of SLE (by criteria of the American Rheumatism Association), a chronic widespread blistering eruption on either sun-exposed skin or nonsun-exposed skin, subepidermal blistering with a neutrophil-rich infiltrate in the upper dermis, and immune deposits at the DEJ. The onset is usually in young adults. Blisters may arise on clinically normal-appearing (nonerythematous) skin but are often preceded by erythema on the trunk and flexural sites. They are usually tense and not easily ruptured, but when ruptured they can leave erosions and crusts. Pruritus may be severe. Histology of skin biposy shows subepidermal blister formation with a neutrophil-rich infiltrate in the upper dermis. Direct IF of both involved and uninvolved skin demonstrates granular deposits of immunoreactants at the DEJ (lupus band).

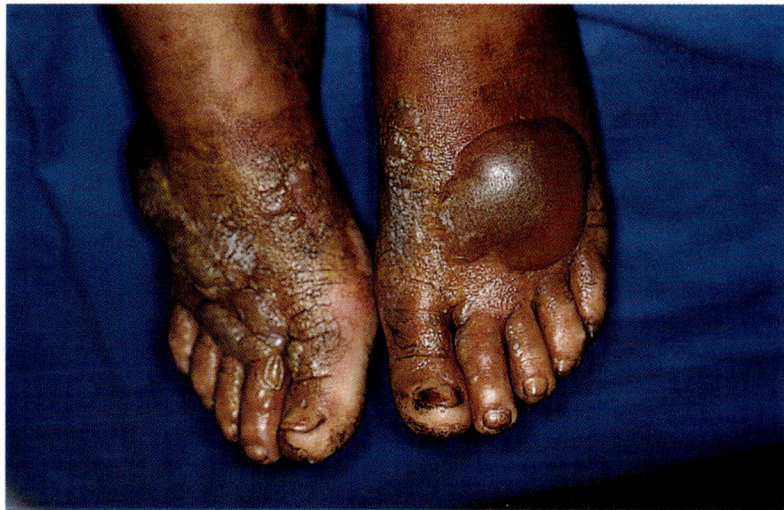

FIGURE 6-31. Tense, large blisters on dorsum of feet in acute contact dermatitis.

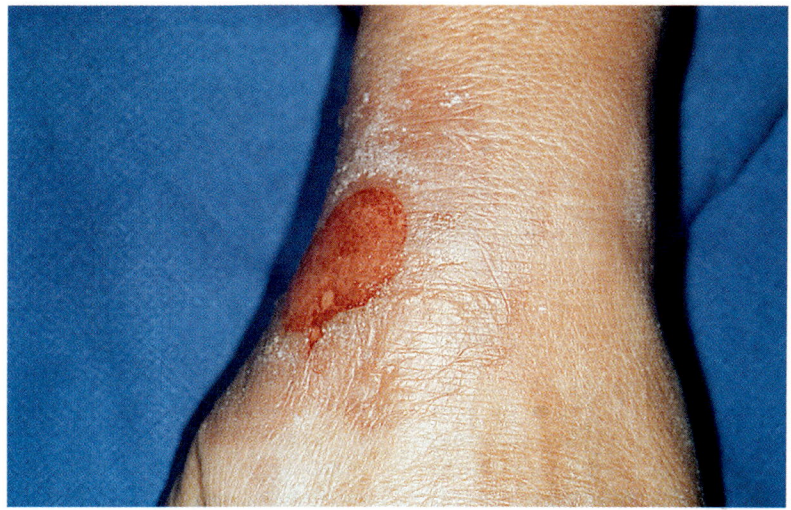

FIGURE 6-32. Erosions on dorsum of hand in bullous drug eruption.

Erythema multiforme is characterized by acute, self-limiting but often recurrent, episodes of erythematous, maculopapular lesions that may develop into classic target or iris lesions or may blister. A history of recent recurrence of herpes simplex, other infectious diseases, and drug exposure should be sought. The lesions are typically distributed symmetrically on the extremities, especially on the dorsum of the hands and extensor aspects of the forearms and legs. The frequency of mucosal involvement varies widely between 2% and 60%. Tense bullae, clear or hemorrhagic, arise in the centre of target lesions and are usually less than 1 cm in diameter. There are no specific laboratory findings in erythema multiforme, although direct IF of early lesions may show immunoreactants within the walls of dermal vessels. Histology of a bullous lesion demonstrates a subepidermal blister with overlying vacuolation of the epidermis. In severe lesions there is necrosis of the whole epidermis.

Direct and indirect IF are the most reliable laboratory techniques for differentiating pemphigoid gestationis from other subepidermal blistering diseases and other diseases that clinically resemble it (Table 6-4). The importance of correct diagnosis is emphasized when it comes to advice regarding the likelihood of involvement of future pregnancies.

Table 6-4. *IF Findings for Differential Diagnosis of Pemphigoid Gestationis*

Diagnosis	Direct IF	Indirect IF
Pemphigoid gestationis	Linear IgG (25%-30%) and C3 (100%) at BMZ	Circulating IgG (20%) against BMZ; pemphigoid gestationis in 25%-50%
Bullous pemphigoid	Linear IgG (50%-90%) and C3 (80%-100%) at BMZ	Circulating IgG (70%) against BMZ
Dermatitis herpetiformis	Granular papillary deposition of IgA (100%)	No circulating IgA but 70% have anti-smooth muscle autoantibody
Linear IgA bullous dermatosis (adult and childhood)	Linear deposition of IgA at BMZ (90%)	Circulating IgA against BMZ (adult 50%, childhood 75%)
Pemphigus	Intercellular IgG	Circulating intercellular IgG

IF, Immunofluorescence; *C3*, third component of complement; *BMZ*, basement membrane zone.

Treatment

The goal of therapy in patients with pemphigoid gestationis is to relieve pruritus, suppress blister formation, and prevent erosions, secondary infection, and scarring of lesional sites. In mild cases of pemphigoid gestationis, judicious but aggressive use of topical fluorinated corticosteroids combined with emollients and systemic antihistamines are adequate. However, once bullae develop it is usually necessary to use systemic steroids.[1] A good response to prednisolone (e.g., 40 mg daily) with control of pruritic symptoms, cessation of new vesicle formation, and clearing within 10 days is common. Some patients receive greater symptomatic relief from divided doses of daily corticosteroids. Once the disease is controlled, single-morning doses of corticosteroids can be prescribed. If no new lesions develop after 3 days of 40 mg prednisolone, the dose should be held constant for 1 to 2 weeks and then gradually decreased. If new lesions continue to develop after 3 days, doubling the dose and following the guidelines as previously stated are recommended. Some degree of disease activity, e.g., one or two new lesions developing every few days, is allowable because much higher doses of prednisolone may be required to completing suppress all disease activity. Thus patients should be tried on ever-lower doses of medication once their disease is controlled. The minimal effective dose of systemic corticosteroids should be used. It is important to remember that many patients actually improve during the latter part of pregnancy, only to have a recurrence at the time of delivery. Doses higher than 80 mg prednisolone are exceptional. The initial dose can often be reduced rapidly to maintenance levels (e.g., 10 mg daily). Since postpartum exacerbations are frequent, it is usual to anticipate this by increasing the steroid dose temporarily immediately postpartum. Some patients may require reinstitution of their medication postpartum after quiescence of their disease during the latter part of the third trimester of pregnancy. Although systemic steroids do not appear to affect fetal prognosis, the mother must be carefully monitored since diabetes mellitus and hypertension may appear.

If pemphigoid gestationis should prove unresponsive to corticosteroids or if they are contraindicated in a particular patient, then plasmapheresis may be considered. It has been used with apparent success in a patient during pregnancy and also in a patient with pemphigoid gestationis persisting postpartum, thereby supporting claims for a circulating pathogenic factor in pemphigoid gestationis. There are no major technical difficulties in performing plasmapheresis during pregnancy, and it has an established role in the treatment of rhesus disease for the removal of maternal rhesus antibodies.

Other treatments have been tried in pemphigoid gestationis, including pyridoxine, dapsone, and ritodrine. Such approaches have not been entirely empiric. For example, pemphigoid gestationis was first thought to be the result of pyridoxine deficiency when treatment of nausea and vomiting with pyridoxine in a patient with pemphigoid gestationis coincided with improvement in the skin disease. Pyridoxine was then used prospectively in three patients with apparent success; these findings were not supported with biochemical confirmation of pyridoxine deficiency.[24] Dapsone is unhelpful and is now contraindicated during pregnancy because it can cause hemolytic disease of the newborn. MacDonald and Raffle in 1984 reported a case of complete remission of severe pemphigoid gestationis when ritodrine, a beta-sympathomimetic drug, was used for the treatment of premature labour.[25]

Alternative drugs, such as gold, methotrexate, and cyclophosphamide, have been reported in the literature. None is useful before term, and the experience with each has been variable at best. Goserelin, a luteinizing hormone–releasing hormone (LHRH) analogue, has recently been used in severe, long-standing beta with chemical oophorectomy, leading to complete remission.[26] Intravenous IgG immunoglobulin has been used with apparent success in a few isolated patients. Pulsed-dose intravenous cyclophosphamide recently produced an excellent clinical response in a patient who had severe and persistent beta refractory to high-dose systemic steroids.[27] The use of second line "steroid-sparing" drugs during pregnancy is not advisable because of the possible teratogenic effects. Systemic corticosteriods, therefore, remain the mainstay of treatment.

Skin lesions in affected infants of patients with pemphigoid gestationis are transient and resolve as maternal autoantibodies are catabolized. Lesions in these infants usually require no specific therapy other than simple wound care. Infants of patients with pemphigoid gestationis who were treated with systemic steroids during pregnancy, however, should be assessed by a neonatologist for evidence and adrenal insufficiency.

Most patients with pemphigoid gestationis require treatment with moderate doses of systemic glucocorticosteriods for control of pruritus and lesion formation at some point in the course of their disease. All patients should be followed carefully and treated aggressively if postpartum flares of disease occur. Although lesions in infants are self-limited, pemphigoid gestationis may be associated with an increased incidence of fetal risk. For this reason, patients with pemphigoid gestationis and their offspring should be coordinately managed by dermatologists, obstetricians and neonatologists. Patients who require treatment postpartum should be advised about appropriate breast-feeding practices.

REFERENCES

1. Jenkins RE, Shornick JK, Black MM: Pemphigoid gestationis, *J Eur Acad Dermatol Venereol* 2:163, 1993.
2. Shornick JK, Stastny P, Gilliam JN: High frequency of histocompatibility antigens HLA-DR3 and DR4 in herpes gestationis, *J Clin Invest* 68:553, 1981.
3. Shornick JK, Jenkins RE, Artlett CM, et al: Class II MHC typing in pemphigoid gestationis, *Clin Exp Dermatol* 20:123, 1995.
4. Shornick JK, Artlett CM, Jenkins RE, et al: Complement polymorphism in herpes gestationis: Association with C4 null allele, *J Am Acad Dermatol* 29:545, 1993.
5. Jenkins RE, Vaughan Jones SM, Black MM: Conversion of pemphigoid gestationis to bullous pemphigoid; two refractory cases highlighting this association, *Br J Dermatol* 135:595, 1996.
6. Berkowitz RS, Goldstein DP: Chorionic tumors, *N Engl J Med* 335:1740, 1996.
7. Kolodny RC: Herpes gestationis. A new assessment of incidence, diagnosis, and fetal prognosis, *Am J Obst Gynecol* 104:39, 1969.
8. Lawley TJ, Stingl G, Katz SI: Fetal and maternal risk factors in herpes gestationis, *Arch Dermatol* 114:552, 1978.
9. Holmes RC, Black MM: The fetal prognosis in pemphigoid gestationis (herpes gestationis), *Br J Dermatol* 110:67, 1984.
10. Shornick JK, Black MM: Fetal risks in herpes gestationis, *J Am Acad Dermatol* 26:63, 1992.
11. Shornick JK, Black MM: Secondary autoimmune diseases in herpes gestationis (pemphigoid gestationis), *J Am Acad Dermatol* 26:563, 1992.
12. Hashimoto T, Amagai M, Murakami H, et al: Specific detection of anti-cell surface antibodies in herpes gestationis sera, *Exp Dermatol* 5:96, 1996.
13. Vaughan Jones SA, Bhogal BS, Black MM, et al: A typical case of pemphigoid gestationis with a unique pattern of intercellular immunofluorescence, *Br J Dermatol* 136:245, 1997.
14. Stanley JR, Hawley-Nelson P, Yuspa SH, et al: Characterization of bullous pemphigoid antigen: a unique basement membrane protein of stratified squamous epithelia, *Cell* 24:897, 1981.
15. Labib RS, Anhalt GJ, Patel HP, et al: Molecular heterogeneity of the bullous pemphigoid antigens as detected by immunoblotting, *J Immunol* 136:1231, 1986.
16. Sawamura D, Nomura K, Sugita Y, et al: Bullous pemphigoid antigen (BPAG1): cDNA cloning and mapping of the gene to the short arm of chromosome 6, *Genomics* 8:722, 1990.
17. Li K, Sawamura D, Guidice GJ, et al: Genomic organization of collagenous domains and chromosomal assignment of human 180-kDa bullous pemphigoid antigen-2, a novel collagen of stratified squamous epithelium, *J Biol Chem* 266:24064, 1991.
18. Li K, Tamai K, Tan EML, et al: Cloning of type XVII collagen, *J Biol Chem* 268:8823, 1993.
19. Kitajima Y: Adhesion molecules in the pathophysiology of bullous diseases, *Eur J Dermatol* 6:399, 1996.
20. Vince GS, Johnson PM: Materno-fetal immunobiology in normal pregnancy and its possible failure in recurrent spontaneous abortion? *Hum Reprod* 10:107, 1995.
21. Kelly SE, Fleming S, Bhogal BS, et al: Immunopathology of the placenta in pemphigoid gestationis and linear IgA disease, *Br J Dermatol* 120:735, 1989.
22. Shornick JK, Jenkins RE, Briggs DC, et al: Anti-HLA antibodies in pemphigoid gestationis (herpes gestationis), *Br J Dermatol* 129:257, 1993.
23. Roger D, Vaillant L, Fignon A, et al: Specific pruritic diseases of pregnancy, *Arch Dermatol* 130:734, 1994.
24. Fosnaugh RP, Bryan HG, Orders RL: Pyridoxine in the treatment of herpes gestationis, *Arch Dermatol* 84:90, 1961.
25. MacDonald KJS, Raffle EJ: Ritodrine therapy associated with remission of pemphigoid gestationis, *Br J Dermatol* 111:630, 1984.
26. Garvey MP, Handfield-Jones SE, Black MM: Pemphigoid gestationis: response to chemical oophorectomy with goserelin, *Clin Exp Dermatol* 17:443, 1992.
27. Castle SP, Mather-Mondrey M, Bennion S, et al: Chronic herpes gestationis and antiphospholipid antibody syndrome successfully treated with cyclophosphamide, *J Am Acad Dermatol* 34:333, 1996.

Dermatitis Herpetiformis

Bita Bagheri
Russell P. Hall III

Etiology and Pathogenesis

Dermatitis herpetiformis is a chronic, usually lifelong disease, with an intensely pruritic papulovesicular eruption that was first described by Duhring in 1884.[1] The skin lesions seen in patients with dermatitis herpetiformis are characteristically distributed on the extensor surfaces of the arms and legs, the upper back, and buttocks. In 1966 Marks and coworkers reported that patients with dermatitis herpetiformis had an associated small bowel villous atrophy that was subsequently determined to be gluten sensitivity and identical to that seen in patients with isolated gluten-sensitive enteropathy (GSE).[2] Subsequently, it was determined that patients with dermatitis herpetiformis also had an increased frequency of the histocompatibility antigen HLA-B8, similar to that seen in patients with isolated GSE.[3] In most patients the GSE is asymptomatic, although approximately 10% of patients may have some degree of gastrointestinal symptoms.[2] In 1966 Cormane reported the presence of immunoreactants in the skin of patients with dermatitis herpetiformis that were subsequently determined to be immunoglobulin A (IgA).[4] These associations highlight the following three important factors in the pathogenesis of dermatitis herpetiformis.

1. Granular IgA deposits are demonstrated by direct immunofluorescence (IF) at the dermal-epidermal junction (DEJ) in all patients with dermatitis herpetiformis. Characterization of the cutaneous IgA found in the skin of patients with dermatitis herpetiformis demonstrates that it is polyclonal and predominantly IgA1.[6] Some investigators demonstrated that J chain, seen in polymeric IgA commonly of mucosal origin, is present in the cutaneous IgA deposits. Other investigators, however, have not confirmed this finding.[7,8] Secretory piece, which is present on secretory IgA, is not present in the cutaneous IgA deposits found in patients with dermatitis herpetiformis.[9] Despite the inability to absolutely confirm the mucosal origin of the cutaneous IgA deposits, the presence of the associated GSE in patients with dermatitis herpetiformis and the important role of IgA in the mucosal immune response led to the hypothesis that the IgA in the skin of these patients arises from the gastrointestinal mucosa. This has not been clearly documented, and the mechanism of the deposition of the IgA in the skin of patients with dermatitis herpetiformis, as well as its source, is not known.

2. Patients with dermatitis herpetiformis have an associated GSE[2] that is most often symptomatic but has histologic features identical, albeit often less severe, to those seen in patients with isolated GSE. Patients with isolated GSE, however, do not have cutaneous disease or cutaneous IgA deposits. Gluten is a protein found in various grains such as wheat, rye, and oats. It has been well documented that patients with dermatitis herpetiformis who are placed on a gluten-free diet are able to control the cutaneous manifestations of the disease and that the villous atrophy present in the small bowel mucosa resolves. Although the mechanism by which the gastrointestinal disease results in cutaneous disease is not fully understood, the response of both the gastrointestinal abnormality and the skin disease to strict avoidance of dietary gluten provides strong evidence of the importance of the associated GSE in the pathogenesis of dermatitis herpetiformis.[10,11]

3. Patients with dermatitis herpetiformis have an increased frequency of the human histocompatibility antigen haplotype, HLA-A1, -B8, -DR3, -DQ2. Further classification of this HLA association demonstrated an increased frequency of the HLA DQ alleles DQB1*0201 and DQA1*0501 and HLA-DR allele DRB1*0301. This HLA association is present in 95% to 100% of patients with dermatitis herpetiformis and is essentially identical to that seen in patients with isolated GSE.[12,13] Although the HLA association is clearly critical in the pathogenesis of dermatitis herpetiformis, it is not sufficient, since the majority of individuals with these HLA alleles do not have either dermatitis herpetiformis or isolated GSE.

DERMATITIS HERPITIFORMIS SUMMARY

ETIOLOGY
The fundamental mechanisms important in the pathogenesis of dermatitis herpetiformis are unknown. Three elements are critical in the development of the disease (1) granular deposits of IgA at the DEJ of normal-appearing perilesional skin; (2) an associated, most often asymptomatic, GSE; and (3) an increased frequency of the HLA-B8, -DR3, -DQ2 haplotype. The well-documented observation that patients on a gluten-free diet can control the cutaneous manifestations provides strong evidence of the critical role of the associated GSE in the pathogenesis of the disease.

CLINICAL FEATURES
The classic clinical manifestation are erythematous papules and vesicles, symmetrically distributed on extensor surfaces of the extremities, scapula, sacrum, and neck. These lesions are extremely pruritic, often resulting in only crusted erosions being noted on presentation. Less commonly, patients may present with urticarial plaques or bullae.

PATHOLOGY
Routine biopsy of early lesions reveals collections of neutrophils and neutrophil fragments with fibrin in papillary tips with a mild perivascular infiltrate of lymphocytes and monocytes. Direct IF of normal-appearing, perilesional skin shows granular deposits of IgA at the DEJ.

DIAGNOSIS
Diagnosis is based on the presence of granular IgA deposits at the DEJ of normal-appearing, perilesional skin by direct IF.

TREATMENT
Cutaneous eruption can be treated with medical therapy using dapsone or adhering to a gluten-free diet.

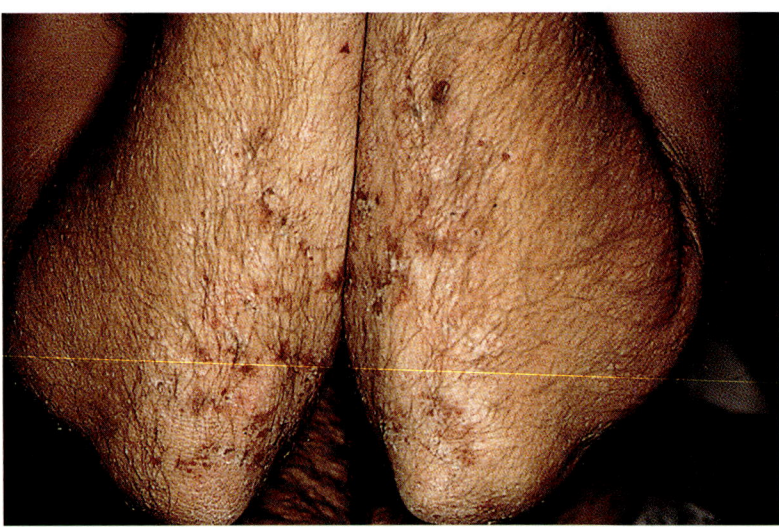

FIGURE 7-1. Patient with dermatitis herpetiformis with crusted papules on the extensor surface of the elbows.

Incidence and Prevalence

Studies of North European populations demonstrated a point prevalence of dermatitis herpetiformis between 1.2 to 39.2 per 100,000 population with incidence of between 0.86 to 1.45 per 100,000 population.[14] Dermatitis herpetiformis is seen more frequently in the northern European populations of Scandinavia, Ireland, and Great Britain and is rarely seen in individuals of African or Asian descent. This incidence is most likely related to the lower frequency of the HLA-A1, -B8, -DR3, -DQ2 haplotypes in these populations. Although onset of dermatitis herpetiformis can occur at any age, the majority of patients present between the second and fourth decade of life. Males are affected slightly more frequently than females.[15]

Clinical Features

Cutaneous Manifestations

The primary lesions seen in patients with dermatitis herpetiformis are erythematous papules or vesicles. These lesions are intensely pruritic, often resulting in patients presenting with multiple erosions with or without crusts (Figures 7-1 and 7-2). Patients can often predict the site

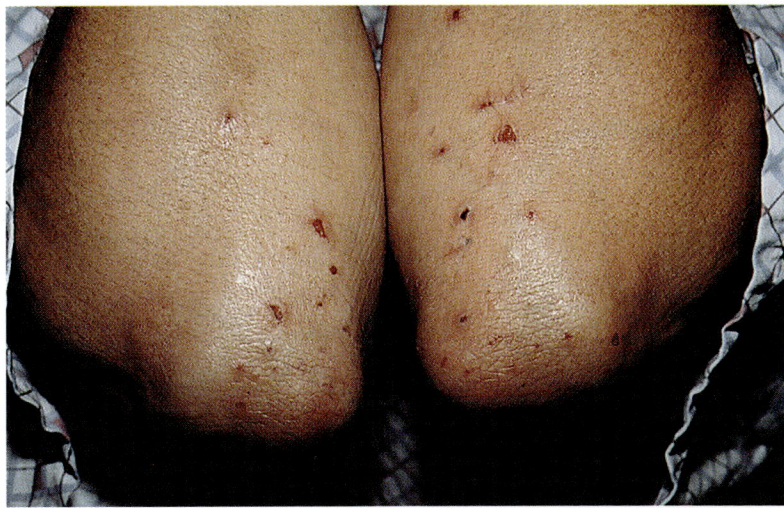

FIGURE 7-2. Patient with dermatitis herpetiformis with erythematous papules and crusted erosions on the extensor surface of the elbows.

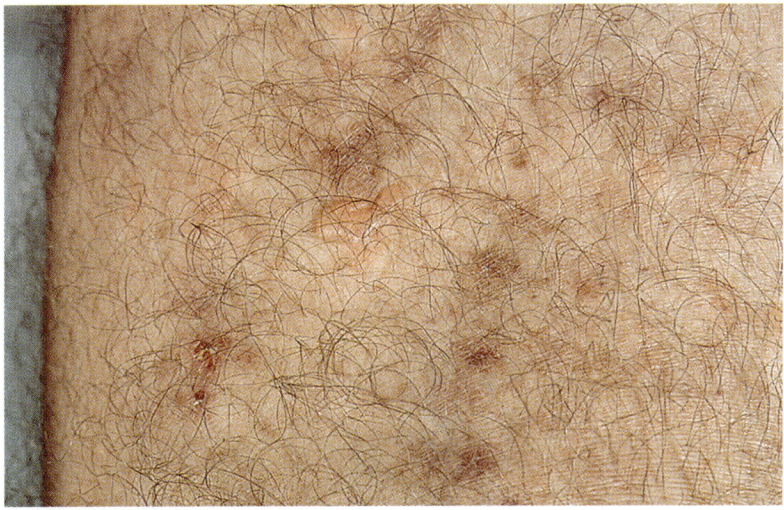

FIGURE 7-3. Patient with dermatitis herpetiformis with an isolated intact vesicle and crusted erosions on the extensor surface of the elbow.

of the cutaneous eruption 8 to 24 hours before the appearance of lesions because of the severe burning and stinging present at the site. Occasionally, patients may present with urticarial plaques or more rarely bullae (Figures 7-3 to 7-5). Larger bullous lesions most frequently occur in patients with long-standing disease who have discontinued their treatment with dapsone.

The skin lesions are characteristically symmetrically distributed on extensor surfaces, especially elbows, knees, shoulders, sacrum, buttocks, and the posterior nuchal area. Patients may also develop lesions on the scalp, face, or groin. When lesions are on the hands, they may present as hemorrhagic vesicles. Mucous membrane lesions are rare and when they are present they are most often asymptomatic.

Lesions can be grouped in a herpetiform configuration or can present as individually dispersed papules, vesicles, and crusted erosions. Individual lesions most often heal without scarring, but pigmentary changes can be seen. Scarring may occur, however, if the lesions develop a secondary infection due to the intense scratching of the patients.[16-18]

The severity of the clinical manifestations of dermatitis herpetiformis is often quite variable. Some pa-

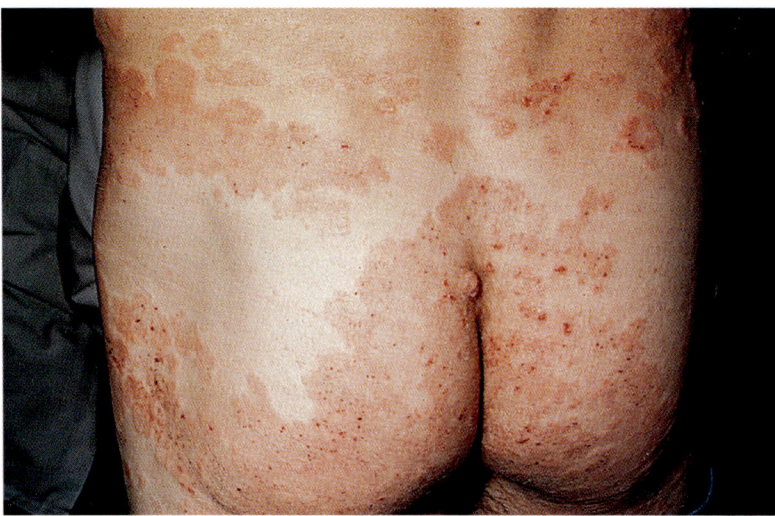

FIGURE 7-4. Patient with dermatitis herpetiformis with urticarial plaques on the buttocks and scattered crusted erosions.

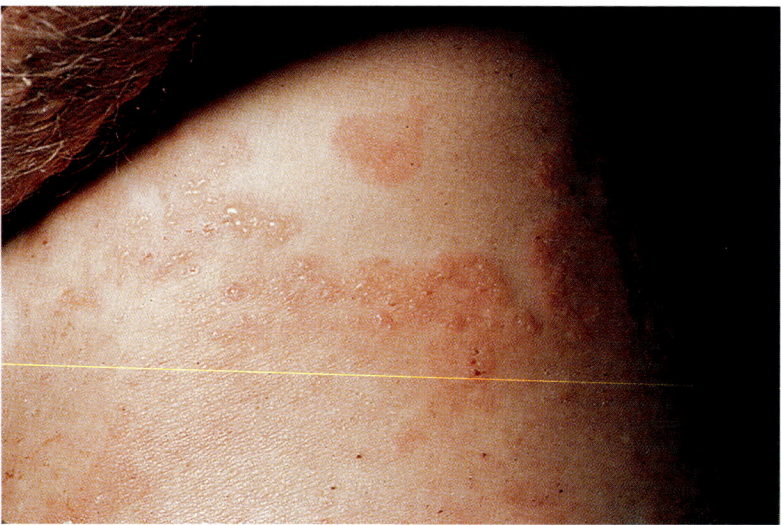

FIGURE 7-5. Patient with dermatitis herpetiformis with urticarial plaque with small vesicles and crusted erosions.

tients suffer severe disease with lesions distributed over wide areas of the skin, whereas others may present with a few isolated papules or vesicles located only on the elbows or knees. In a similar manner, some patients have numerous exacerbations of disease, with no apparent inciting event, while others experience only a few lesions per month and may not even require medical or diet therapy. Some patients report that they suffer exacerbations of disease after ingesting shellfish or iodized salt, which suggests a sensitivity to iodides or other halogens, although this is not consistently observed. Clinical exacerbation of the skin disease when taking nonsteroidal antiinflammatory drugs, such as indomethacin or ibuprofen, has been described in some patients with dermatitis herpetiformis.

Gastrointestinal Manifestations

Patients with dermatitis herpetiformis have an associated, most often asymptomatic, GSE. Unlike patients with isolated GSE, the clinical manifestations of gastrointestinal disease are minimal in patients with dermatitis herpetiformis. Approximately 5% to 10% of patients with dermatitis herpetiformis may experience gastrointestinal symptoms such as diarrhea, bloating, or

BOX 7-1. DISEASE ASSOCIATIONS WITH DERMATITIS HERPETIFORMIS

> GSE
> Autoimmune thyroid disease
> Atrophic gastritis, achlorhydria, and pernicious anemia
> Small bowel lymphoma, malignancy
> Autoimmune diseases: dermatomyositis, Sjögren's syndrome, SLE, rheumatoid arthritis

abdominal pain consistent with a symptomatic GSE. A slightly higher proportion of patients, although clinically asymptomatic, have evidence of functional abnormalities of the small bowel, such as mild malabsorption; steatorrhea; and abnormal D-xylose, iron, folate, glucose, water, and bicarbonate absorption.[19,20] In contrast, patients with isolated GSE often have severe gastrointestinal symptoms of diarrhea, abdominal pain, and significant malabsorption. It is important to note that patients with isolated GSE do not have cutaneous IgA deposits or the cutaneous manifestations seen in patients with dermatitis herpetiformis.

Patients with dermatitis herpetiformis have increased incidence of atrophic gastritis and achlorhydria, which are also seen in patients with isolated GSE.[21] Recent studies also suggest that patients with dermatitis herpetiformis have a small increased risk of developing malignancies, including small bowel lymphoma, although the true magnitude of this risk is not well established.[22]

Other Associated Diseases

Patients with dermatitis herpetiformis also have an increased frequency of other autoimmune diseases (Box 7-1). Approximately 39% of patients have elevated thyroid antimicrosomal antibodies and clinical manifestations of thyroid diseases, including hypothyroidism, hyperthyroidism, thyroid nodules, and malignancies.[23] Other associated diseases include rheumatoid arthritis, dermatomyositis, myasthenia gravis, systemic lupus erythematous (SLE), and Sjögren's syndrome.[24] These associations are thought to be due to the increased frequency of the HLA A1, -B8, -DR3, -DQ2 haplotype associations found in patients with dermatitis herpetiformis.

Pathology

Cutaneous

Skin biopsy of an early erythematous papular lesions of dermatitis herpetiformis reveals the characteristic neutrophilic microabcess. Neutrophils are present within the dermal papillae with fibrin, leukocytoclastic debris, and edema (Figure 7-6). A perivascular, lymphohistiocytic infiltrate is often present in the upper and middle

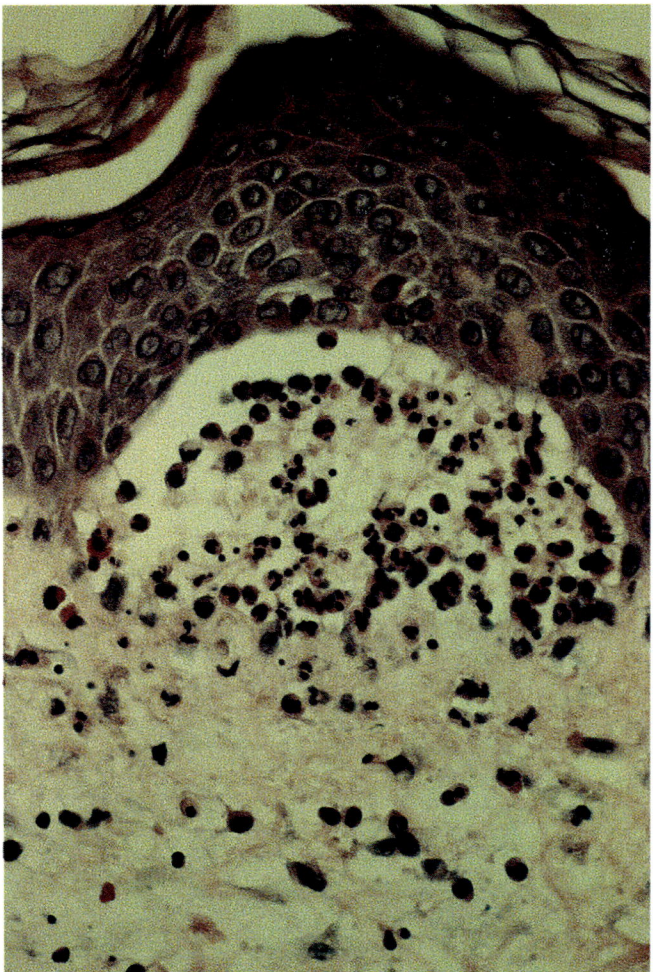

FIGURE 7-6. Routine histology of early lesion of dermatitis herpetiformis showing collection of neutrophils in the papillary tips with leukocytoclasis, fibrin deposition, edema, and dermal-epidermal separation.

dermis. At the sites of neutrophil accumulation, vacuoles and clefts appear, which coalesce to become the clinically evident vesicles and bullae.

Skin biopsy of a well-established blister (vesicle or bullae) will reveal a neutrophil-predominant infiltrate with subepidermal blister formation, which can be difficult to separate from other subepidermal blistering diseases. Similar histology can be seen in other diseases, including bullous pemphigoid, cutaneous vasculitis, bullous LE, and other inflammatory diseases.[25]

The diagnosis of dermatitis herpetiformis is based on the immunopathology found by direct IF of normal-appearing, perilesional skin. Direct IF of normal-appearing, perilesional skin of a patient with dermatitis herpetiformis shows the diagnostic granular deposits of IgA (Figure 7-7). These deposits are most characteristically present in the papillary dermis along the DEJ, often accentuated in the dermal papillary tips. IgA de-

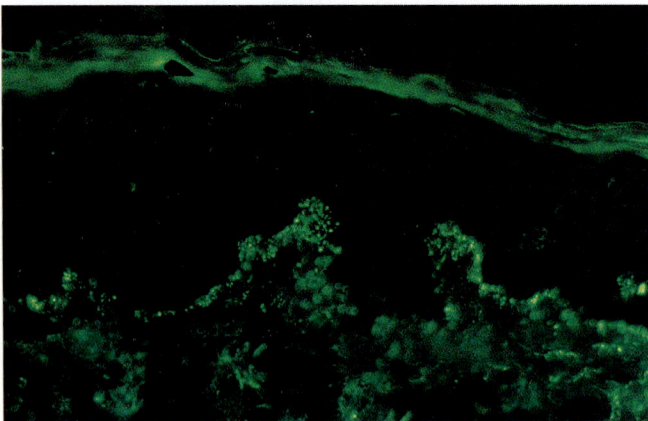

FIGURE 7-7. Direct IF of normal appearing, perilesional skin of patient with dermatitis herpetiformis. IgA deposits are present in a granular pattern at the DEJ with accentuation in the dermal papillary tips.

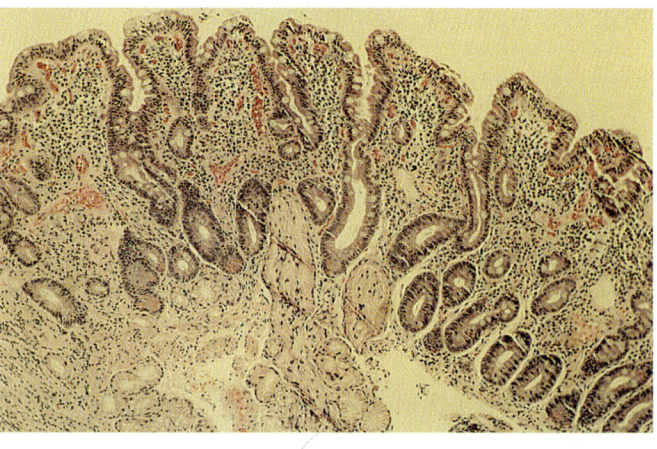

FIGURE 7-8. Small bowel biopsy from a patient with dermatitis herpetiformis on a normal diet containing gluten shows villous atrophy with increased intraepithelial lymphocytes and a lamnia propria infiltrate of lymphocytes and eosinophils.

posits can be found all along the DEJ in a granular pattern or occasionally in a fibrillar and granular pattern in the papillary dermis. In addition to IgA, patients may have granular deposits of the third component of the complement cascade, C3, and much less frequently other immunoglobulins such as IgG and IgM. Although the original description of the direct IF findings in patients thought to have dermatitis herpetiformis included patients with linear deposits of IgA, it is clear that these patients have a different disease, linear IgA dermatosis, with a different pathogenetic mechanism. The diagnosis of dermatitis herpetiformis is reserved for those patients with a consistent clinical presentation and granular deposits of IgA at the DEJ.

Direct IF studies of lesional skin may result in false-negative results due to the presence of the intense inflammatory infiltrate. In a similar manner, immunohistochemistry studies of formalin-fixed tissue may also give false-negative results, making it important to submit fresh tissue for frozen-section direct IF studies. Finally, Zone et al reported that in some patients, direct IF of skin never involved with the clinical lesions of dermatitis herpetiformis may not have detectable IgA deposits.[26] These observations suggest that to maximize the diagnostic utility of the direct IF the biopsy should be obtained from normal-appearing, perilesional skin and processed for frozen-section analysis of the immunoreactants.

Gastrointestinal Pathology

The histologic appearance of the small bowel is similar in both patients with dermatitis herpetiformis and those with isolated GSE. Small bowel biopsies taken distal to the duodeno-jejunal junction show intestinal villi blunting, elongation of epithelial crypts, and flattening of the jejunal mucosa (Figure 7-8). An inflammatory infiltrate consisting mainly of lymphocytes in the lamina propria with a resultant increase in number of intraepithelial lymphocytes can be seen. The severity of the changes can range from subtotal villous atrophy to severe flattening of the intestinal mucosa.[19]

Diagnosis

The diagnosis of dermatitis herpetiformis is confirmed by direct IF of perilesional, normal-appearing skin showing the typical granular deposits of IgA at the DEJ, most often without any other immunoglobulins present in a patient with consistent clinical features of the disease. The differential diagnosis of the clinical presentation seen in patients with dermatitis herpetiformis includes linear IgA dermatosis, bullous eruption of LE, bullous pemphigoid, scabies, neurotic excoriations, papular urticaria, transient acantholytic dermatosis, erythema multiforme, and folliculitis.[16] The histologic differential diagnosis of skin biopsies obtained from lesions of patients with dermatitis herpetiformis includes linear IgA bullous dermatosis, bullous eruption of LE, and rarely bullous pemphigoid, leukocytoclastic vasculitis, herpes gestationis, bullous drug eruption, and the inflammatory type of epidermolysis bullosa acquisita.[16]

Treatment

The two mainstays of therapy for dermatitis herpetiformis are medical therapy or dietary therapy (Box 7-2).

> **BOX 7-2. TREATMENT OF DERMATITIS HERPETIFORMIS**
>
> **MEDICAL THERAPY**
> Dapsone
> Sulfapyridine
> **DIETARY THERAPY**
> Gluten-free diet
> **TYPICAL DOSAGE**
> 100-200 mg/day
> 500-2000 mg/day

Medical Therapy

Medical therapy with dapsone is the most common form of treatment in the United States. Cutaneous symptoms and the development of new lesions can be controlled in most patients with a dosage of dapsone ranging from 100 to 200 mg per day.[27,28] Patients usually experience symptomatic relief from the burning and itching within 24 hours of taking dapsone, with a cessation in the appearance of new lesions. Dapsone does not, however, alter the morphology or any symptoms of the associated GSE found in patients with dermatitis herpetiformis. While the control of the cutaneous lesions of dermatitis herpetiformis that occurs with dapsone is remarkable, it is not diagnostic and similar responses can be seen in other diseases. It should also be noted that patients may note small breakthroughs of clinical disease, which should not result in an increase of the dosage of dapsone. Indeed the potential dose-related adverse events associated with dapsone therapy makes it very important that patients be maintained on the lowest possible dose of medication possible. In addition, it is important that the patient be made aware of the possible side effects, which are pharmacologic and idiosyncratic, and of the danger of changing their dose of dapsone without their physician's knowledge and input.

Dapsone causes a dose-related hemolysis and methemoglobinemia.[29] The hemolysis that occurs may be severe in patients that are glucose-6-phosphate dehydrogenase (G6PD) deficient. Because of this, patients are often tested before therapy for G6PD deficiency, especially those patients of Mediterranean descent, Asians, and African-Americans. G6PD deficiency is not an absolute contraindication to dapsone therapy, but extreme caution should be exercised if patients with this deficiency are to be treated with dapsone. Methemoglobinemia also occurs to some degree in all patients that take dapsone. The clinical significance of the methemoglobinemia relates to the absolute level of methemoglobin, the total hemoglobin level of the individual patient, and the patient's general health. For example, a patient that develops 10% methemoglobin with a total hemoglobin of 13 gm/dl has an effective oxygen-carrying capacity of approximately 11.7 gm/dl hemoglobin (13 gm/dl − 1.3 gm/dl), a level rarely associated with symptoms. If, however, that patient had a total hemoglobin level of 10 gm/dl, then the effective oxygen-carrying capacity of that patient would be 9 gm/dl, with the very real possibility of symptoms developing. In addition, the degree of symptoms relates to the patient's underlying health. If in the first example the patient had severe coronary artery disease, decreasing the oxygen-carrying capacity a relatively small amount could result in significant symptoms. The clinician who uses dapsone should be well aware of the patient's underlying health and be familiar with the pharmacologic side effects of dapsone.

In addition to the pharmacologic side effects of dapsone, there are number of idiosyncratic side effects that can occur in patients taking dapsone. Agranulocytosis can occur in patients on dapsone therapy. Agranulocytosis has been estimated to occur at a rate of approximately 1 case per 3000 patient years of exposure.[30] It is important to note that this is not a dose-related effect; the average dose is 100 mg/day. In addition, this is usually an early event in dapsone therapy, occurring an average of 7 weeks into therapy.[30]

Patients with dapsone can also develop abnormalities of liver function, including hepatitis with an infectious mononucleosis-like syndrome sometimes being seen.[27,28,31] Patients on dapsone have also developed distal motor neuropathy; only rarely, patients have an associated sensory component. This adverse event appears to be dose-related and most often occurs later in the course of therapy or in patients who take very high doses of dapsone.[28,31,32]

Dapsone is associated with a wide variety of other side effects, including skin rashes, some of which can be severe and life-threatening. The reader is referred to comprehensive review articles on the use of dapsone.[27,28,31]

The wide variety of both pharmacologic and idiosyncratic side effects associated with the use of dapsone (Box 7-3) mandate that the patient taking dapsone be followed by a clinician who has experience using the drug with appropriate laboratory and clinical testing.[28,31] Knowledge of these side effects can help the clinician develop a structure for evaluating a patient before therapy with dapsone and for monitoring the patient during therapy. The potential hematologic complications dictate that a complete blood count (CBC) with differential, as well as a G6PD level, be obtained before the initiation of therapy especially in individuals at high risk for G6PD deficiency, e.g., African-Americans, Asians, and those of Mediterranean descent. The CBC with differential should be repeated weekly for the initial 4 to 6 weeks of dapsone therapy to assess the degree of he-

BOX 7-3. SELECTED ADVERSE EFFECTS OF DAPSONE

PHARMACOLOGIC	Cholestatic jaundice
Hemolytic anemia	Morbilliform eruption
Methemoglobinemia	Exfoliative erythroderma
IDIOSYNCRATIC	Toxic epidermal necrolysis
Headache	Psychosis
Gastric irritation	Leukopenia/agranulocytosis
Anorexia	Peripheral neuropathy (motor predominant)
Hepatitis, infectious mononucleosis-like syndrome	Hypoalbuminemia

molysis and to monitor the white blood cell count for the development of agranulocytosis. Further testing should be performed on a bimonthly basis for the next 6 to 8 weeks of therapy, followed by additional testing every 2 to 4 months for the remainder of therapy. Routine determination of methemoglobin levels is not valuable unless the clinical symptoms of the patient suggest elevated methemoglobinemia (fatigue, headaches, malaise, and so on). The potential for hepatic dysfunction suggests that liver function tests should be obtained before therapy and monitored every 3 to 4 months while on dapsone and when clinically indicated. Since dapsone is also partially excreted via the kidney, renal function should be assessed before therapy and followed as clinically indicated in the individual patients.[27,28,31] The possibility of development of a motor neuropathy provides an indication for a good pretreatment neurologic examination, focusing on distal motor strength, and follow-up neurologic examinations for the development of signs of distal muscle weakness. Finally, a complete history and physical examination, focusing on potential problems that may develop because of the predicted development of anemia and methemoglobinemia should be performed before the institution of therapy and at regular intervals during follow-up care, as clinically indicated.

Recently, several modalities have been described that may lessen the pharmacologic side effects in patients taking dapsone. These include the use of cimetidine, methylene blue, vitamin C, or vitamin E. While many of these treatments may lessen the laboratory changes seen with dapsone, without diminishing the therapeutic effectiveness of the drug, the extent of their value in decreasing the symptoms from these changes in patients is still not clear.[33,34]

Sulfapyridine is also useful in controlling the clinical manifestations of dermatitis herpetiformis.[28,31] Sulfapyridine is not currently available in the United States. This drug is often less effective in the management of patients with dermatitis herpetiformis, most likely due to its being more poorly absorbed from the gastrointestinal tract than dapsone.

Dietary Therapy

The clinical signs and symptoms of dermatitis herpetiformis can also be controlled by the use of a gluten-free diet.[10,35,36] Patients with dermatitis herpetiformis on a gluten-free diet not only control their cutaneous lesions but also experience the alleviation of their gastrointestinal disease. Dietary therapy also seems to reverse the IgA deposition in the DEJ after long-term therapy, which is an average of 12 years on a gluten-free diet.[37] Most patients require from 12 to 18 months on a gluten-free diet to be able to reduce their dapsone dose by greater than 50%. Some patients that immediately begin a gluten-free diet at the time of initial diagnosis appear to be able to control their disease more quickly than those in whom the disease has been present for a number of years. In addition, although a partial gluten-free diet may help decrease dapsone use, it usually is not successful in controlling the disease. Although a gluten-free diet can be quite effective in controlling dermatitis herpetiformis, the difficult nature of the diet given the normal American lifestyle often limits its usefulness in patients with dermatitis herpetiformis. Although there is some evidence that a gluten-free diet may decrease the risk of small bowel lymphoma in patients with isolated GSE, this has not been clearly documented to be the case in patients with dermatitis herpetiformis.

When patients attempt a gluten-free diet to control dermatitis herpetiformis, it is important that the clinician is absolutely certain that the patient has dermatitis herpetiformis with granular IgA deposits and not linear IgA dermatosis, since this disorder is not associated with gluten sensitivity and does not respond to a gluten-free diet.[38] In addition, the wide-spread presence of gluten in the normal diet makes it necessary for patients to consult with a dietitian before beginning the diet, so chances for success can be maximized.

REFERENCES

1. Duhring LA: Landmark article, Aug 30, 1884: Dermatitis herpetiformis, *JAMA* 250:212-216, 1997.
2. Marks J, Shuster S, Watson AJ: Small bowel changes in dermatitis herpetiformis, *Lancet* 1:1280-1282, 1966.
3. Katz SI, Hertz KC, Rogentine N, et al: HLA-B8 and dermatitis herpetiformis in patients with IgA deposits in skin, *Arch Dermatol* 113:155-156, 1977.
4. Cormane RH: Immunofluorescent studies of the skin in lupus erythematosus and other diseases, *Pathologica Eur* 2:170-187, 1967.
5. van der Meer JB: Granular deposits of immunoglobulins in the skin of patients with dermatitis herpetiformis: An immunofluorescent study, *Br J Dermatol* 81:493-503, 1969.
6. Hall RP, Lawley TJ: Characterization of circulating and cutaneous IgA immune complexes in patients with dermatitis herpetiformis, *J Immunol* 135:1760-1765, 1985.
7. Barghuthy FS, Kumar V, Valeski E, et al: Identification of IgA subclasses in skin of dermatitis herpetiformis patients, *Int Arch All Appl Immunol* 85:268-271, 1988.

8. Unsworth DJ, Payne AW, Leonard JN, et al: IgA in dermatitis-herpetiformis skin is dimeric, *Lancet* 1:478-479, 1982.
9. Katz SI, Strober WI: The pathogenesis of dermatitis herpetiformis (review), *J Invest Dermatol* 70:63-75, 1978.
10. Fry L, McMinn RMH, Cowan J, et al: Effect of gluten free-diet on dermatological, intestinal and haematological manifestations of dermatitis herpetiformis, *Lancet* 1:557-561, 1968.
11. Shuster S, Watson AJ, Marks J: Coeliac syndrome in dermatitis herpetiformis, *Lancet* 1:1101-1106, 1968.
12. Otley CC, Wenstrup RJ, Hall RP: DNA sequence analysis and restriction fragment length polymorphism (RFLP) typing of the HLA-DQw2 alleles associated with dermatitis herpetiformis, *J Invest Dermatol* 97:318-322, 1991.
13. Kagnoff MF, Harwood JI, Bugawan TL, et al: Structural analysis of the HLA-DR, -DQ, and -DP alleles on the celiac disease-associated HLA-DR3(DRw17) haplotype, *Proc Natl Acad Sci USA* 86:6274-6278, 1989.
14. Mobacken H, Kastrup W, Nilsson LA: Incidence and prevalence of dermatitis herpetiformis in western Sweden, *Acta Derm Venereol* 64:400-404, 1984.
15. Gawkrodger DJ, Blackwell JN, Gilmour HM, et al: Dermatitis herpetiformis: Diagnosis, diet and demography, *Gut* 25:151-157, 1984.
16. Katz SI: Clinical and histological overview. In Katz SI (moderator): Dermatitis herpetiformis: The skin and the gut, *Ann Intern Med* 93:857-874, 1980.
17. Hall RP: The pathogenesis of dermatitis herpetiformis: Recent advances, *J Am Acad Dermatol* 16:1129-1144, 1987.
18. Buckley DB, English J, Molloy W, et al: Dermatitis herpetiformis: A review of 119 cases, *Clin Exp Dermatol* 8:477-487, 1983.
19. Brow JR, Parker F, Weinstein WM: The small intestinal mucosa in dermatitis herpetiformis, *Gastroenterology* 60:355-361, 1971.
20. Fry L, Keir P, McMinn RMH: Small intestinal structure and function and haematological changes in dermatitis herpetiformis, *Lancet* 1:729, 1967.
21. Gillberg R, Kastrup W, Mobacken H, et al: Gastric morphology and function in dermatitis herpetiformis and in coeliac disease, *Scand J Gastroenterol* 20:133-140, 1985.
22. Leonard JN, Tucker WF, Fry JS, et al: Increased incidence of malignancy in dermatitis herpetiformis, *Br Med J* 286:16-18, 1983.
23. Gaspari AA, Huang CM, Davey RJ, et al: Prevalence of thyroid abnormalities in patients with dermatitis herpetiformis and in control subjects with HLA-B8/-DR3, *Am J Med* 88:145-150, 1990.
24. Hall RP: Dermatitis herpetiformis (review), *J Invest Dermatol* 99:873-881, 1992.
25. Blenkinsopp WK, Haffenden GP, Fry L, et al: Histology of linear IgA disease, dermatitis herpetiformis, and bullous pemphigoid, *Am J Dermatopathol* 5:547-554, 1983.
26. Zone JJ, Meyer LJ, Petersen MJ: Deposition of granular IgA relative to clinical lesions in dermatitis herpetiformis, *Arch Dermatol* 132:912-918, 1996.
27. Katz SI: Treatment: Drugs and diet. In Katz SI (moderator): Dermatitis herpetiformis: The skin and the gut, *Ann Intern Med* 93:857-874, 1980.
28. Lang PG: Sulfones and sulfonamides in dermatology today, *J Am Acad Dermatol* 1:479-492, 1979.
29. Jollow DJ, Bradshaw TP, McMillan DC: Dapsone-induced hemolytic anemia, *Drug Metab Rev* 27:107-124, 1995.
30. Hornsten P, Keisu M, Wiholm BE: The incidence of agranulocytosis during treatment of dermatitis herpetiformis with dapsone as reported in Sweden, 1972 through 1988, *Arch Dermatol* 126:919-922, 1990.
31. Uetrecht J: Dapsone and sulfapyridine, *Clin Dermatol* 7:111-120, 1989.
32. Daneshmend TK: The neurotoxicity of dapsone, *Adv Drug React Ac Pois Rev* 3:43-58, 1984.
33. Coleman MD, Rhodes LE, Scott AK, et al: The use of cimetidine to reduce dapsone-dependent methaemoglobinaemia in dermatitis herpetiformis patients, *Br J Clin Pharmacol* 34:244-249, 1992.
34. Prussick R, Ali MA, Rosenthal D, et al: The protective effect of vitamin E on the hemolysis associated with dapsone treatment in patients with dermatitis herpetiformis, *Arch Dermatol* 128:210-213, 1997.
35. Fry L, Seah PP, Riches DJ, et al: Clearance of skin lesions in dermatitis herpetiformis after gluten withdrawal, *Lancet* 1:288-291, 1973.
36. Fry L, Leonard JN, Swain F, et al: Long term follow-up of dermatitis herpetiformis with and without dietary withdrawal, *Br J Dermatol* 107:631-640, 1982.
37. Fry L, Leonard JN, Swain F, et al: Long term follow-up of dermatitis herpetiformis with and without dietary gluten withdrawal, *Br J Dermatol* 107:631-640, 1982.
38. Leonard JN, Griffiths CE, Powles AV, et al: Experience with a gluten free diet in the treatment of linear IgA disease, *Acta Derm Venerol (Stockh)* 67:145-148, 1987.

Linear IgA Bullous Dermatosis

Pamela G. Nemzer
Conleth A. Egan
John J. Zone

Etiology

Linear IgA bullous dermatosis is an autoimmune bullous dermatosis that affects adults of any age. It is considered a separate entity based on unique immunopathology of linear IgA deposition along the cutaneous basement membrane zone (BMZ).[1,2,3] Linear IgA bullous dermatosis can be idiopathic, drug-induced, or associated with infection or internal disease, including malignancies.[1] Drug-induced linear IgA dermatosis has been described most often with vancomycin, but captopril, lithium, and diclofenac have also been implicated.[1] Associated infections include varicella, herpes zoster, and upper respiratory infections.[1] A recent infection history can frequently be elicited, but the significance is not known,[4] although it has been postulated that the infectious agent may have triggered the autoimmune response.[1] An attractive mechanism for this includes the stimulation of an initial immune response through the IgA mucosal defense system, which eventuates into an IgA-predominant autoimmune response.[1] Implicated autoimmune diseases include ulcerative colitis, Crohn's disease, systemic lupus erythematosus (SLE), dermatomyositis, thyrotoxicosis, autoimmune hemolytic anemia, rheumatoid arthritis, and one case of glomerulonephritis.[1] Internal malignancies reportedly associated with linear IgA bullous dermatosis include lymphoma, chronic lymphocytic leukemia, and carcinomas of the bladder, thyroid, and esophagus, as well as case reports of plasmacytoma and ocular melanoma.[1]

When immunopathology identical to linear IgA bullous dermatosis is present in children, it is termed *chronic bullous disease of childhood*.[4,5] Chronic bullous disease of childhood demonstrates characteristic clinical findings with annular vesicobullae favoring intertriginous and flexural areas.

This work was supported by the Department of Veterans Affairs Medical Research Funds and in part by the Department of Dermatology, University of Utah Health Sciences Center.

Clinical Features

Linear IgA Bullous Dermatosis

The incidence of linear IgA bullous dermatosis is approximately 1:200,000 with an average age of onset after 60 years (mean 52 years).[1] Clinical features of linear IgA bullous dermatosis are widely variable. Patients typically demonstrate the appearance of widespread or localized subepidermal vesicles and bullae arising on normal skin or less commonly within urticarial plaques (Figures 8-1 and 8-2). The distribution favors the trunk, but involvement of extremities commonly occurs and can be similar to dermatitis herpetiformis or bullous pemphigoid (Figures 8-3 to 8-5). Linear IgA bullous dermatosis lesions tend to be less symmetric and more widespread than dermatitis herpetiformis. Although linear IgA bullous dermatosis lesions can be clinically identical to bullous pemphigoid lesions, they are easily distinguished by perilesional direct immunofluorescence (IF) examination. An annular, polycyclic, or targetlike appearance is frequently described in both linear IgA bullous disease and chronic bullous disease of childhood. However, facial and perineal involvement, which is nearly universal in chronic bullous disease of childhood, is seen in less than one third of adult patients with linear IgA bullous dermatosis[4] (Figures 8-6 and 8-7). More frequent mucous membrane involvement in linear IgA bullous dermatosis can also be helpful in distinguishing it from bullous pemphigoid.[1,4]

Chronic Bullous Disease of Childhood

Chronic bullous disease of childhood usually presents in early childhood at a mean age of 4.5 years with a female preponderance of close to 2:1.[4] Perineal and perioral involvement is very common, as well as the nearly-universal trunk and limb lesions. There is a tendency for more widespread bullous pemphigoid-like lesions in older children and adolescents[4] (Figures 8-8 and 8-9). Like linear IgA bullous dermatosis, individual lesions often have an annular or polycyclic appearance.[1,4] Grouped annular

LINEAR IGA BULLOUS DERMATOSIS SUMMARY

ETIOLOGY
Idiopathic or drug-induced autoimmune bullous dermatosis

CLINICAL FEATURES
Cutaneous vesicular or bullous lesions and mucocutaneous and ocular involvement

PATHOLOGY
Classic subepidermal vesicobullae with predominantly neutrophilic inflammation

DIAGNOSIS
Clinical features, skin biopsy, direct and indirect IF

TREATMENT
Dapsone, sulfapyradine, systemic steroids, and immunosuppression

DIFFERENTIAL DIAGNOSIS
Bullous pemphigoid, dermatitis herpetiformis, cicatricial pemphigoid, bullous LE, erythema multiforme, and epidermolysis bullosa acquisita

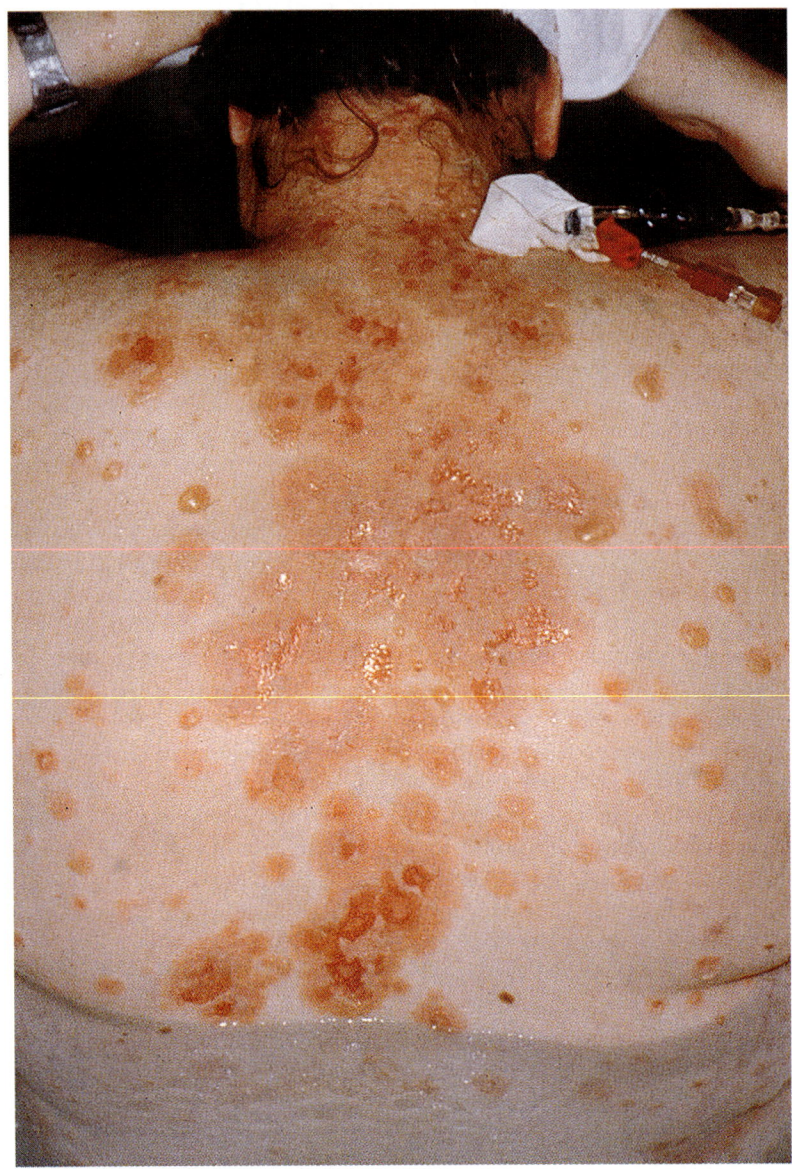

FIGURE 8-1. Vesicles and bullae of linear IgA bullous dermatosis on the back. Note that the lesions are arising on an urticarial plaque.

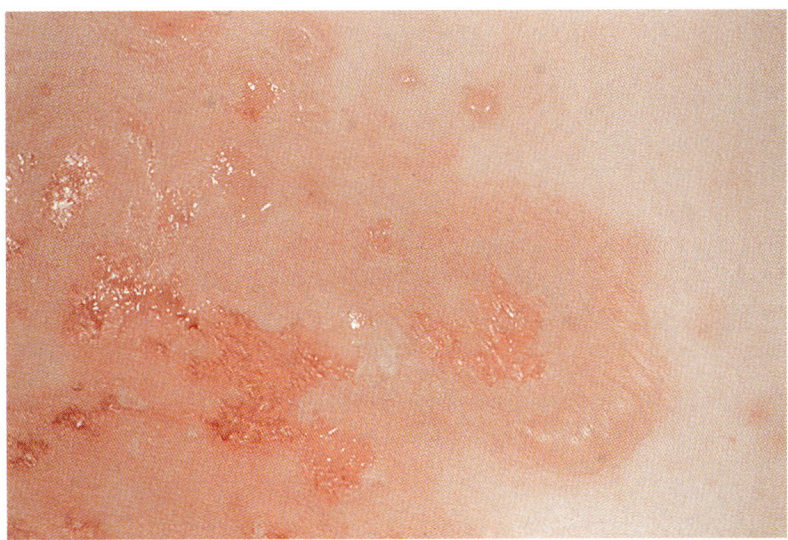

FIGURE 8-2. Close-up of Figure 8-1 showing bullae, vesicles, erosions, and urticarial lesions of linear IgA bullous dermatosis.

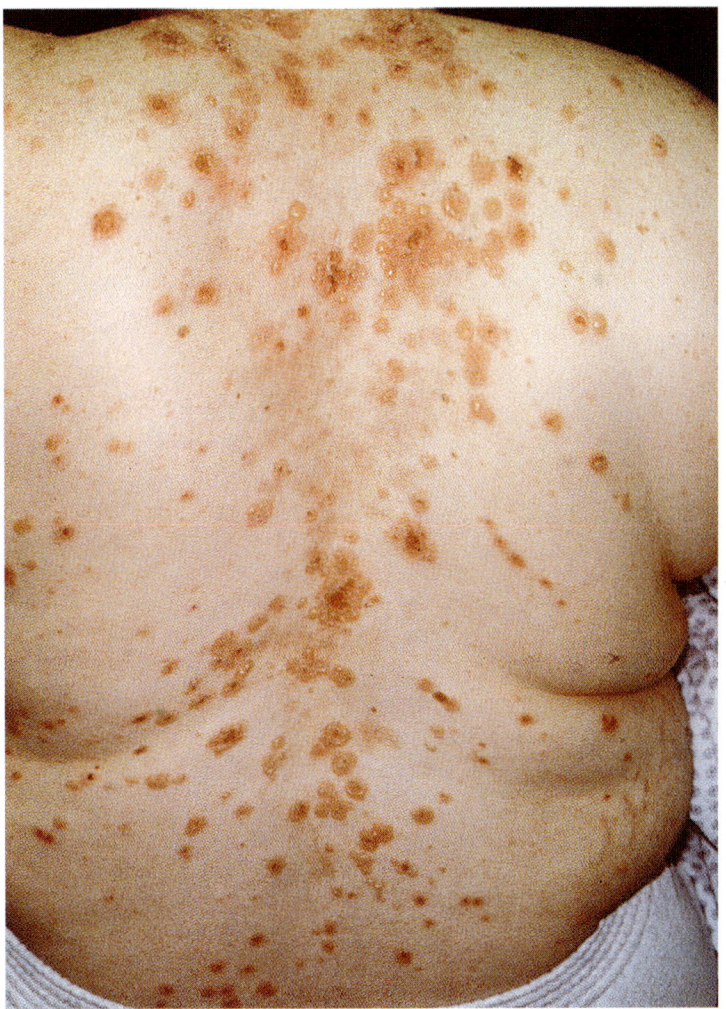

FIGURE 8-3. Typical smaller vesicles and bullae of linear IgA bullous dermatosis on a patient's back that resemble those of dermatitis herpetiformis and bullous pemphigoid.

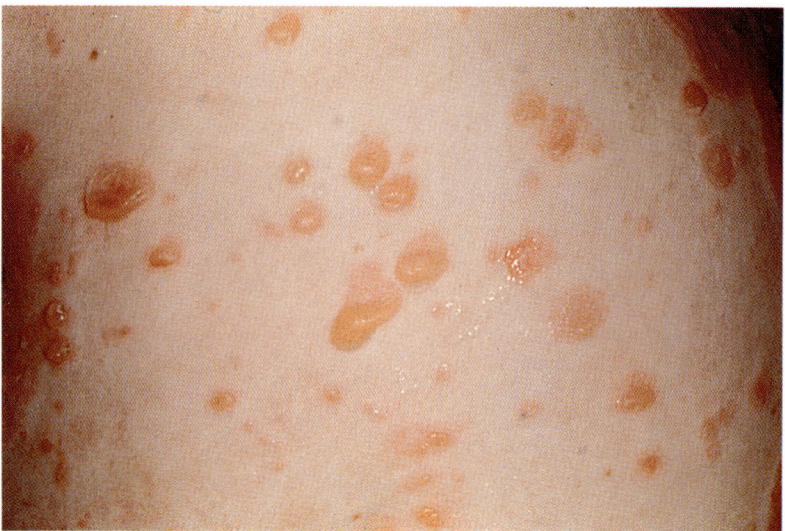

FIGURE 8-4. Close-up of isolated vesicles and bullae of linear IgA bullous dermatosis on a patient's lateral trunk that are indistinguishable from bullous pemphigoid. Note the annular bulla in the upper left side of the photograph.

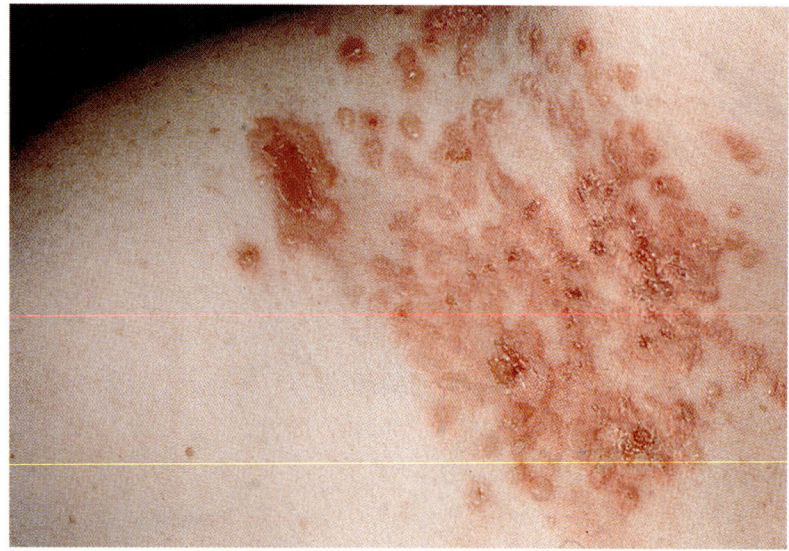

FIGURE 8-5. Close-up of clustered vesicles, bullae, and crusted erosions in a patient's axilla.

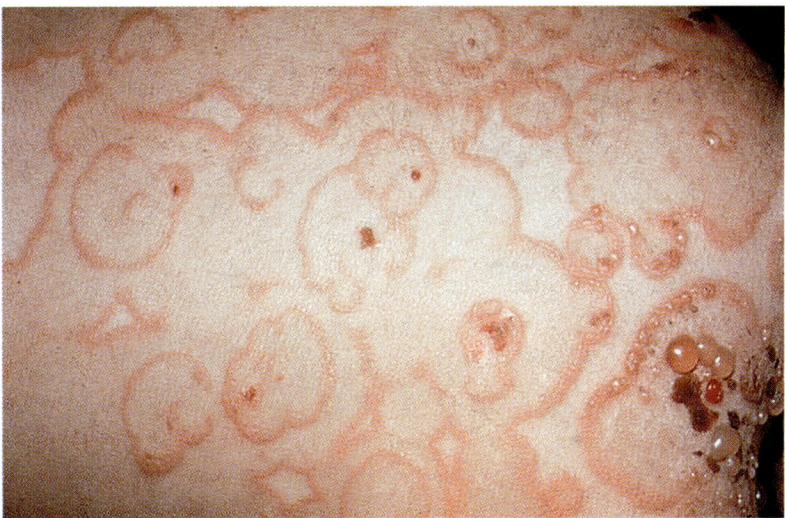

FIGURE 8-6. Annular plaques with peripheral bullae in a patient with chronic bullous disease of childhood. *(Courtesy Steven Eyre, MD.)*

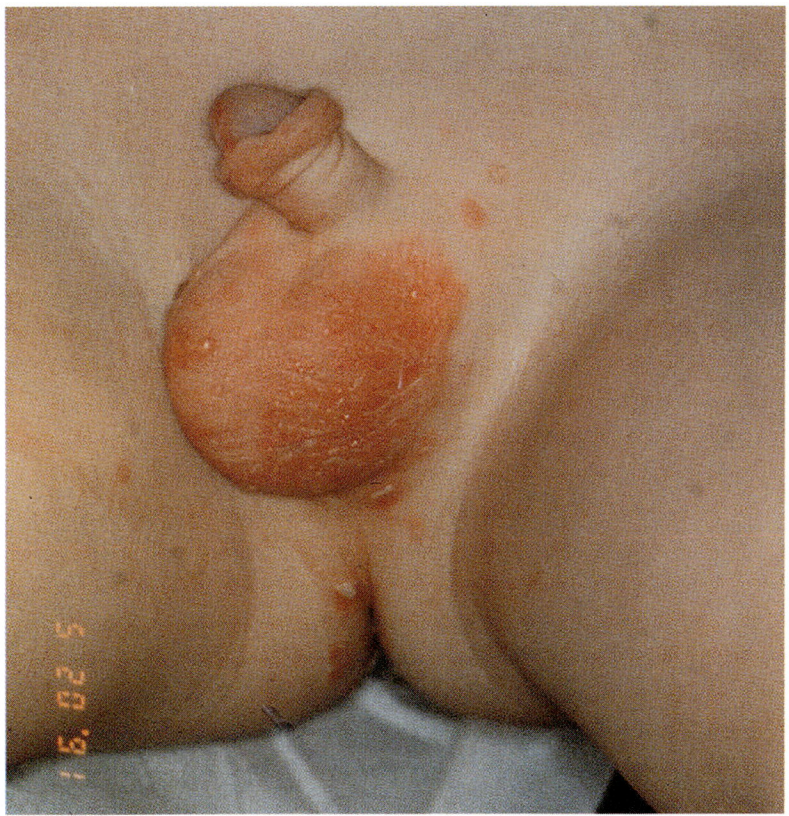

FIGURE 8-7. Scrotal vesicles and erosions in a patient with chronic bullous disease of childhood.

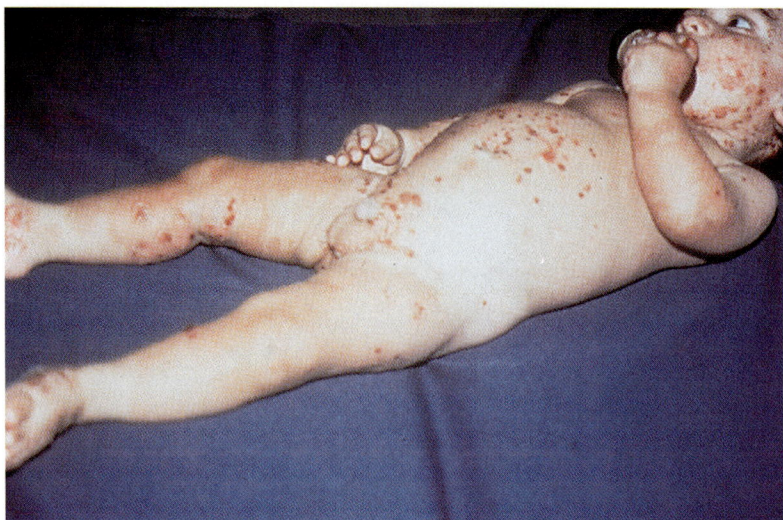

FIGURE 8-8. Diffusely located vesicles and bullae in a patient with chronic bullous disease of childhood. Note the prominent facial and perineal involvement. *(Courtesy Steven Eyre, MD.)*

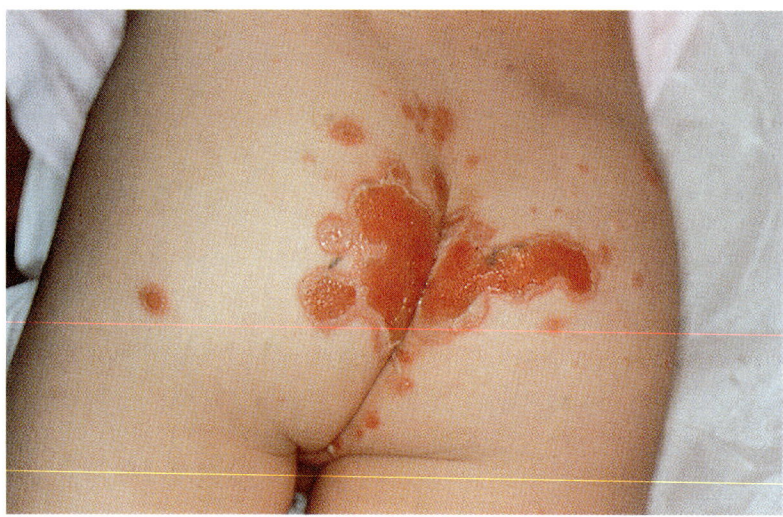

FIGURE 8-9. Prominent involvement of buttocks with perianal lesions in chronic bullous disease of childhood. Note the characteristic annular configuration, peripheral bullae, and central erosions.

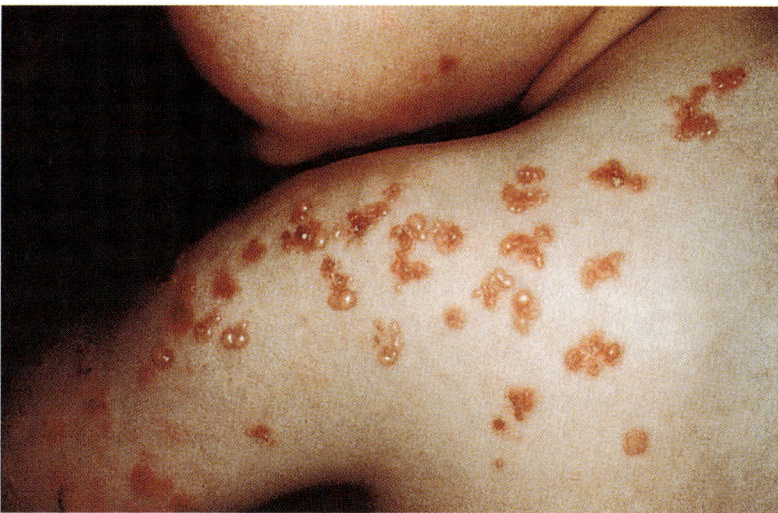

FIGURE 8-10. "Cluster of jewels" configuration in chronic bullous disease of childhood on a patient's shoulder.

vesicular and bullous lesions often have the appearance of a "string of pearls" or "cluster of jewels," which is a widely described sign in chronic bullous disease of childhood[1,4] (Figures 8-10 to 8-12). Mucous membrane, as well as ocular, involvement is frequent with reports of ocular scarring in both adults and children.[4,6]

Drug-Induced Linear IgA Bullous Dermatosis

A clear relationship between the occurrence of clinical, pathologic, and immunofluorescent findings of linear IgA bullous dermatosis has been reported with many drugs, including captopril, lithium, diclofenac, trimethoprim-sulfamethoxazole, somatostatin, and most often vancomycin[1,7] (Figures 8-13 to 8-16). In the drug-induced form of linear IgA bullous dermatosis, classic skin lesions are abrupt in onset, which occurs between 1 and 3 weeks after administration of the offending agent.[7,8,9] Resolution of the eruption frequently occurs as soon as 7 to 14 days after drug withdrawal without treatment.[7,8,9] The majority of reported cases in which localization of circulating IgA antibody was investigated demonstrated dermal or sublamina densa binding to 1 M NaCl-split normal human skin.[7,8] This demonstration may be helpful in differentiating between the idiopathic and drug-induced variants of linear IgA bullous dermatosis, but one patient demonstrated IgA antibody specific to the 97 kD lamina lucida antigen, which is a component of BPAG2 (180 kD), and another demonstrated IgA antibody specific to BPAG1 (230 kD), respectively.[9]

Pathology and Immunopathology

Linear IgA bullous dermatosis is a neutrophil-rich subepidermal bullous disease that shares many pathologic features with dermatitis herpetiformis.[1,10] A spectrum of pathology is seen from a vacuolar interface dermatitis with neutrophils along the dermal-epidermal junction (DEJ) in early lesions to neutrophil-rich multilocular abscesses at the dermal papillary tips or within a large subepidermal bulla[1,10] (Figures 8-17 to 8-19). The presence of fibrin and neutrophilic nuclear debris (leukocytoclasis) in the dermal papillary tips is more specific for linear IgA bullous dermatosis than dermatitis herpetiformis[10] (Figures 8-20 to 8-22). Increasingly, numerous eosinophils are often present in both diseases over time.[1] Because of the similarities, a definitive diagnosis can only be made with direct IF examination.[1,10] All patients with characteristic histopathologic findings should have direct IF examination, since patients with granular IgA (dermatitis herpetiformis) are likely to respond to dietary gluten restriction and patients with linear IgA bullous dermatosis are at risk for ocular and esophageal scarring.

Immunoelectron microscopy of linear IgA bullous dermatosis reveals three patterns of IgA deposition. The largest group has immunoglobulin in the lamina lucida, a second group shows deposition in the sublamina densa, while a third group demonstrates IgA in both locations. Both adults and children with lamina lucida IgA share a common 97-kD antigen, which is a fragment of the BPAG2 (BP180).[2,5] Consequently, from an immuno-

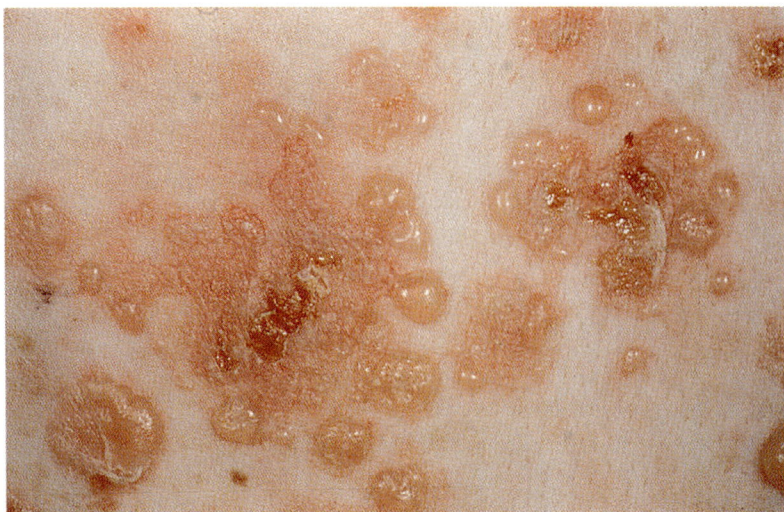

FIGURE 8-11. Close-up of "cluster of jewels" or "string of pearls" configuration in chronic bullous disease of childhood.

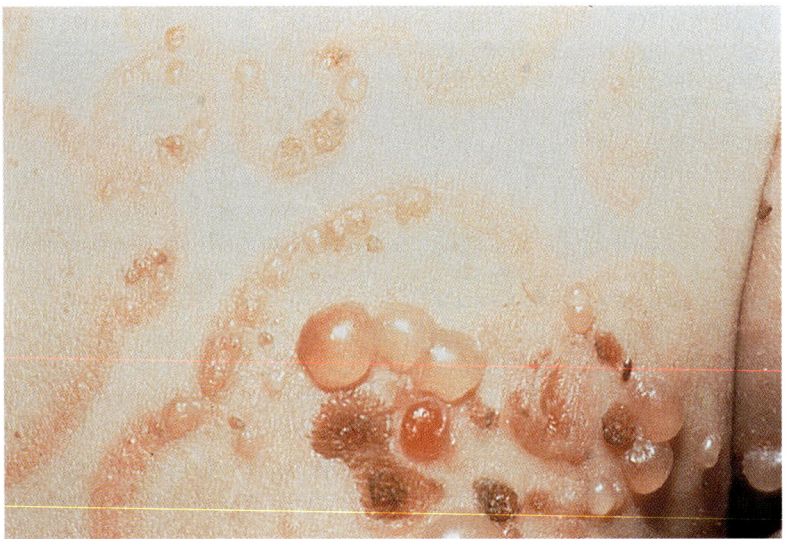

FIGURE 8-12. Close-up of "string of pearls" configuration in chronic bullous disease of childhood; linear vesicles located at the annular rim of this lesion. *(Courtesy Steven Eyre, MD.)*

pathologic perspective, linear IgA bullous dermatosis and chronic bullous disease of childhood appear to be identical but simply occur in different age groups. In addition, a selected group of eleven patients with clinical, histologic, and immunofluorescent findings of linear IgA bullous dermatosis reacted exclusively to one of the bullous pemphigoid antigens.[11] Another group has implicated a 285-kD upper dermal antigen, which has yet to be characterized.[4] Zambruno et al reported a case of sublamina densa disease with IgA autoantibodies to the 290-kD dermal-anchoring fibril protein, which is type VII collagen.[12] They concluded that this case was most likely an IgA variant of epidermolysis bullosa acquisita.

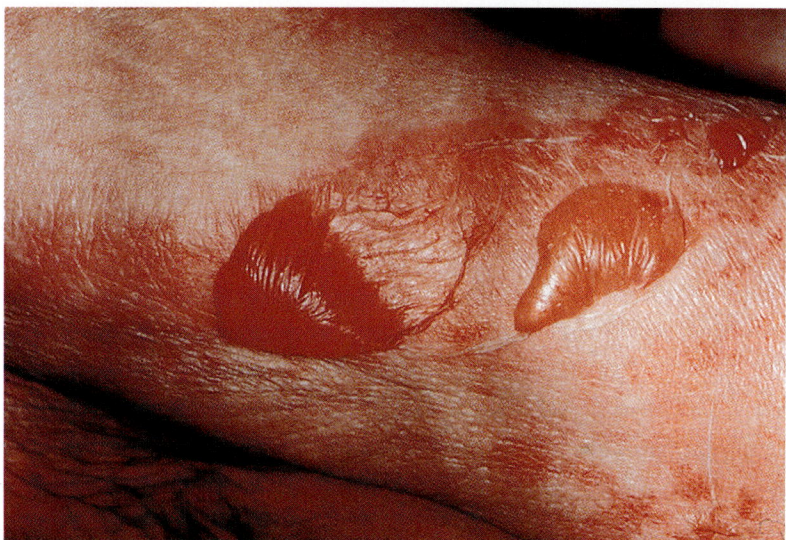

FIGURE 8-13. Large bullae on the thigh of a patient with drug-induced linear IgA bullous dermatosis.

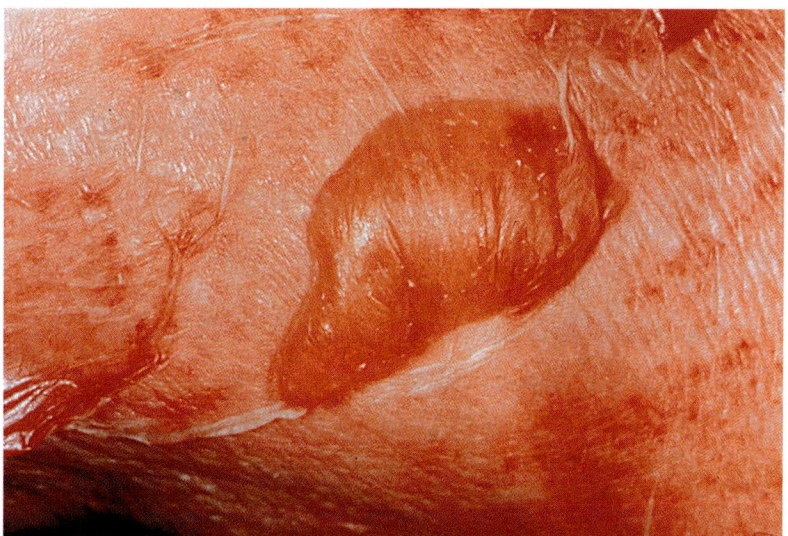

FIGURE 8-14. Close-up of one bulla from Figure 8-13; drug-induced linear IgA bullous dermatosis.

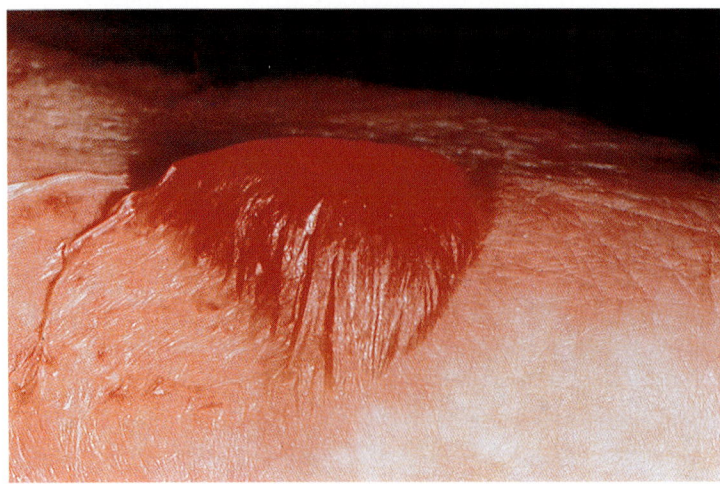

FIGURE 8-15. Close-up of one bulla from Figure 8-13; drug-induced linear IgA bullous dermatosis.

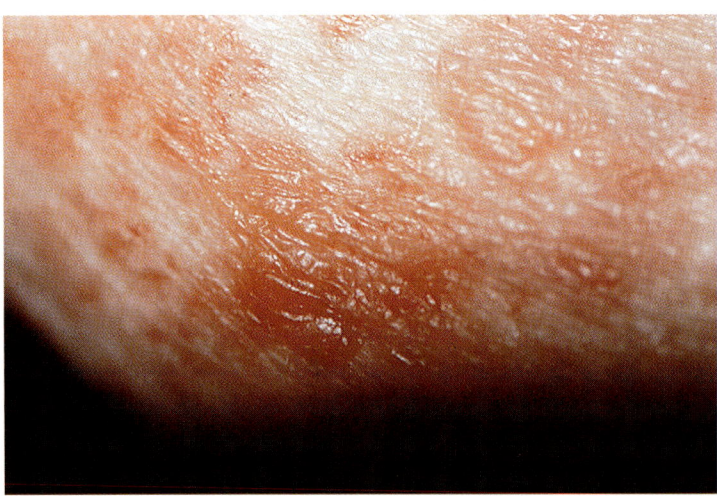

FIGURE 8-16. Urticarial plaques and bullae on the leg of a patient with drug-induced linear IgA bullous dermatosis.

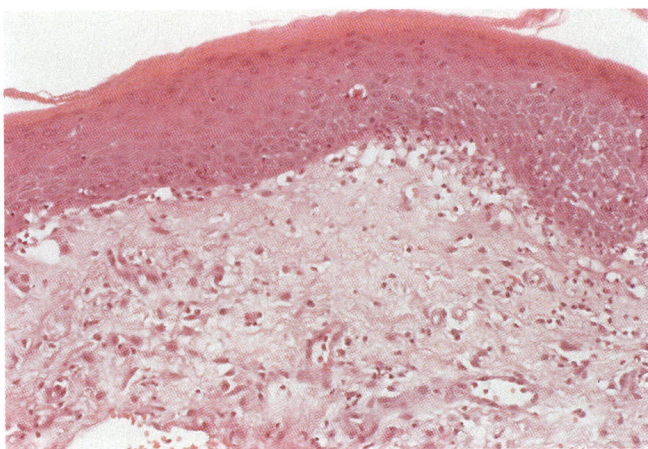

FIGURE 8-17. Involved (lesional) skin biopsy of a patient with drug-induced linear IgA bullous dermatosis demonstrating a dramatic vacuolar interface change at the dermal-epidermal junction. (H&E, ×400.)

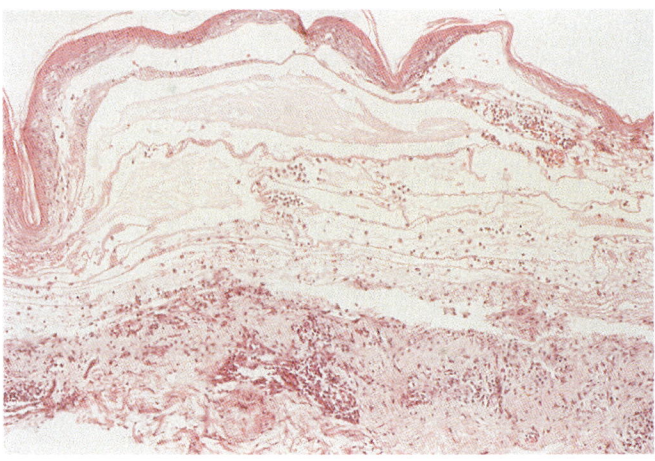

FIGURE 8-18. Lesional skin biopsy of a patient with drug-induced linear IgA bullous dermatosis demonstrating a subepidermal bulla filled with fibrinous debris. The upper dermis at the base of this micrograph is infiltrated with numerous inflammatory cells. (H&E, ×100.)

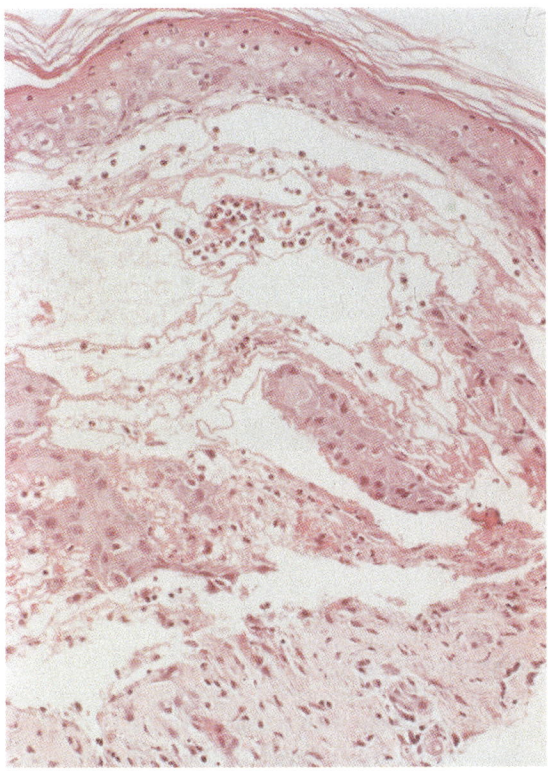

FIGURE 8-19. Lesional skin biopsy of a patient with drug-induced linear IgA bullous dermatosis demonstrating a subepidermal bulla filled with fibrinous debris and inflammatory cells including neutrophils. The upper dermis is seen at the base of this micrograph. (H&E, ×200.)

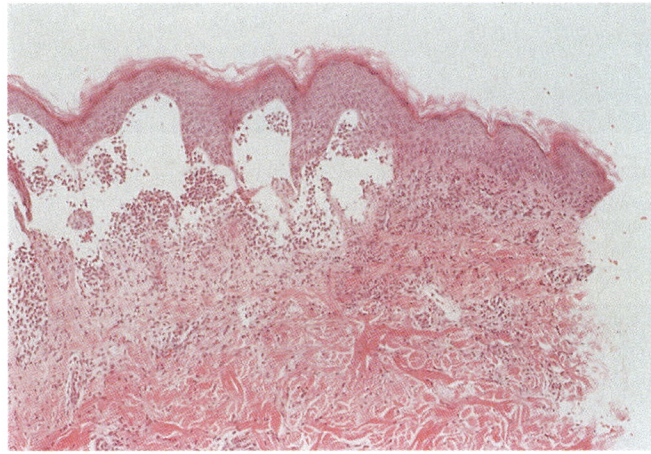

FIGURE 8-20. Lesional skin biopsy of a patient with classic idiopathic linear IgA bullous dermatosis. On the right edge, intact epidermis is seen with a subepidermal vesicle to the left. Numerous inflammatory cells are seen within the vesicle cavity and in the upper dermis. (H&E, ×100.) NOTE: Clinical and immunopathologic photographs of this patient appear in Figures 8-1 to 8-5, 8-23, 8-24, 8-27, and 8-28.

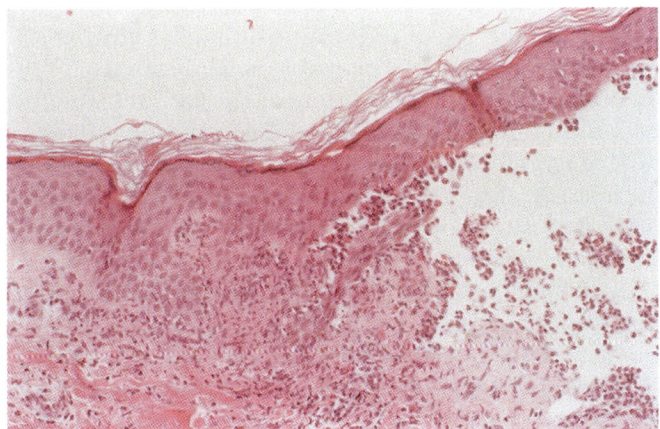

FIGURE 8-21. A close-up view of the patient in Figure 8-20 shows the intense neutrophilic infiltrate within the vesicle cavity and the upper dermis. (H&E, ×200.)

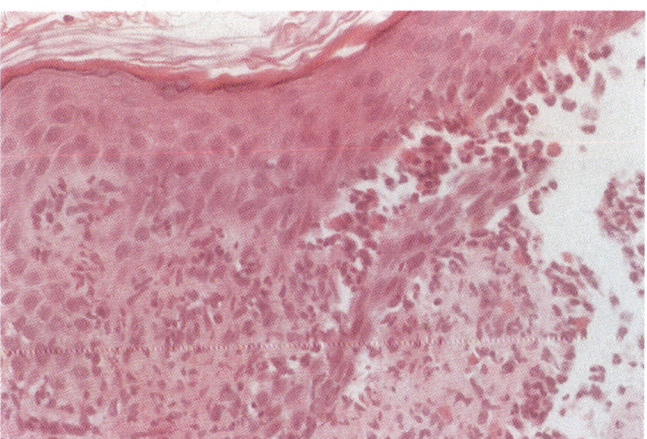

FIGURE 8-22. A closer view of Figure 8-21 clearly shows the intense neutrophilic infiltrate within the vesicle cavity and the upper dermis. An island of reepithelialization is seen jutting into the edge of the vesicle cavity. (H&E, ×400.)

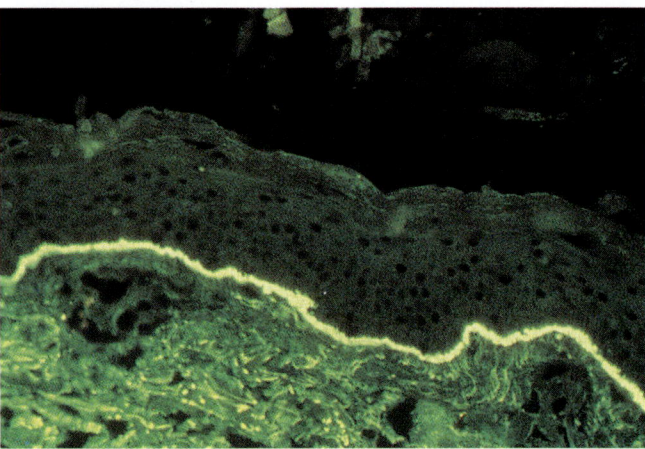

FIGURE 8-23. Direct IF of perilesional skin in a patient with linear IgA bullous dermatosis. (×400.)

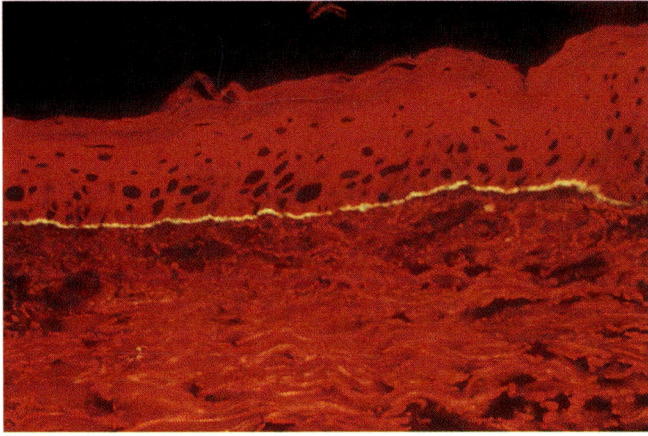

FIGURE 8-24. Direct IF of perilesional skin in a patient with linear IgA bullous dermatosis counterstained with Evans blue. (×400.)

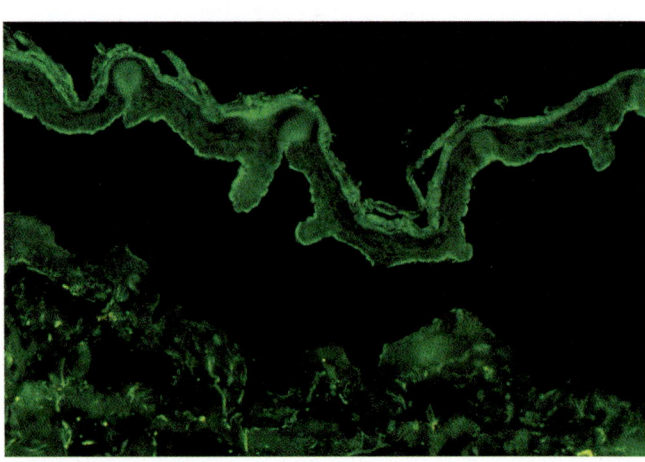

FIGURE 8-25. Indirect IF demonstrating binding of serum containing epidermal BMZ antibody to the roof of BMZ-split skin. (×200.)

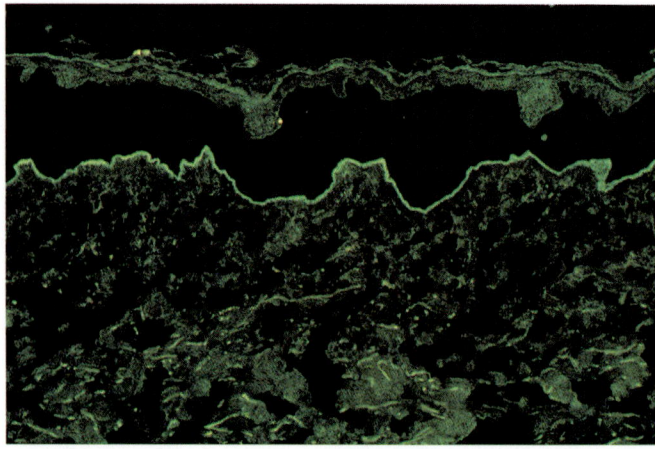

FIGURE 8-26. Indirect IF demonstrating binding of serum containing epidermal BMZ antibody to the base of BMZ-split skin. (×100.)

Diagnosis

A diagnosis of linear IgA bullous dermatosis is made with a combination of the clinical examination, skin biopsy, and direct IF results. Other useful supplemental information includes indirect IF and immunomapping.

IF examination can be performed by two standard methods, both of which give different clinically useful information for diagnosis and management. Direct IF is performed on fresh, perilesional unfixed tissue for the detection of in vivo bound autoantibodies and proteins, including IgG, IgA, IgM, C3, and less commonly fibrinogen.[13] Indirect IF is performed on a suitable substrate, such as a fresh-frozen human donor 1MNaCl-split skin in the lower laminda lucida, or EDTA for the detection and titering of serum autoantibodies directed toward BMZ antigens.[13] This gives the clinician useful information about the location of the antigen for the patient's autoantibodies.[13] By definition, linear deposition of IgA along the BMZ is seen in linear IgA bullous dermatosis, although the additional presence of less intense deposition of IgG, IgM, and complement can be seen in 20% to 30% of patients[1] (Figures 8-23 and 8-24). Detectable circulating levels of IgA antibodies can be demonstrated in 60% to 70% of sera of patients with linear IgA bullous dermatosis, which is similar to demonstration of circulating IgG in sera of patients with bullous pemphigoid[1] (Figure 8-25). Because lamina lucida antigens are located in the roof of the split skin, both linear IgA bullous dermatosis and bullous pemphigoid demonstrate binding to the roof.[2,13] This binding is in contrast to the dermal binding of antibodies in bullous diseases such as epidermolysis bullosa acquisita, bullous lupus erythematosus (LE), and the less common sublamina densa variant of linear IgA bullous dermatosis[13] (Figure 8-26).

Table 8-1. *Differential Diagnosis of Linear IgA Bullous Disease*

Diagnostic Method	Linear IgA bullous disease	Dermatitis herpetiformis	Bullous pemphigoid
Clinical	Small vesicles or large bullae; urticarial plaques	Pruritic papules and small vesicles in a grouped or herpetiform configuration	Widespread large tense bullae; urticarial plaques
Distribution	Trunk, extremities, mucosal surfaces—similar to dermatitis herpetiformis or bullous pemphigoid	Extensor surfaces, symmetric—especially elbows, knees, buttocks, and neck	Trunk, extremities, mucosal surfaces
Direct IF	Linear IgA at BMZ; possibly IgG and C3	Granular IgA in dermal papillae	Linear IgG and C3 at BMZ
Indirect IF	Linear IgA at BMZ in 70% of sera	Negative	Linear IgG at BMZ in 70% of sera
Enteropathy	0%-24%	>85%	None
Sulfone responsiveness	Good, may also require corticosteroids	Excellent	Minimal

BMZ, Basement membrane zone.
Adapted from Smith E, Zone J: Linear IgA bullous dermatosis. In Arndt K et al, eds: *Cutaneous medicine and surgery*, Philadelphia, 1996, WB Saunders.

Differential Diagnosis

Linear IgA bullous dermatosis is difficult to diagnose clinically because of the similar presentation of both bullous pemphigoid and dermatitis herpetiformis (Table 8-1). They can be separated primarily based on results of direct IF examination of perilesional skin. Other bullous diseases that should be considered are erythema multiforme and bullous LE, both of which can present with bullae arising within urticarial plaques. Erythema multiforme usually demonstrates a nonspecific direct IF; bullous LE will have mixed linear and granular deposition of immunoglobulins along the DEJ as opposed to the fine linear pattern seen in linear IgA bullous dermatosis.[1]

Linear IgA bullous dermatosis has not been consistently associated with a gluten-sensitive enteropathy as is characteristic in dermatitis herpetiformis. Although circulating IgG anti-gliadin antibodies are universally found in patients with untreated dermatitis herpetiformis, titers measured in patients with linear IgA bullous dermatosis and chronic bullous disease of childhood were similar to controls.[14] In the same study, one patient of ten with linear IgA bullous disease had biopsy-proved jejunal mucosal changes on a normal diet.[14] The presence of intestinal enteropathy is not a typical feature of linear IgA bullous dermatosis or chronic bullous disease of childhood.

Treatment

Linear IgA bullous dermatosis responds well to treatment with dapsone or sulfapyridine, often as early as 48 to 72 hours after initiation of therapy[1] (Figures 8-27

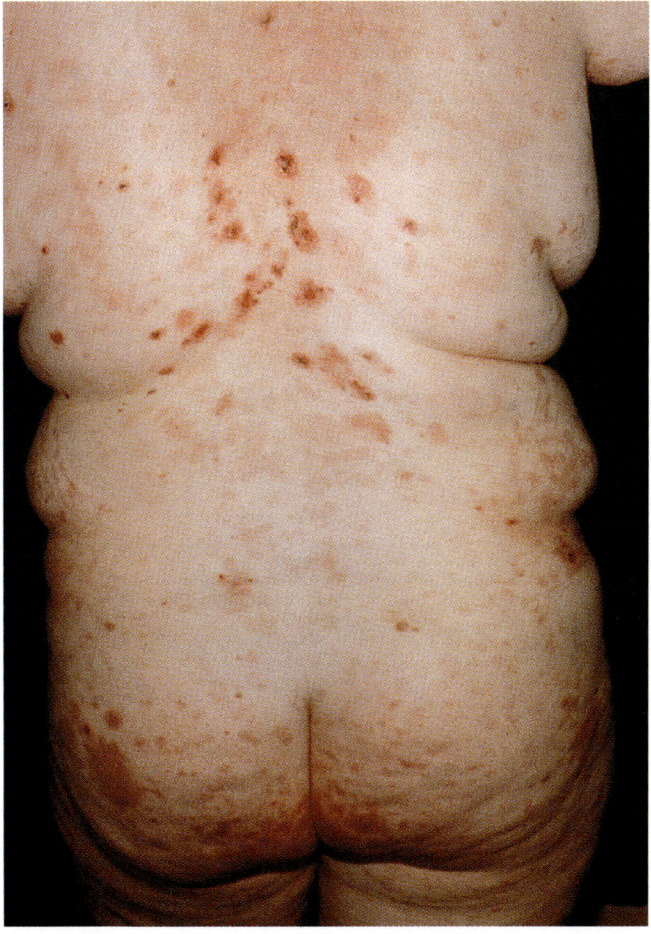

FIGURE 8-27. Follow-up of the back of the patient with linear IgA bullous dermatosis in Figure 8-1 showing improvement on therapy with very few new bullae and erosions.

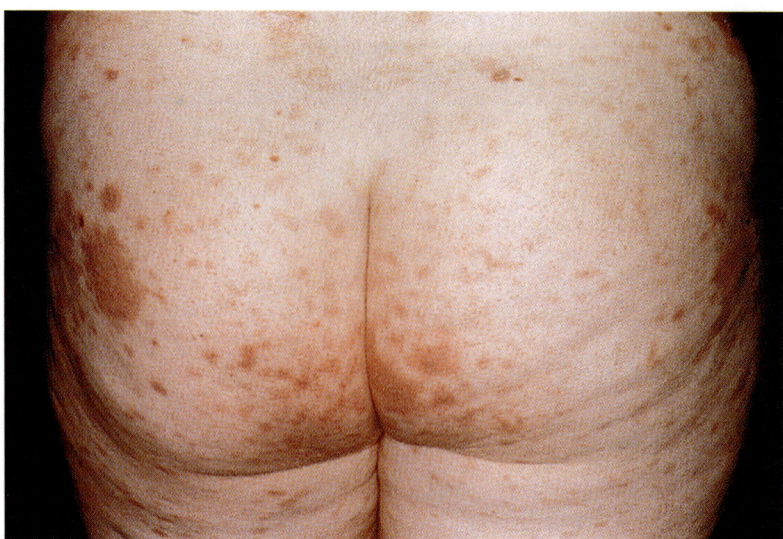

FIGURE 8-28. Follow-up of the buttocks of the patient with linear IgA bullous dermatosis in Figure 8-1 showing improvement on therapy. Erythematous macules and patches remain, as well as mild scarring in an area of previously intense disease activity.

Table 8-2. *Treatment of Linear IgA Bullous Disease and Chronic Bullous Disease of Childhood*

DISEASE	MEDICATION	LABORATORY EVALUATION
Linear IgA bullous disease	Dapsone 100-300 mg daily; start 25 mg, increase every 1-2 weeks until control of lesions	Baseline CBC and liver function tests Weekly CBC × 4 weeks Monthly CBC × 5 months and liver function tests every 6 weeks
	Prednisone 10-60 mg daily	Blood glucose level and blood pressure
Chronic bullous disease of childhood	Sulfapyridine 70 mg/kg per day in divided doses, not to exceed 100 mg/kg per day	Baseline CBC and liver function tests Monthly CBC × 5 months and liver function tests every 6 weeks
	Dapsone 1-2 mg/kg per day, not to exceed 3-4 mg/kg per day	Baseline CBC and liver function tests Weekly CBC × 4 weeks Monthly CBC × 5 months and liver function tests every 6 weeks

CBC, Complete blood count.
Adapted from Smith E, Zone J: Linear IgA bullous dermatosis. In Arndt K et al, eds: *Cutaneous medicine and surgery,* Philadelphia, 1996, WB Saunders.

and 8-28). Chronic bullous dermatosis of childhood responds equally well to either sulfapyridine or dapsone, but sulfapyridine is preferred in children because of the fewer side effects when compared to dapsone[1] (Table 8-2). Although the average dose of dapsone in an adult is 100 mg daily, doses up to 300 mg daily may be needed.[1] Most toxicity, however, is dose-dependent, and efforts to minimize dapsone doses should continually be made. Careful monitoring of laboratory parameters should be done, including a complete blood count (CBC) to assess the degree of hemolysis and exclude the occurrence of agranulocytosis. Liver function tests should be evaluated for drug-inducted hepatitis. Addition of oral prednisone in doses up to 1 mg/kg daily may be necessary in some patients to achieve a full remission.[1] Resistant cases may require immunosuppression as is done in bullous pemphigoid and pemphigus vulgaris.

REFERENCES

1. Smith E, Zone J: Linear IgA bullous dermatosis. In Arndt K et al, eds: *Cutaneous medicine and surgery,* Philadelphia, 1996, WB Saunders Co.
2. Zone J, Taylor T, Kadunce D, et al: Identification of the cutaneous basement membrane zone antigen and isolation of antibody in linear immunoglobulin A bullous dermatosis, *J Clin Invest* 85:812-820, 1990.
3. Chorzelski T, Jablonska S, Beutner E, et al: Linear IgA bullous dermatosis. In Buetner E, Chorzelski T, Bean S, eds: *Immunopathology of the skin,* New York, 1979, John Wiley and Sons.
4. Wojnarowska F, Marsden R, Bhogal B, et al: Chronic bullous disease of childhood, childhood cicatricial pemphigoid and linear IgA disease of adults, *J Am Acad Dermatol* 1988, 19(5):792-805, 1988.
5. Zone J, Taylor T, Kadunce D, et al: IgA antibodies in chronic bullous disease of childhood react with a 97 kDa basement membrane zone protein, *J Invest Dermatol* 106:1277-1280, 1996.
6. Smith E, Taylor T, Meyer L, et al: Identification of a basement membrane zone antigen reactive with circulating IgA antibody in ocular cicatricial pemphigoid, *J Invest Dermatol* 101(4):619-623, 1993.
7. Kuechle M, Stegemir E, Maynard B, et al: Drug-induced linear IgA bullous dermatosis: Report of six cases and review of the literature, *J Am Acad Dermatol* 30(2):187-192, 1994.
8. Carpenter S, Berg D, Sudhu-Malik N, et al: Vancomycin-associated linear IgA dermatosis, *J Am Acad Dermatol* 26(1):45-8, 1992.
9. Paul C, Wolkenstein P, Prost C, et al: Drug-induced linear IgA disease: Target antigens are heterogenous, *Br J Dermatol* 136(3):406-411, 1997.
10. Blenkinsopp W, Fry L, Haffenden G, et al: Histology of linear IgA disease, dermatitis herpetiformis, and bullous pemphigoid, *Am J Dermatopath* 5(6):547-554, 1983.
11. Ghohestani R, Nicolas J, Kanitakis J, et al: Linear IgA Bullous dermatosis with IgA antibodies exclusively directed against the 180- or 230-kDa epidermal antigens, *J Invest Dermatol* 108(6):854-858, 1997.
12. Zambruno G, Manca V, Kanitakis J, et al: Linear IgA bullous dermatosis with autoantibodies to a 290kd antigen of anchoring fibrils, *J Am Acad Dermatol* 31(5):884-888, 1994.
13. Gammon W, Fine J-D, Forbes M, et al: Immunofluorescence on split skin for the detection and differentiation of basement membrane zone autoantibodies, *J Am Acad Dermatol* 27(1):79-87, 1992.
14. Ciclitira P, Ellis H, Venning V, et al: Circulating antibodies to gliadin subfactions in dermatitis herpetiformis and linear IgA dermatosis of adults and children, *Clin Exp Dermatol* 11:502-509, 1986.

Epidermolysis Bullosa Acquisita

Edel A. O'Toole
David T. Woodley

Etiology

Epidermolysis bullosa acquisita is a chronic, subepidermal blistering disease associated with autoimmunity to the collagen (type VII collagen) within anchoring fibril structures that are located at the dermal-epidermal junction (DEJ). Although it is an acquired disease that usually begins in adulthood, it was placed in the category of "epidermolysis bullosa" approximately 100 years ago because physicians were struck by how similar the lesions were to those seen in children with hereditary dystrophic forms of epidermolysis bullosa.[1]

In the early 1970s, Roenigk et al[2] summarized the world literature of epidermolysis bullosa acquisita, reported three new cases, and suggested the following as the first diagnostic criteria: (1) a negative family and personal history for a previous blistering disorder, (2) an adult-onset of the eruption, (3) spontaneous or trauma-induced blisters that resemble those of hereditary dystrophic epidermolysis bullosa, and (4) the exclusion of all other bullous diseases.

The etiology of epidermolysis bullosa acquisita is unknown, but most of the evidence to date suggests an autoimmune etiology. Direct IF of perilesional skin biopsies from patients with epidermolysis bullosa acquisita reveals IgG deposits at the DEJ.[3,4] Epidermolysis bullosa acquisita autoantibodies bind to type VII collagen within anchoring fibrils.[5] Anchoring fibrils are wheat stacklike structures that emanate from the lamina densa in a perpendicular fashion and stretch about 200 to 300 µm into the papillary dermis where they associate with globular structures called *anchoring plaques*. The anchoring plaques contain type IV collagen, a component shared with the lamina densa zone of the BMZ between the epidermis and dermis (Figure 9-1). Anchoring fibrils anchor the epidermis and its underlying basement membrane to the papillary dermis.

The type VII collagen alpha chain has a molecular mass between 250 to 320 kilodaltons (kD). Each type VII collagen molecule consists of a homotrimer of three identical alpha chains. Each alpha chain consists of a large globular noncollagenous amino terminus called the *noncollagenous 1* (NC1) domain; this domain comprises approximately half the entire mass of the alpha chain. Next, within each alpha chain, there is a helical domain with typical glycine-X-Y repeats. At the carboxyl terminus is a second globular noncollagenous domain (NC2) that is approximately 20 kD. Epidermolysis bullosa acquisita autoantibodies bind to type VII collagen alpha chains; this is associated with decreased anchoring fibrils, yet the pathway leading to this reduction is unknown. It may be that type VII collagen alpha chains that are newly synthesized, but decorated with epidermolysis bullosa acquisita autoantibodies, cannot form triple helical structures and stable anchoring fibrils. The paucity of anchoring fibrils causes poor epidermal-dermal adherence, skin fragility, and blister formation. Lapiere et al[6] demonstrated that epidermolysis bullosa acquisita autoantibodies recognize four predominant antigenic epitopes within the NC1 domain. Therefore the antigenic targets for the epidermolysis bullosa acquisita autoantibodies in adults are largely confined to the NC1 domain. However, Tanaka et al recently described three children with autoantibodies to the collagenous triple helical domain of type VII collagen.[7]

Evidence for the pathogenic role of epidermolysis bullosa acquisita antibodies also comes from the observation that when patients with systemic lupus erythematosus (SLE) develop autoantibodies to the epidermolysis bullosa acquisita antigen, they develop skin blisters and fall into a subset of LE called *bullous LE*.[8] Patients with SLE do not usually have skin fragility or blisters, but when patients with SLE make autoantibodies to anchoring fibril collagen (the epidermolysis bul-

---

This work was supported in part by grant AR 33625-09 and Career Development Award K04-AR1540 from the National Institutes of Health, Bethesda, Maryland. Dr. O'Toole is a Howard Hughes Medical Institute Physician Postdoctoral Fellow.

EPIDERMOLYSIS BULLOUS ACQUISITA SUMMARY

ETIOLOGY
Epidermolysis bullous acquisita is a chronic, subepidermal blistering disease associated with autoimmunity to anchoring fibril collagen (type VII collagen).

CLINICAL FEATURES
Erosions and blisters in trauma-prone areas. Lesions heal with scarring and formation of milia.

PATHOLOGY
Subepidermal blistering with a mixed inflammatory infiltrate in the dermis.

DIAGNOSIS
Routine immunofluorescence, immunoelectron microscopy, indirect salt-split skin immunofluorescence, Western blotting, and ELISA.

TREATMENT
Cyclosporine, colchicine, photopheresis, intravenous immunoglobulin, and supportive therapy.

DIFFERENTIAL DIAGNOSIS
Porphyria cutanea tarda, cicatricial pemphigoid, bullous pemphigoid.

---

losa acquisita antigen), a widespread blistering eruption of the skin ensues. This "experiment of nature" suggests that epidermolysis bullosa acquisita autoantibodies are pathogenic and capable of inducing disadherence between the epidermis and dermis. Nevertheless, consistent induction of blisters in an animal by the passive transfer of epidermolysis bullosa acquisita IgG autoantibodies into the animal has not been achieved despite numerous attempts.

Although epidermolysis bullosa acquisita is not a genetic disease with a Mendelian inheritance pattern, patients with epidermolysis bullosa acquisita do have a genetic predisposition to autoimmunity. African-American patients in the southeastern United States who have either epidermolysis bullosa acquisita or bullous SLE have a high incidence of the HLA-DR2 phenotype. The calculated relative risk for epidermolysis bullosa acquisita in HLA-DR2 positive individuals is 13.1 in African-Americans.[9]

Clinical Features

Although the clinical spectrum of epidermolysis bullosa acquisita is still being defined, it appears that there are at least four clinical presentations (Box 9-1). All patients with epidermolysis bullosa acquisita have autoimmunity to type VII collagen.[10] The classic presentation is a noninflammatory bullous disease with an acral distribution that heals with scarring and milia formation (Figure 9-2). When mild, this presentation is reminiscent of porphyria cutanea tarda; when severe, it is reminiscent of hereditary, recessive, dystrophic epidermolysis bullosa. Classic epidermolysis bullosa acquisita is a mechanobullous disease marked by skin fragility. These patients have erosions, blisters, and scars over trauma-prone surfaces such as the back of the hands, knuckles, elbows, knees, sacral area, and toes. Intact tense blisters appear within noninflamed skin or areas of scarring. Some blisters may be hemorrhagic or develop scales, crusts, or erosions. A

BOX 9-1. CLINICAL PRESENTATIONS OF EPIDERMOLYSIS BULLOSA ACQUISITA

CLASSIC NONINFLAMMATORY (65%)
Noninflammatory blistering in an acral distribution
Scarring and milia formation
BULLOUS PEMPHIGOID–LIKE (25%)
Widespread inflammatory vesiculobullous eruption involving trunk, skin folds, and extremities
Lesions surrounded by inflamed or even urticarial skin
CICATRICIAL PEMPHIGOID–LIKE (10%)
Erosions and scars on the mucosal surfaces of the mouth, upper esophagus, conjunctiva, anus, or vagina
BRUNSTING-PERRY CICATRICIAL PEMPHIGOID–LIKE (VERY RARE)
Recurrent vesiculobullous eruption localized to the head and neck with residual scarring

scarring alopecia and some degree of nail dystrophy may be seen. The lesions heal with scarring and frequently with the formation of pearllike, milia cysts within the scarred areas (Figure 9-3). Although this presentation may be reminiscent of porphyria cutanea tarda, these patients do not have the other hallmarks of porphyria cutanea tarda such as hypertrichosis, a clear photodistribution, or scleroderma-like changes; urinary porphyrin studies of these patients are normal.

Although not as severe as patients with hereditary forms of recessive dystrophic epidermolysis bullosa, patients with the classic form of the disease may have many of the same sequelae such as scarring, loss of hair on the scalp, loss of nails, fibrosis of the hands and fingers, and esophageal stenosis.

A second clinical presentation is a widespread, inflammatory vesiculobullous eruption involving the

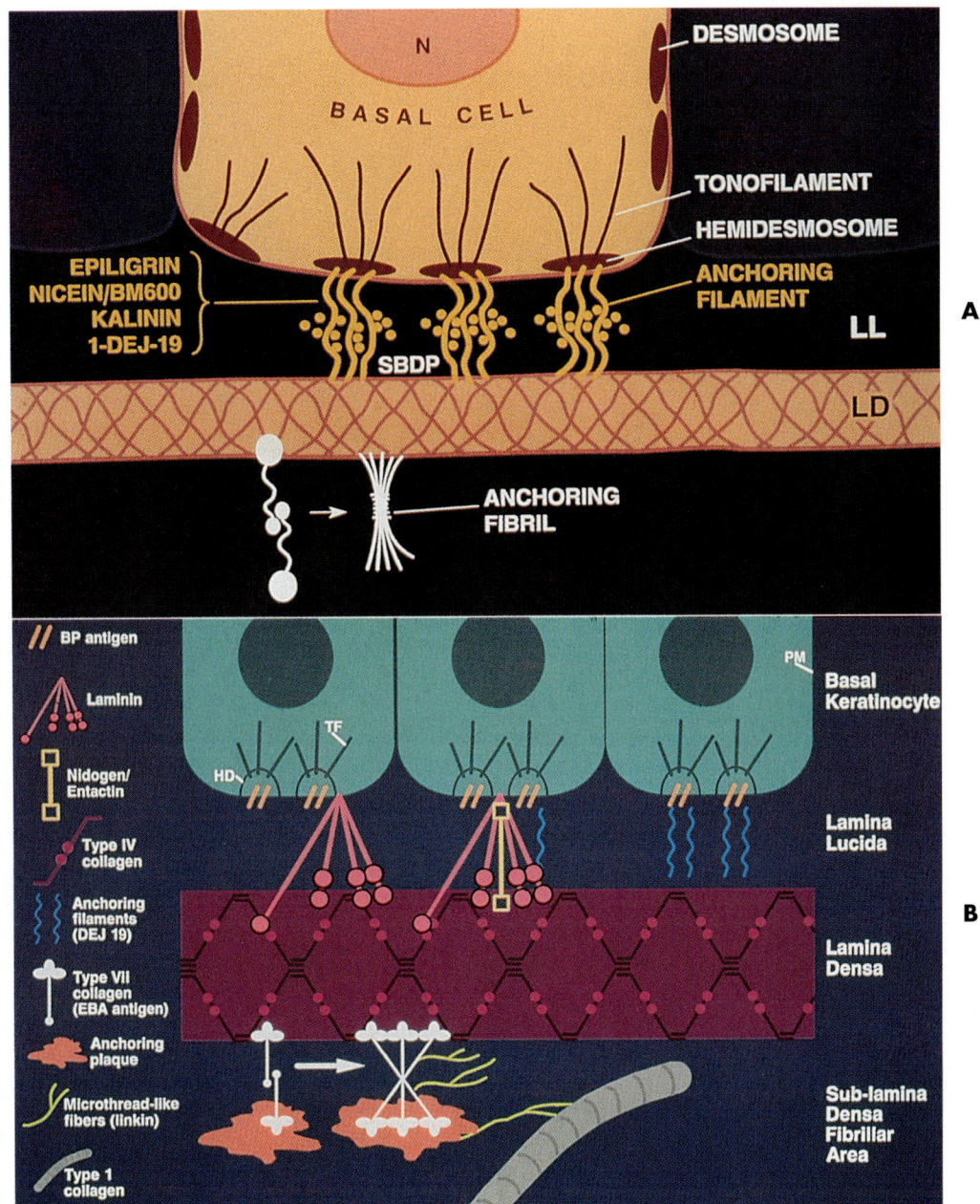

FIGURE 9-1. Schematic diagrams of the BMZ beneath basal keratinocytes. **A,** Simplified schematic that shows anchoring filaments emanating beneath hemidesmosomes and traversing the lamina lucida zone in contrast to anchoring fibrils that emanate vertically from the lamina densa zone. Anchoring filaments contain laminin-5, which has also been called epiligrin, nicein, and BM 600. Anchoring filaments also contain 1 DEJ 19. **B,** More complete schematic demonstrating the major components of the BMZ.

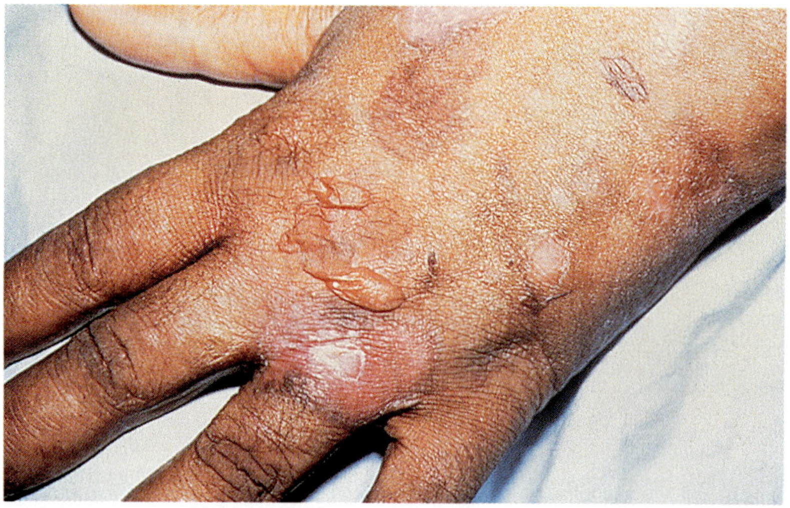

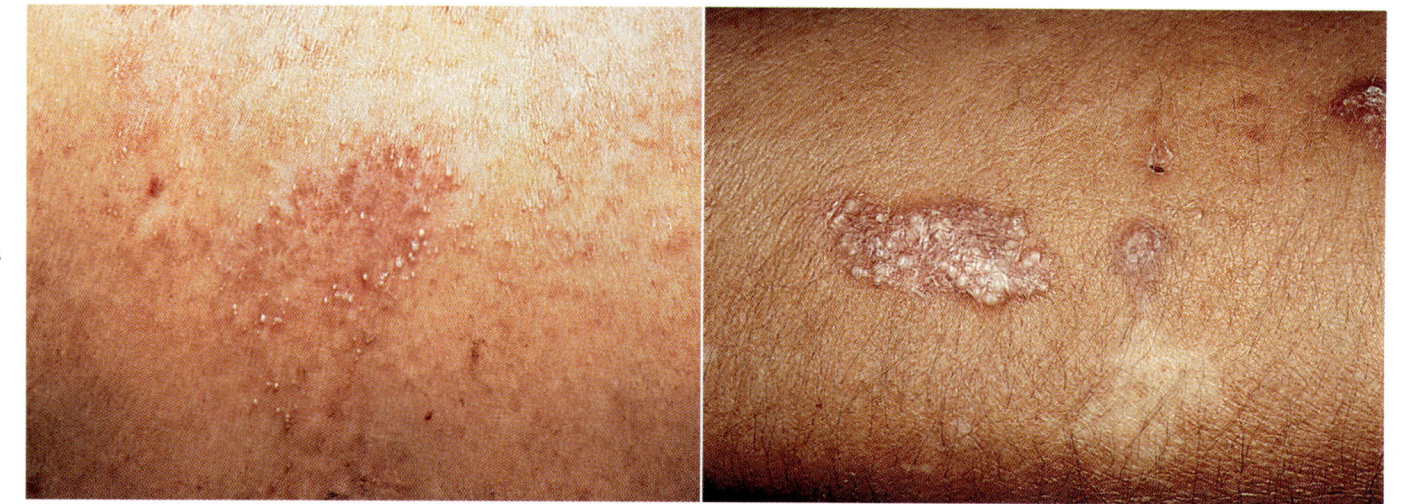

FIGURE 9-2. A patient with epidermolysis bullosa acquisita who has severe blistering, erosions, scarring, and milia formation on her hand.

FIGURE 9-3. **A,** Milia formation around a scar in a patient with epidermolysis bullosa acquisita. **B,** A large cluster of milia in an area of repeated blistering on patient's arm.

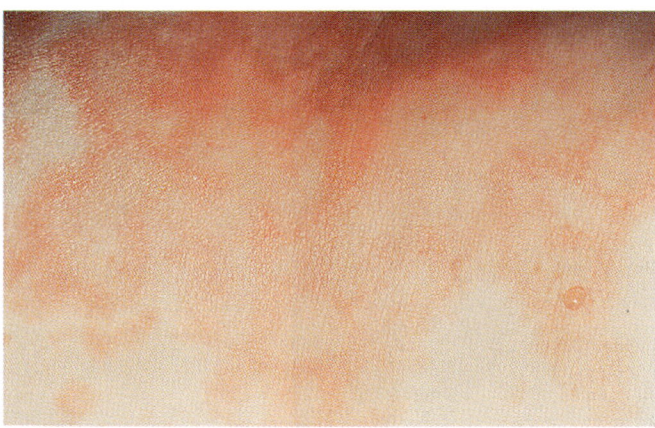

FIGURE 9-4. A patient with epidermolysis bullosa acquisita and autoantibodies to type VII collagen who presented with an inflammatory widespread vesiculobullous disease reminiscent of bullous pemphigoid.

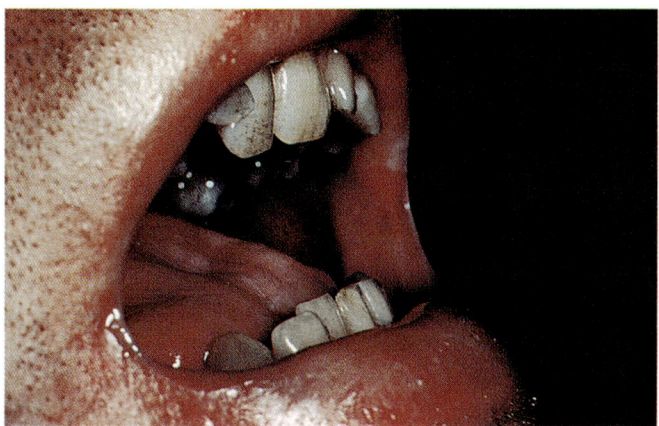

FIGURE 9-5. Mucosal erosions on the tongue and lip of a patient with epidermolysis bullosa acquisita whose clinical presentation resembled cicatricial pemphigoid.

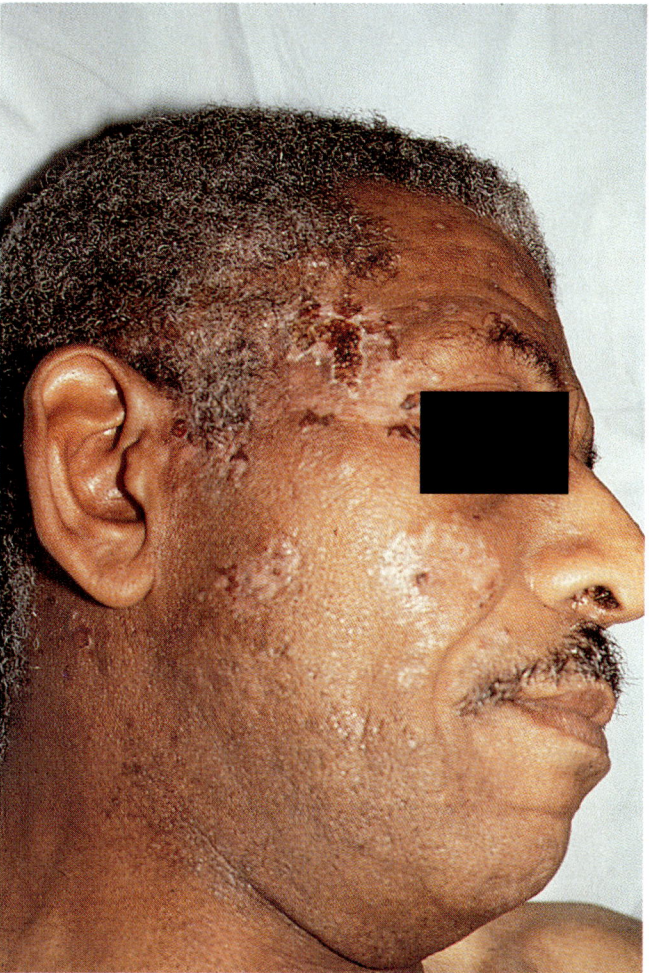

FIGURE 9-6. A patient with the clinical presentation of Brunsting-Perry pemphigoid but with autoantibodies to type VII collagen and the true diagnosis of epidermolysis bullosa acquisita.

trunk, central body, and skin folds in addition to the extremities.[11] The bullous lesions are tense and surrounded by inflamed or even urticarial skin. Large areas of inflamed skin may be seen without blisters at all, and only erythema or urticarial plaques are seen. These patients often complain of pruritus and do not demonstrate prominent skin fragility, scarring, or milia formation. This clinical constellation is more reminiscent of bullous pemphigoid than a mechanobullous disorder (Figure 9-4). Like bullous pemphigoid, the distribution of the lesions may accent the flexural areas and skin folds.

Both the classic and bullous pemphigoid–like forms may have involvement of mucosal surfaces. However, epidermolysis bullosa acquisita also may present with such predominant mucosal involvement that the clinical appearance is reminiscent of cicatricial pemphigoid.[12] These patients usually have erosions and scars on the mucosal surfaces of the mouth, upper esophagus, conjunctiva, anus, or vagina with or without similar lesions on the glabrous skin (Figure 9-5). Epidermolysis bullosa acquisita in childhood is rare. However, mucosal involvement may be severe in children.

Brunsting-Perry cicatricial bullous pemphigoid is a chronic, recurrent vesiculobullous eruption localized to the head and neck. Clinically, this condition is characterized by residual scars, subepidermal bullae, IgG deposits at the DEJ, and minimal or no mucosal involvement. The antigenic target for the IgG autoantibodies in this form of cicatricial pemphigoid, however, have not been defined. Three additional patients with the features of Brunsting-Perry pemphigoid and autoantibodies directed to type VII collagen have been documented (Figure 9-6). Therefore it appears that this clinical phe-

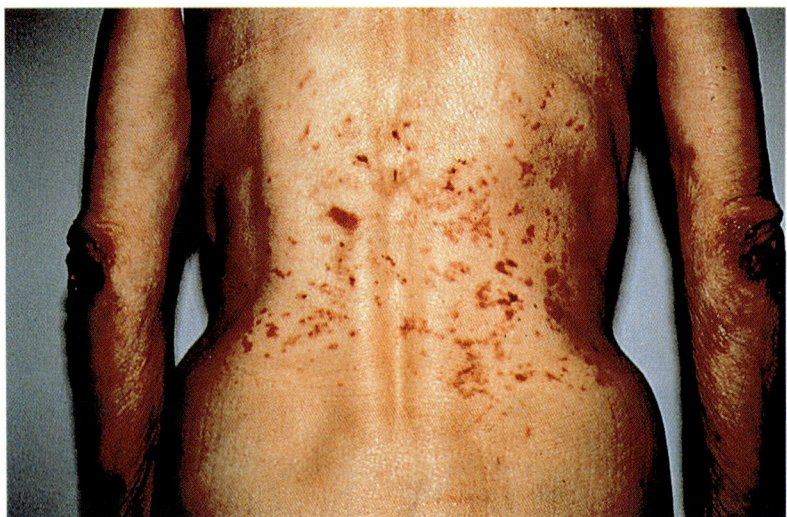

FIGURE 9-7. A patient with epidermolysis bullosa acquisita demonstrating two presentations of the disease. First, the classic mechanobullous presentation with erosions, scarring, and milia over extensor surfaces such as the elbows, knees, and knuckles. Second, the more inflammatory bullous pemphigoid–like lesions on the trunk.

BOX 9-2. SYSTEMIC DISEASES ASSOCIATED WITH EPIDERMOLYSIS BULLOSA ACQUISITA

- Inflammatory bowel disease
- SLE
- Amyloidosis
- Thyroiditis
- Multiple endocrinopathy syndrome
- Rheumatoid arthritis
- Pulmonary fibrosis
- Chronic lymphocytic leukemia
- Thymoma
- Diabetes

notype may be within the spectrum of epidermolysis bullosa acquisita.

About 10% to 15% of patients with epidermolysis bullosa acquisita may have the bullous pemphigoid–like clinical appearance (unpublished observation). The disease of many of these patients eventually smolders into a more noninflammatory mechanobullous form. However, both the classic and bullous pemphigoid–like forms of the disease may coexist in the same patient (Figure 9-7). The clinical phenotype of epidermolysis bullosa acquisita that is reminiscent of pure cicatricial pemphigoid is probably more rare and occurs in less than 10% of all epidermolysis bullosa acquisita cases.

A number of published reports suggest that epidermolysis bullosa acquisita may be associated with various systemic diseases (Box 9-2). However, epidermolysis bullosa acquisita is a relatively rare disease, and most of these reports are anecdotal. It is interesting, however, that a number of the systemic diseases associated with cases of epidermolysis bullosa acquisita are diseases in which an autoimmune pathogenesis has been implicated such as SLE, inflammatory bowel disease, and thyroiditis. The combined experience of the University of North Carolina, Stanford, and Northwestern following over 60 patients points to inflammatory bowel disease as the systemic disease most frequently associated with epidermolysis bullosa acquisita.

Pathology

Histopathology and Routine Electron Microscopy

Routine histologic examination of lesional skin obtained from patients with epidermolysis bullosa acquisita shows a subepidermal blister and a clean separation between the epidermis and dermis. The degree of inflammatory infiltrate within the dermis usually reflects the degree of inflammation of the lesion observed by the clinician. Lesions that are reminiscent of the hereditary, recessive, and dystrophic form of epidermolysis bullosa or porphyria cutanea tarda usually have a notable scarcity of inflammatory cells within the dermis. Lesions that are clinically reminiscent of bullous pemphigoid usually have significantly more inflammatory cells within the dermis, and these cells may be a mixture of lymphocytes, monocytes, neutrophils, and eosinophils (Figure 9-8). The histology of epidermolysis bullosa acquisita skin specimens obtained from bullous pemphigoid–like lesions may be difficult to distinguish from bullous pemphigoid itself.

Ultrastructural studies of epidermolysis bullosa acquisita skin demonstrated a paucity of anchoring fibrils

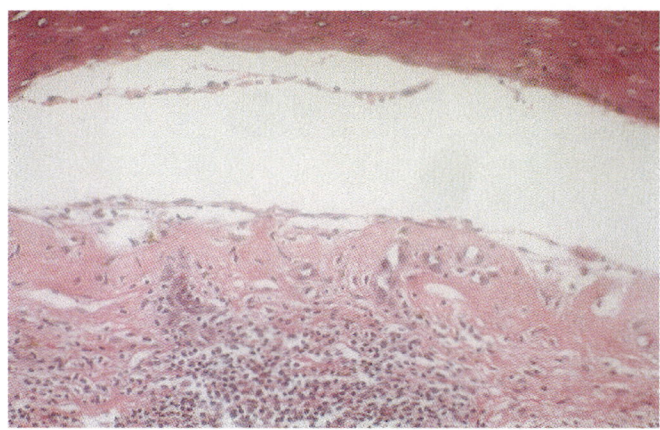

FIGURE 9-8. Routine histologic examination of lesional skin from a patient with epidermolysis bullosa acquisita demonstrating a subepidermal blister and a clean separation between the epidermis and the dermis.

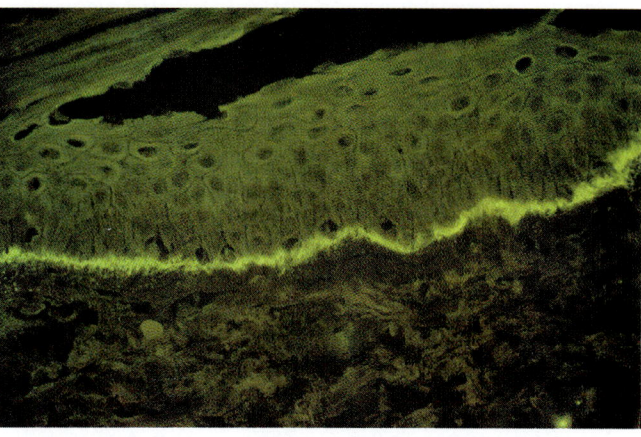

FIGURE 9-9. Direct IF staining for IgG deposits in perilesional skin of a patient with epidermolysis bullosa acquisita. Note the dense deposits within the DEJ.

and an amorphous, electron-dense band just beneath the lamina densa. The cleavage plane of the blister may be within the sublamina densa space of the BMZ. Immunomapping studies, however, have shown that these blisters frequently separate above the immune deposits within the lamina lucida. Therefore the cleavage plane of the blister is *not* a good way to discriminate epidermolysis bullosa acquisita from a number of other subepidermal bullous diseases.

Routine Immunofluorescence

Patients with epidermolysis bullosa acquisita have IgG deposits within the DEJ of their skin.[4] This is best detected by direct IF of a biopsy specimen obtained from a perilesional site (Figure 9-9). IgG is the predominant immunoglobulin class, but deposits of complement, IgA, IgM, factor B, and properdin may also be detected. The direct IF staining demonstrates an intense, linear fluorescent band at the DEJ.

Patients with porphyria cutanea tarda (a syndrome that clinically may mimic epidermolysis bullosa acquisita) frequently have IgG and complement deposits at the DEJ just like patients with epidermolysis bullosa acquisita. However, the direct IF feature that distinguishes porphyria cutanea tarda from epidermolysis bullosa acquisita is that porphyria cutanea tarda skin also demonstrates immune deposits around the dermal blood vessels.

Diagnosis

The diagnostic criteria developed by Yaoita et al[4] for the diagnosis of epidermolysis bullosa acquisita still stand. These criteria with slightly updated modifications are outlined in Box 9-3.

BOX 9-3. DIAGNOSIS OF EPIDERMOLYSIS BULLOSA ACQUISITA

- A bullous disorder within the clinical spectrum outlined
- No family history of a bullous disorder
- Histology showing a subepidermal blister
- Deposition of IgG deposits within the DEJ, i.e., a positive direct IF of perilesional skin
- The IgG deposits are localized to the lower lamina densa or sublamina densa zone of the DEJ when perilesional skin is examined by direct immunoelectron microscopy.
- Alternatives for direct immunoelectron microscopy are indirect or direct salt-split skin IF, Western blotting, and ELISA.

ELISA, Enzyme-linked immunoabsorbent assay.

Indirect Immunofluorescence

Patients with epidermolysis bullosa acquisita may have autoantibodies in their blood directed against the DEJ.[9] These antibodies can be detected by indirect IF of the patient's serum on a substrate of monkey or rabbit esophagus or human skin and will react with the DEJ in a linear fashion that may be indistinguishable from bullous pemphigoid sera. Anti-BMZ antibodies in the sera of patients with epidermolysis bullosa acquisita will label basement membranes beneath stratified squamous epithelium (skin, upper esophagus, and mucosa of the mouth and vagina); they will not bind to basement membranes within most mesenchymal organs such as blood vessels, liver, and kidney. Therefore the labeling pattern and distribution of epidermolysis bullosa acquisita antibodies is identical to bullous pemphigoid antibodies.

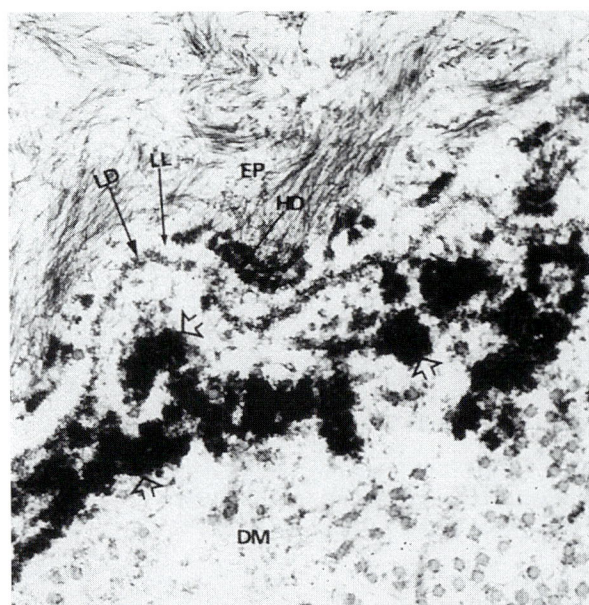

FIGURE 9-10. Immunoelectron microscopy of perilesional skin from a patient with epidermolysis bullosa acquisita. Note the dense IgG deposits *(black arrows)* that lie beneath the lamina densa *(LD)* of the BMZ. In this case the blister formation is occurring within the sublamina densa area.

Immunoelectron Microscopy

The localization of the immune deposits within the DEJ of the skin of patients with epidermolysis bullosa acquisita by immunoelectron microscopy is the "gold standard" for the diagnosis.[4] Patients with epidermolysis bullosa acquisita have immune deposits within the sublamina densa zone of the cutaneous BMZ (Figure 9-10). This localization is clearly distinct from the deposits in bullous pemphigoid, which are higher up in the hemidesmosome area or lamina lucida area of the basement membrane. It is also distinct from cicatricial pemphigoid, which has antigenic targets confined to the lamina lucida.

Indirect Salt-Split Skin Immunofluorescence

When human skin is incubated in 1 M NaCl, the DEJ fractures cleanly through the lamina lucida zone. This fracture places the bullous pemphigoid antigen on the epidermal side of the split, and all other basement membrane components on the dermal side of the separation.[13] Salt-split skin substrate can be used to distinguish epidermolysis bullosa acquisita and bullous pemphigoid sera. If the serum antibody is IgG and labels the epidermal roof, the patient does not have epidermolysis bullosa acquisita, and bullous pemphigoid should be considered.

If the antibody labels the dermal side of the separation, the patient usually has either epidermolysis bullosa

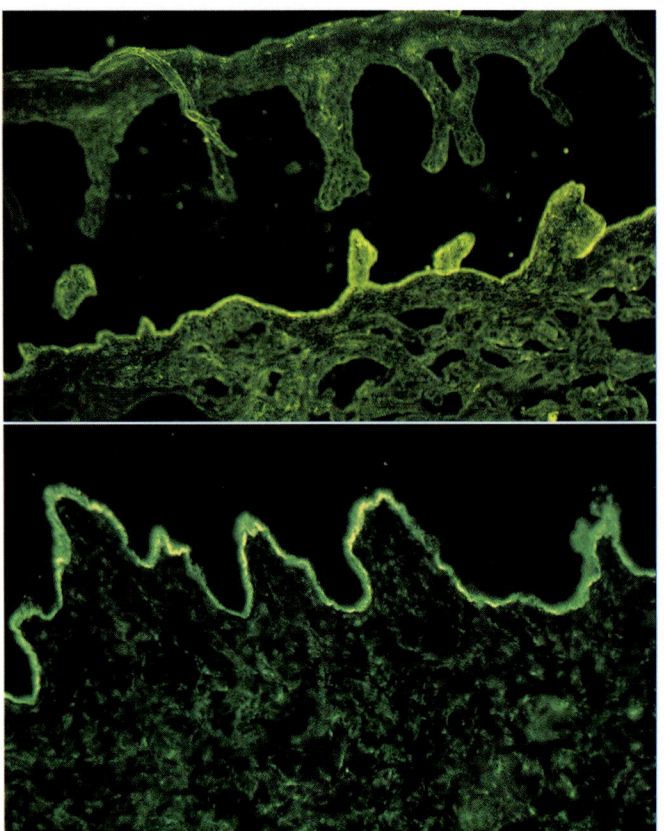

FIGURE 9-11. **A,** Patient with epidermolysis bullosa acquisita had a skin biopsy on normal-appearing skin 1 half-inch away from a blister; the specimen was incubated in cold 1 M NaCl for 92 hours before being processed for routine direct IF. The incubation in salt causes the epidermis to separate from the dermis at the level of the lamina lucida. In epidermolysis bullosa acquisita, the IgG deposits visualized by direct IF remain with the dermal floor side of the separated skin as shown in **A.** In contrast, in bullous pemphigoid, the IgG deposits would remain with the epidermal roof after the separation induced by an incubation in cold salt water. **B,** Normal human skin was separated by incubation in 1M NaCl. Indirect IF was performed on this tissue using a serum from a patient with epidermolysis bullosa acquisita containing autoantibodies to type VII (anchoring fibril) collagen. Note that the serum antibodies strongly label the dermal floor of the separated skin.

acquisita or bullous LE (Figure 9-11). The latter can be ruled out by other serology and clinical criteria.

Until recently, it was thought that only epidermolysis bullosa acquisita and bullous LE gave dermal labeling when salt-split skin IF technology was used. There are two rare blistering diseases that may also cause this pattern of dermal fluorescence on salt-split skin. The first new disease is a subset of patients with cicatricial pemphigoid who have autoantibodies against laminin-5, a noncollagenous component of anchoring filaments within the lamina lucida compartment.[14] The second

> **BOX 9-4. TREATMENT OF EPIDERMOLYSIS BULLOSA ACQUISITA**
>
> **CLASSIC MECHANOBULLOUS FORM**
> Cyclosporine
> Colchicine
> Intravenous gammaglobulin
> Photopheresis
> **INFLAMMATORY BULLOUS PEMPHIGOID–LIKE FORM**
> Systemic corticosteroids
> Azathioprine
> Methotrexate
> Cyclophosphamide
> **INFLAMMATORY FORM WITH PREDOMINANTLY NEUTROPHILIC INFILTRATE**
> Dapsone

new disease is a bullous pemphigoid–like disease in which the patients have autoantibodies to a 105-kD lamina lucida glycoprotein that is unrelated to laminin-5.[15] In both diseases, the immune deposits are within the lower lamina lucida and salt-split skin IF gives a dermal floor pattern of staining identical to epidermolysis bullosa acquisita because laminin-5 and the 105-kD protein go down with the dermis when the skin BMZ is fractured by salt and a variety of other laboratory methods.

Direct Salt-Split Skin Immunofluorescence

Gammon and colleagues[16] showed that direct IF on perilesional skin that has been incubated in 1 M NaCl can be useful for making the diagnosis of epidermolysis bullosa acquisita. In this procedure, a 4-mm biopsy of perilesional skin is placed for 3 to 4 days in cold 1 M NaCl, embedded, sectioned on a cryotome, and then stained by routine direct IF methods with fluorescein-tagged, anti-human IgG. When cut on the cryotome, the salt-incubated skin is fractured through the DEJ, which effectively places the bullous pemphigoid antigen (and any associated immune deposits) on the epidermal roof and the epidermolysis bullosa acquisita antigen (and any associated immune deposits) on the dermal floor of the separation. If the patient has epidermolysis bullosa acquisita, immune deposits are detected on the dermal side of the separation with the fluorescein-conjugated antibody.

Western Immunoblotting

The serum of patients who have anti-BMZ antibodies by indirect IF can be used to make the definitive diagnosis of epidermolysis bullosa acquisita in a Western blotting procedure. Human skin basement membrane proteins containing type VII (anchoring fibril) collagen are separated on a sodium dodecyl sulfate-polyacrylamide slab gel. The proteins are "blotted" onto nitrocellulose paper and incubated with the patient's serum. Antibodies in epidermolysis bullosa acquisita sera will bind to a 290-kD band, whereas sera from all other primary blistering diseases will not. This band is the alpha chain of type VII collagen.[5] Often a second band of 145 kD will be labeled with epidermolysis bullosa acquisita antibodies. The 145-kD band is the aminoterminal globular NC1 domain of the type VII collagen alpha chain, which is rich in carbohydrate and contains the predominant antigenic epitopes for epidermolysis bullosa acquisita autoantibodies, bullous LE autoantibodies, and monoclonal antibodies against type VII collagen.

Enzyme-linked Immunoabsorbent Assay

Recently, Chen et al produced milligram quantities of purified posttranslationally modified NC1 protein in stably transfected human cells; they used this recombinant NC1 to develop an enzyme-linked-immunoabsorbent assay (ELISA) for autoantibody detection in patients with epidermolysis bullosa acquisita and bullous LE.[17] This new ELISA is more sensitive than IF and Western blotting, and yet it is very specific for antibodies to type VII collagen.

Treatment

Epidermolysis bullosa acquisita is a very difficult disease to treat. Box 9-4 outlines some of the therapeutic options. In general, patients with epidermolysis bullosa acquisita are refractory to high doses of systemic corticosteroids, azathioprine, methotrexate, and cyclophosphamide, especially when they have the classic, mechanobullous form of the disease. These agents are somewhat helpful in controlling epidermolysis bullosa acquisita when it appears as an inflammatory bullous pemphigoid–like disease. Some patients with epidermolysis bullosa acquisita improve on dapsone, especially when neutrophils are present in their dermal infiltrate.

Cyclosporine, a very potent immunosuppressive agent chiefly used for organ transplantation, has been shown to be beneficial in patients with epidermolysis bullosa acquisita. High doses of cyclosporine above 6 mg/kg are needed, however, and the long-term toxicity of the drug makes its use warranted only as a last-resort measure.

There are now several independent reports of patients with epidermolysis bullosa acquisita responding to high doses of colchicine.[18] Colchicine is a good first-line drug because its side effects are relatively benign compared with other therapeutic choices. An example of a successful response to colchicine is illustrated in Figures 9-12 and 9-13. Diarrhea is a common side effect of colchicine, however, which makes it difficult for many patients to achieve a high enough dose to con-

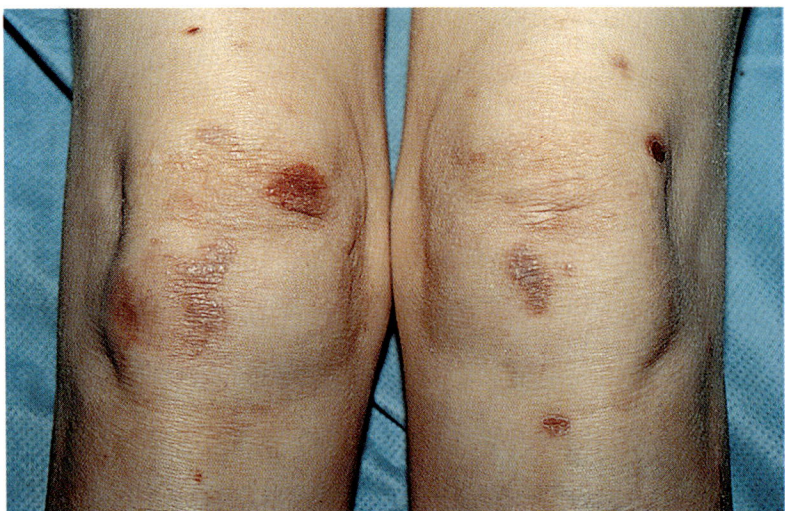

FIGURE 9-12. Painful blisters, erosions, scars, and milia on both knees of a patient with epidermolysis bullosa acquisita before colchicine treatment.

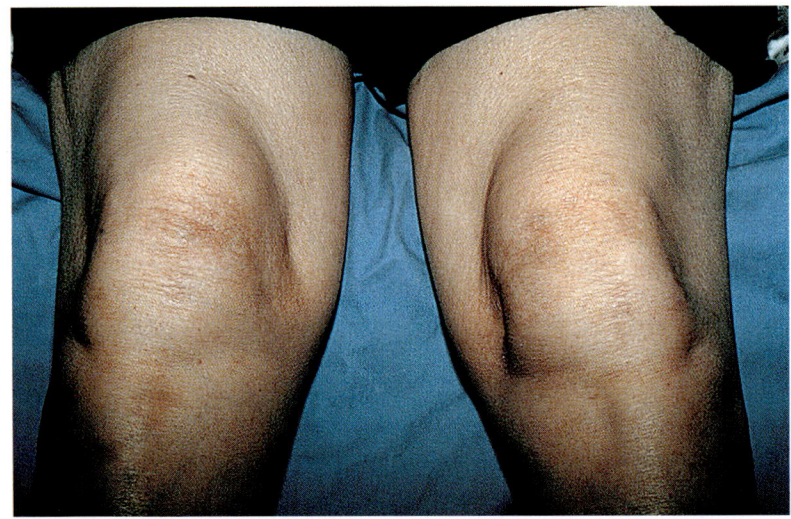

FIGURE 9-13. Knees of the same patient after 4 months of colchicine treatment.

trol the disease. Moreover, because of this side-effect we are hesitant to try colchicine in patients with epidermolysis bullosa acquisita who also have inflammatory bowel disease. In addition, there are patients who do not respond to colchicine. Colchicine is a well-known microtubule inhibitor, but it also may inhibit antigen presentation to T cells, which could downregulate autoimmunity.

Photopheresis has been used in Sezary syndrome, mycosis fungoides, and a variety of autoimmune bullous diseases. Photopheresis had a dramatic effect on one patient with epidermolysis bullosa acquisita in a life-threatening situation. In three other patients with epidermolysis bullosa acquisita, photopheresis improved some clinical parameters and remarkably lengthened the suction blistering times of the patients, suggesting an improvement in their dermal-epidermal adherence (Figures 9-14 to 9-17).[19]

Intravenous immunoglobulin has been used in dermatomyositis, an entity in which autoimmunity may play

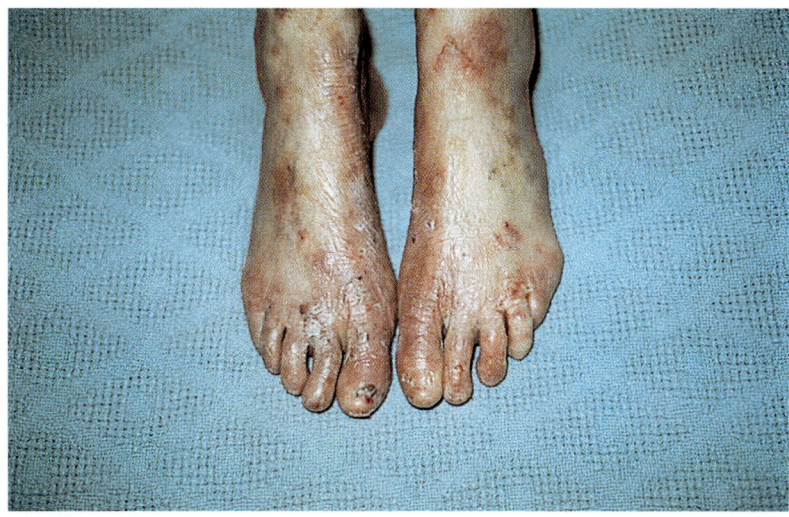

FIGURE 9-14. Feet of a patient with epidermolysis bullosa acquisita before treatment with photopheresis.

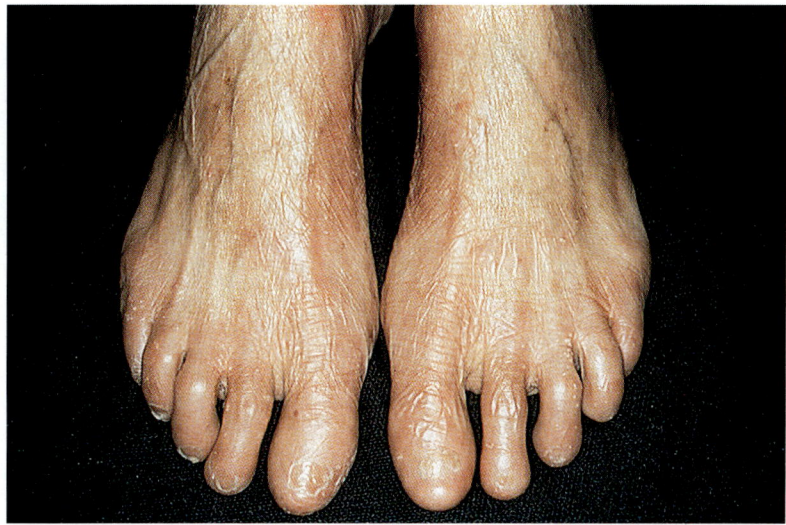

FIGURE 9-15. The feet of the same patient 6 months after final treatment with photopheresis.

a role. Intravenous immunoglobulin has been reported to be effective in some patients with epidermolysis bullosa acquisita and ineffective in at least one patient. The mechanism by which gammaglobulin might invoke a positive response in epidermolysis bullosa acquisita is unknown.

Supportive therapy is warranted in all patients with epidermolysis bullosa acquisita (Box 9-5). This includes instruction in open wound care and strategies for avoiding trauma. Patients should be warned not to overwash, use hot water or harsh soaps too much, and to avoid prolonged or vigorous rubbing of their skin with a washcloth or towel. In some patients, it appears that prolonged sun exposure might aggravate or promote new lesions on the dorsal hands and knuckles. Avoidance of prolonged sun exposure and the use of sunscreens may be helpful. The patient should be educated to recognize localized skin infections and to promptly seek medical care and antibiotic therapy when this occurs.

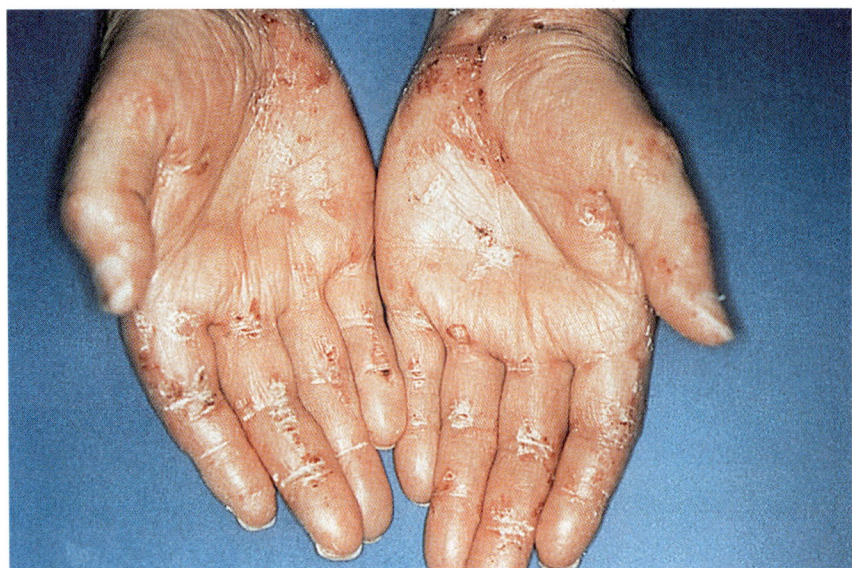

FIGURE 9-16. Hands of a patient with epidermolysis bullosa acquisita before photopheresis.

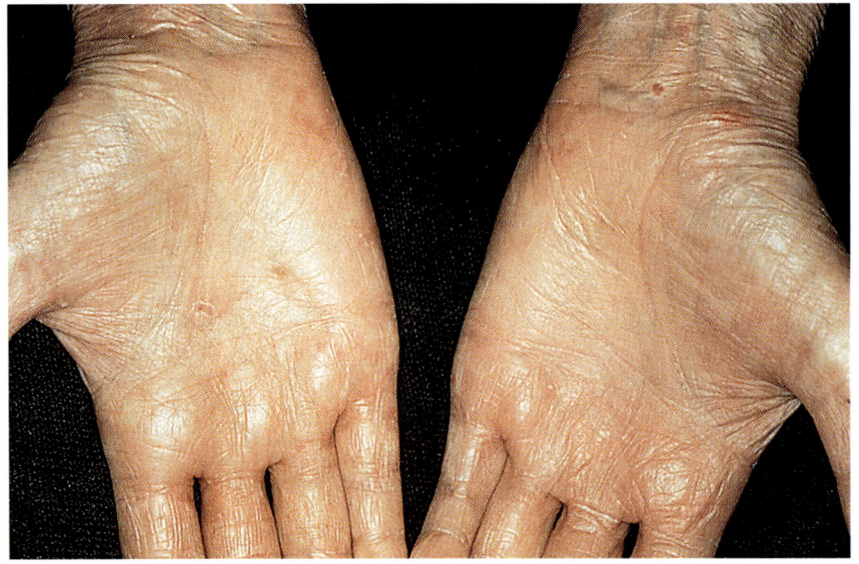

FIGURE 9-17. Hands of the same patient after photopheresis.

BOX 9-5. **SUPPORTIVE THERAPY**

Instruct in open wound care
Avoid trauma
Avoid overly hot water and harsh soaps
Avoid prolonged sun exposure
Use photoprotection
Recognize localized skin infection and seek prompt antibiotic therapy

Differential Diagnosis

Epidermolysis bullosa acquisita must be distinguished from bullous pemphigoid (Figure 9-18), cicatricial pemphigoid (Figure 9-19), and porphyria cutanea tarda (Figure 9-20). The development of specialized investigations, such as the ELISA, to detect autoantibodies to type VII collagen, has simplified the process of arriving at a definitive diagnosis of epidermolysis bullosa acquisita.

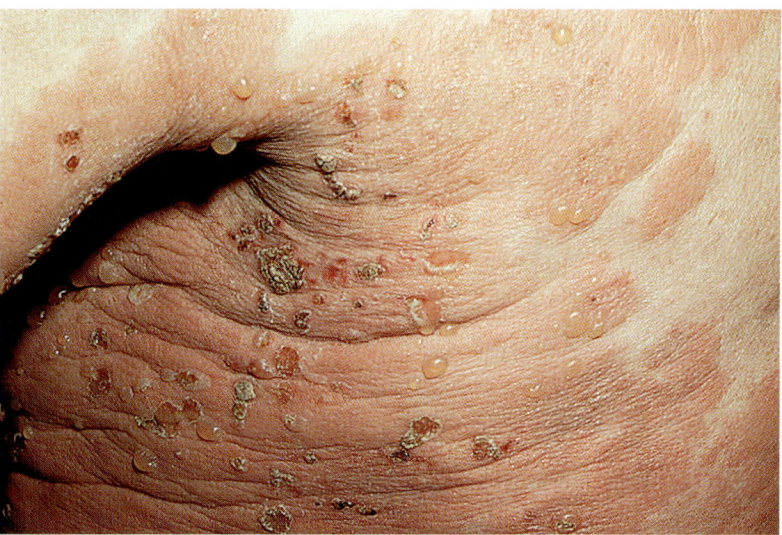

FIGURE 9-18. A patient with a classic case of bullous pemphigoid with the usual widespread, highly inflammatory vesiculobullous eruption and urticarial plaques.

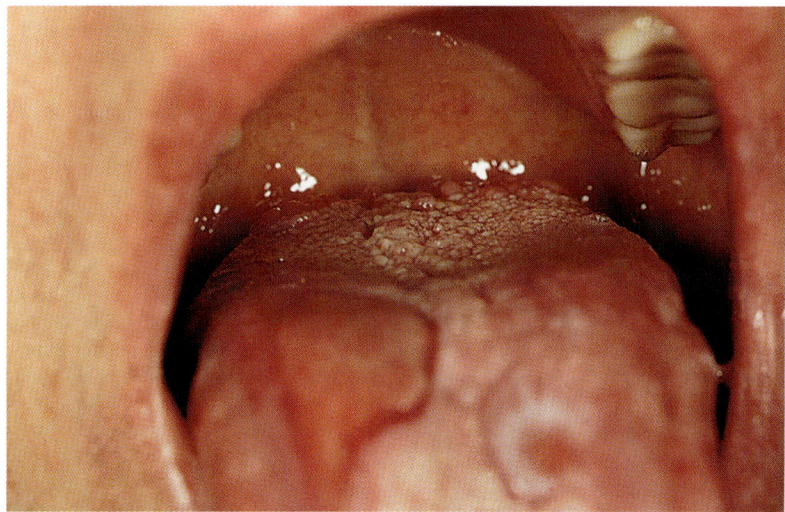

FIGURE 9-19. A patient with cicatricial pemphigoid featuring marked erosions in her oral cavity and conjunctiva.

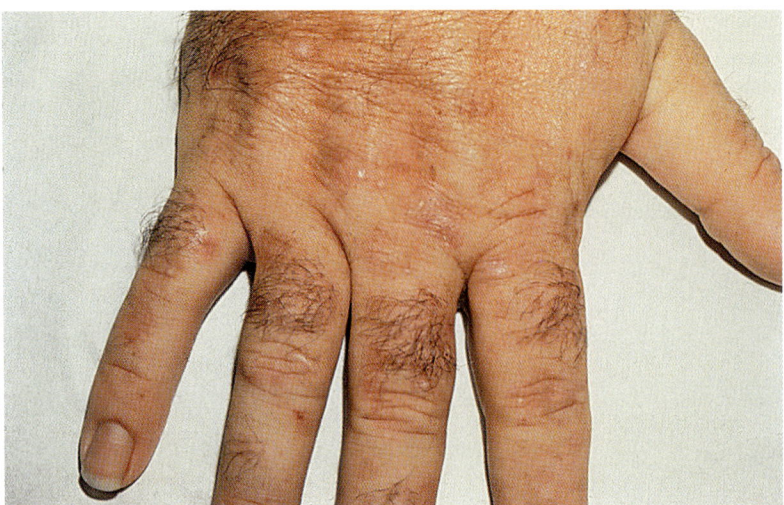

FIGURE 9-20. A patient with porphyria cutanea tarda who presented with chronic blistering, scar formation, and milia on his hands, predominantly over the most trauma-prone areas of his hands.

References

1. Elliott GT: Two cases of epidermolysis bullosa, *J Cutan Genitourin Dis* 13:10, 1895.
2. Roenigk HH Jr, Ryan JG, Bergfeld WF: Epidermolysis bullosa acquisita: Report of three cases and review of all published cases, *Arch Dermatol* 103:1-10, 1971.
3. Kushniruk W: The immunopathology of epidermolysis bullosa acquisita, *Can Med Assoc J* 108:1143-1146, 1973.
4. Yaoita H, Briggaman RA, Lawley TJ, et al: Epidermolysis bullosa acquisita: Ultrastructural and immunological studies, *J Invest Dermatol* 76:288-292, 1981.
5. Woodley DT, Briggaman RA, O'Keefe EJ, et al: Identification of the skin basement membrane autoantigen in epidermolysis bullosa acquisita, *N Engl J Med* 310:1007-1013, 1984.
6. Lapiere J-C, Woodley DT, Parente MG, et al: Epitope mapping of type VII collagen: Identification of discrete peptide sequences recognized by sera from patients with acquired epidermolysis bullosa, *J Clin Invest* 92:1831-1839, 1993.
7. Tanaka H, Ishida-Yamamoto A, Hashimoto T, et al: A novel variant of acquired epidermolysis bullosa with autoantibodies against the central triple-helical domain of type VII collagen, *Lab Invest* 77(6):623-632, 1997.
8. Gammon WR, Woodley DT, Dole KC: Evidence that antibasement membrane zone antibodies in bullous eruption of systemic lupus erythematosus recognize epidermolysis bullosa acquisita autoantigens, *J Invest Dermatol* 84:472-478, 1985.
9. Gammon WR, Heise ER, Burke WA, et al: Increased frequency of HLA DR2 in patients with autoantibodies to EBA antigen: Evidence that the expression of autoimmunity to type VII collagen is HLA class II allele associated, *J Invest Dermatol* 91:228-232, 1988.
10. Woodley DT, Burgeson RE, Lunstrum G, et al: The epidermolysis bullosa acquisita antigen is the globular carboxyl terminus of type VII procollagen, *J Clin Invest* 81:683-687, 1988.
11. Gammon WR, Briggaman RA, Wheeler CE Jr: Epidermolysis bullosa acquisita presenting as an inflammatory disease, *J Am Acad Dermatol* 7:382-387, 1982.
12. Dahl MGC: Epidermolysis bullosa acquisita—a sign of cicatricial pemphigoid? *Br J Dermatol* 101:475, 1979.
13. Woodley D, Sauder D, Talley MJ, et al: Localization of basement membrane components after dermal-epidermal junction separation, *J Invest Dermatol* 81:149, 1983.
14. Domloge-Hultsch N, Gammon WR, Briggaman RA, et al: Epiligrin, the main keratinocyte integrin ligand is target in both an acquired autoimmune and an inherited sub-epidermal blistering disease, *J Clin Invest* 90:1628-1633, 1992.
15. Cotell SL, Lapiere JC, Chen JD, et al: A novel 105 kDa lamina lucida autoantigen associated with bullous pemphigoid, *J Invest Dermatol* 103:78-83, 1994.
16. Gammon WR, Briggaman RA, Inman AO, et al: Differentiating anti-lamina lucida and anti-sublamina densa anti-BMZ antibodies by indirect immunofluorescence on 1.0 M sodium chloride-separated skin, *J Invest Dermatol* 82(2):139-44, 1984.
17. Chen M, Chan LS, Cai X, et al: Development of an ELISA for rapid detection of anti-type VII collagen autoantibodies in epidermolysis bullosa acquisita, *J Invest Dermatol* 108:68-72, 1997.
18. Cunningham BB, Kirchmann TT, Woodley DT: Colchicine for epidermolysis bullosa (EBA), *J Am Acad Dermatol* 34:781-784, 1996.
19. Gordon K, Chan L, Woodley DT: Treatment of refractory epidermolysis bullosa acquisita with extracorporeal photochemotherapy, *Br J Dermatol* 136:415-420, 1997.

Bullous Lupus Erythematosus

Thomas T. Provost

Etiology

Bullous lupus erythematosus (LE) is a heterogeneous disease.[1] Bullous lesions are not a feature of benign cutaneous LE, which is defined as patients with lupus demonstrating discoid lupus lesions in the absence of significant lupus serologies (i.e., antinuclear, anti-dsDNA, anti-Ro [SS-A] antibodies, and so on). Based on immunophenotyping of the inflammatory infiltrate and the occurrence of discoid lesions in the absence of serologic findings, these discoid lupus lesions are thought to result froma T cell autoaggressive mediated-immune response. The exact details of this putative T cell immune response are unknown.

Bullous LE generally occurs in the presence of systemic features, and the following three distinct mechanisms may be responsible.

On unusual occasions, subepidermal bullae may be seen in anti-Ro (SS-A) antibody positive patients with systemic LE (SLE). The bullae emerge from inflammatory skin lesions and are thought to result from a gross extension of the liquefaction degeneration occurring at the dermal-epidermal junction (DEJ) in these lesions.

On unusual occasions, anti-Ro (SS-A) antibody positive patients may develop a toxic epidermal necrolysis (TEN) picture, associated with subepidermal bullae and widespread denuding of the skin (Figures 10-1 and 10-2). Such reactions have been described after excessive ultraviolet (UV) light exposure.[1-3]

These patients are frequently exquisitely photosensitive. In our series, 80% were photosensitive, compared to a 40% sensitivity in anti-U_1RNP positive patients with lupus. Other investigators, evaluating an anti-Ro (SS-A) antibody rheumatologic SLE cohort, have described a 90% frequency of photosensitivity. Furthermore, some of these patients with SLE and positive anti-Ro (SS-A) antibody "burn through window glass," indicating that relatively low energy, long-wave UV light (UVA) is capable of inducing skin disease.

The exact pathogenesis of the bullous lesions in these patients is unknown. However, studies of the neonatal LE syndrome, in which mothers with positive anti-Ro (SS-A) antibody pass this antibody to their fetus, via the placenta, have provided important data. The infant frequently develops cutaneous lesions of neonatal lupus after UV exposure. These data support the hypothesis that the cutaneous lupus lesions in patients with positive anti-Ro (SS-A) antibody are the result of an antibody-dependent cellular cytotoxicity immune mechanism.

A caveat is in order when discussing photosensitivity and anti-Ro (SS-A) antibodies. A direct correlation between anti-Ro (SS-A) antibodies and photosensitivity has not yet been detected. For example, at least 30% of a general cohort of patients with Sjögren's syndrome are anti-Ro (SS-A) antibody positive and are generally not photosensitive unless they develop concomitant features of SLE, which is the Sjögren's syndrome/LE overlap syndrome.[4]

No studies have been done that examine the fine specificity of the anti-Ro (SS-A) antibody response with the presence or absence of photosensitivity nor have any formal studies examined the presence of anti-60 kD Ro (SS-A) versus anti-52 kD Ro (SS-A), or anti-calreticulin antibodies with the presence or absence of photosensitivity. These studies may be fruitful in light of recent data suggesting a pathologic role of some anti-52 kD Ro (SS-A) antibodies in the pathogenesis of isolated congenital heart block in the neonatal lupus syndrome.

The second pathogenesis for bullous LE was described by Hall et al[5] (Figures 10-3 and 10-4). Small blisters were described, predominantly on the sides of the neck, in patients with SLE. The clinical and histologic picture was reminiscent of dermatitis herpetiformis. The subepidermal blisters demonstrated neutrophil microabscesses and nuclear dust at the tips of dermal papillae.

These patients with SLE had significant systemic disease, and their sera generally demonstrated the multiple autoantibodies associated with their disease.

Direct immunofluorescent (IF) examination demonstrated granular deposition of IgG, IgM, IgA, and C3

BULLOUS LUPUS ERYTHROMATOSUS SUMMARY

ETIOLOGY
Antibody-dependent cellular cytotoxicity, immune complexes, and anti-type VII collagen antibodies may be causative in bullous LE.

CLINICAL FEATURES
Subepidermal bullae occur in patients with systemic but not discoid LE.

PATHOLOGY
Subepidermal bullae of three following possible histologic patterns:
1. Extension of severe liquefaction degeneration at the DEJ.
2. Subepidermal bullae associated with microabscess formation at tips of dermal papillae.
3. Subepidermal bullae associated with thick linear immunoglobulin and complement deposition, along skin BMZ.

DIAGNOSIS
Serologic testing for LE, direct IF examination of biopsies.

TREATMENT
Treatment of underlying lupus disease process with steroids or immunosuppressive agents.

DIFFERENTIAL DIAGNOSIS
Dermatitis herpetiformis, linear IgA disease, pemphigus foliaceus, and bullous pemphigoid.

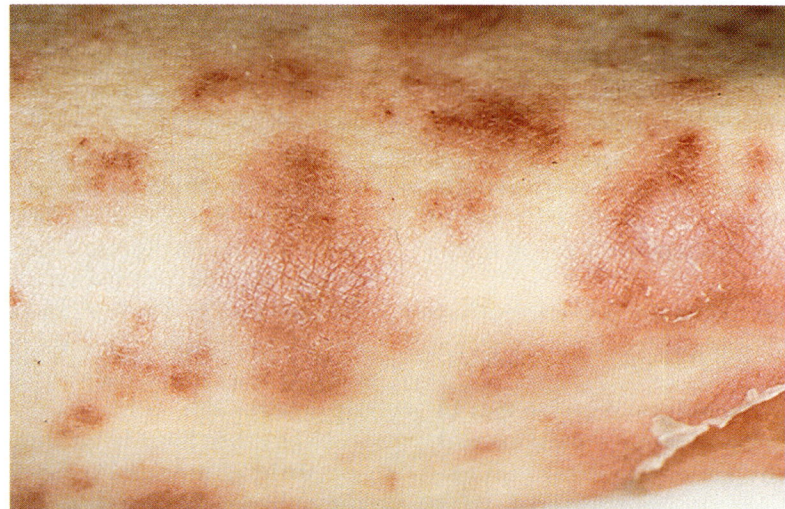

FIGURE 10-1. Widespread bullae (TEN-like picture) in a patient with psorasis with an unrecognized anti-Ro (SS-A) antibody positive treated with UVB therapy.

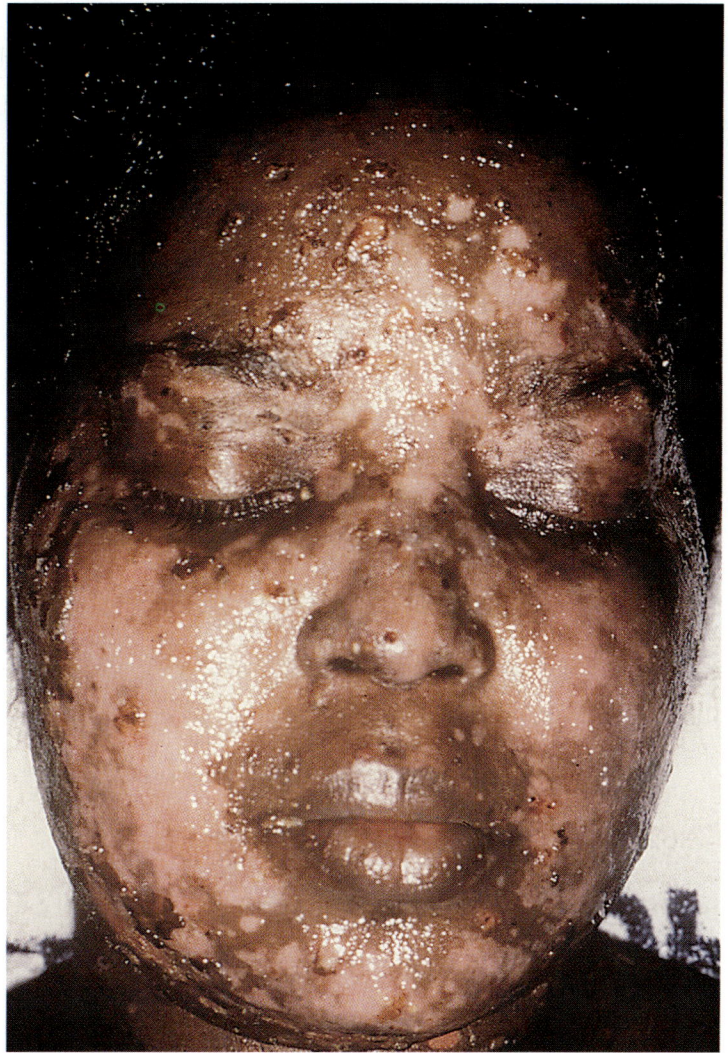

FIGURE 10-2. Widespread denuding of facial skin in an African-American female with bullous LE (Courtesy Robert E. Jordon, MD.)

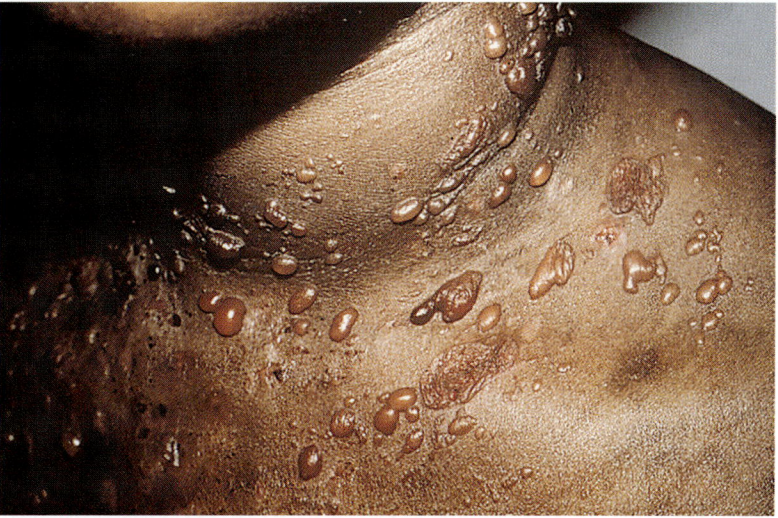

FIGURE 10-3. Bullous LE lesions on the side of neck and upper trunk in an African-American with SLE patient. (Courtesy Raymond Gammon, MD.)

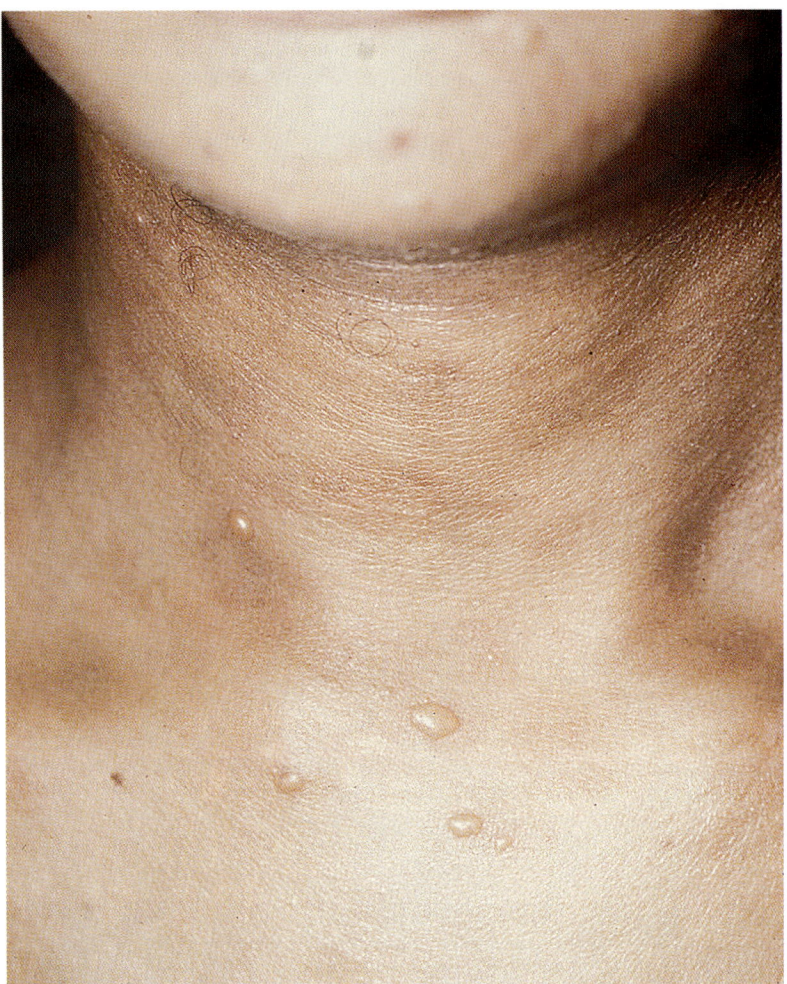

FIGURE 10-4. Bullous LE anterior chest and neck in a patient with SLE. (Courtesy Raymond Gammon, MD.)

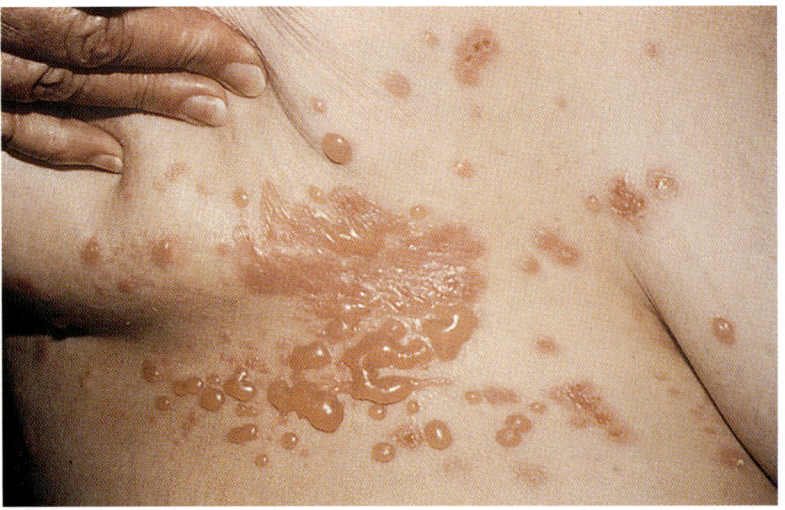

FIGURE 10-5. Bullous LE lesions beneath breast in a patient with SLE. (Courtesy Robert E. Jordon, MD.)

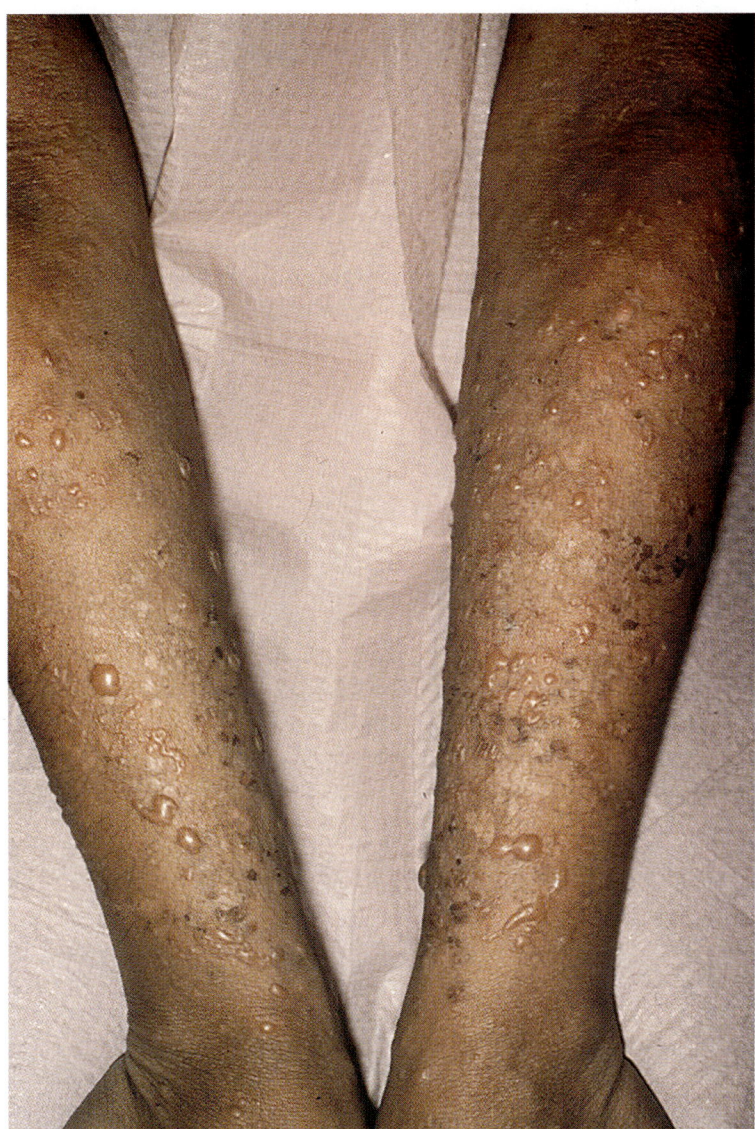

FIGURE 10-6. Bullous LE involving exterior forearms in a patient with SLE.

along the DEJ.[5,6] Granular deposition of C3 may be detected in dermal blood vessels. It is theorized that this form of bullous LE results from a low-grade vasculitis, involving blood vessels high in the dermal papillae. As a result of immune complex–induced inflammation in the affected blood vessels, it is theorized that the integrity of the DEJ is disrupted and blister formation occurs.

The third pathophysiologic mechanism to be detected in the induction of blister formation in SLE is the result of work performed by Gammon and colleagues[7-10] (Figures 10-5 and 10-6). These investigators described a blistering disease involving all areas of the body, with a predilection for the extensor surface of the arms. Oral pharyngeal involvement may occur, and scarring of the lesions has been described on unusual occasions (Figure 10-7).

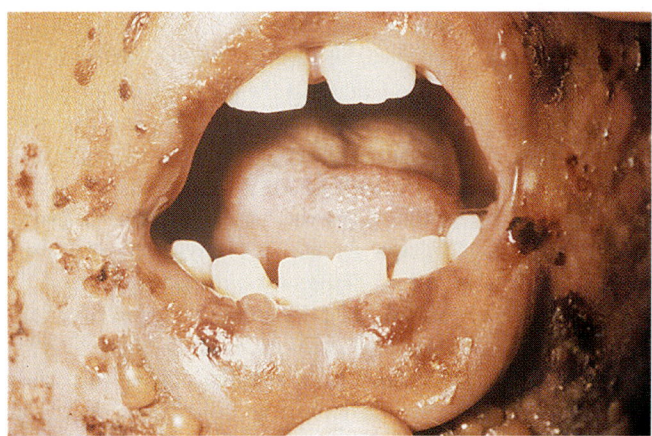

FIGURE 10-7. Mucous membrane bullae in a patient with SLE. (Courtesy Raymond Gammon, MD.)

Direct IF examination of the skin demonstrates a thick, intense, linear deposition of IgG, IgA, and IgM along the basement membrane zone (BMZ).

Immunoreactants on the dermal side of the blister are demonstrated by 1 M NaCl-split skin, indicating the immunoreactants are being deposited below the lamina densa.

Immunoblotting studies indicate that the autoantibodies in this form of bullous SLE react with the 290-kD type VII collagen protein and a 145-kD degradation product. Further studies indicate the epitopes reside in the noncollagenous portion of type VII collagen. These antibodies are capable of activating complement and the inflammation induces a disruption of the type VII collagen (anchoring fibril), producing a subepidermal blister.

Since some of the blisters in patients with SLE with type VII collagen antibodies may occur on noninflamed skin, it is conceivable that noncomplement fixing, anti-type VII collagen antibodies may induce blister formation by binding to type VII collagen (anchoring fibril) and induce an allosteric change, which destroys the integrity of the anchoring fibril, resulting in blister formation.

Immunogenetic studies demonstrate an increased frequency of the HLA-DR2 and DQ1 phenotypes in these patients.[11] Furthermore, some studies suggest an increased frequency of glomerulonephritis and anti-dsDNA antibodies in patients with SLE patients with these HLA phenotypes. Thus it is not surprising that patients with bullous LE, demonstrating anti-type VII collagen antibodies, frequently have been detected to have anti-dsDNA antibodies and glomerulonephritis.

Clinical Features

Bullous lesions in LE are rare. For example, in a series of 143 untreated patients with SLE, only one patient with epidermolysis bullosa acquisita-like lesions and anti-type VII collagen antibodies was detected.

During the same period, two patients with asymptomatic unrecognized positive anti-Ro (SS-A) antibody developed TEN lesions after UVB therapy for psoriasis.

By comparison, 16 of these untreated patients with SLE demonstrated urticaria-like vasculitic lesions. Thus, by these standards, bullous LE lesions are rare.

It should be noted, however, that a number of well-defined primary blistering diseases have been reported in association with LE. These include pemphigus foliaceus, bullous pemphigoid, dermatitis herpetiformis, linear IgA disease, and porphyria cutanea tarda.[12]

The bullae associated with anti-Ro (SS-A) antibody positive SLE are generally detected in association with photosensitivity. Small blisters may arise in the periphery of existing lesions of subacute cutaneous LE, or have an explosive onset after intense UV exposure and present with a TEN-like picture. Blistering, in association with photosensitivity, is the hallmark of this subset of bullous LE.

The vesicular bullous lesions associated with putative immune complex–mediated vasculitis occur as small blisters predominantly but not solely localized to the sides of the neck and axillary regions. These blisters generally occur in patients who are systemically ill. Generally, a direct relationship with UV exposure is not detected.

The blisters in patients with SLE, associated with anti-type VII collagen antibodies, are generally larger than those seen with the immune complex–mediated vasculitis. They generally occur on erythematous skin but occasionally may be detected on normal-appearing skin. These blisters may infrequently occur in the oral pharynx. They generally heal without scarring, but exceptions do exist.

Pathology

Routine hematoxylin and eosin (H&E) biopsies demonstrate subepidermal cleft formation (Figures 10-8 and 10-9). At times, microabscess formation, composed of neutrophils at the tip of papillae, may be seen (Figure 10-10).

Direct IF examination of perilesional skin of immune complex–mediated blisters may demonstrate granular deposition of immunoreactants along the DEJ. Immunoglobulin and complement deposition may be detected in the affected dermal blood vessels.

Direct IF studies of large bullous LE lesions often are associated with anti-type VII collagen antibodies. Direct IF studies of perilesional skin will demonstrate a thick, linear band of immunoglobulin deposition along the DEJ. Studies using 1 M NaCl-split skin will demonstrate that this linear deposition occurs on the dermal side of the cleft formation (Figure 10-11).

Less frequently, serum from this form of bullous LE may demonstrate IgG deposition along the DEJ by direct IF.

The research technique, immunoblotting, will demonstrate binding of IgG antibodies to the 290-kD type VII collagen protein.

As noted, blister formation almost never occurs in patients with chronic cutaneous LE (discoid LE). Serologic testing of patients with bullous LE will frequently reveal valuable information.

The bullous lesions associated with UV light exposure (sunburn, UVB or PUVA therapy) are most likely seen in patients who have positive anti-Ro (SS-A) antibody. The bullous lesions of the putative immune complex and the anti-type VII collagen antibody are frequently seen in patients with SLE with anti-dsDNA, anti-U_1RNP, and anti-Sm antibodies.

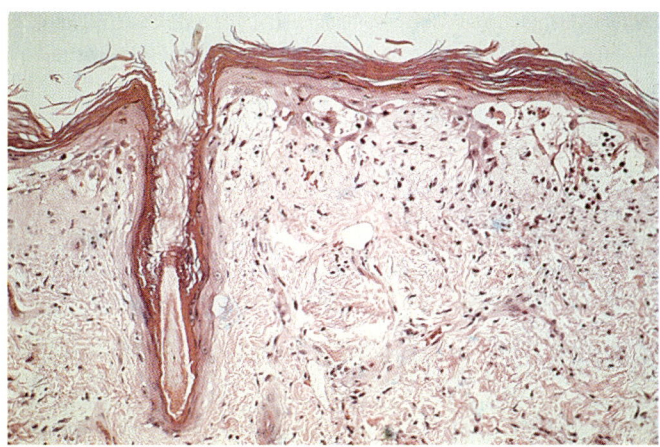

FIGURE 10-8. Biopsy of an-anti Ro (SS-A) antibody positive patient with SLE demonstrating prominent liquifaction degeneration at the DEJ.

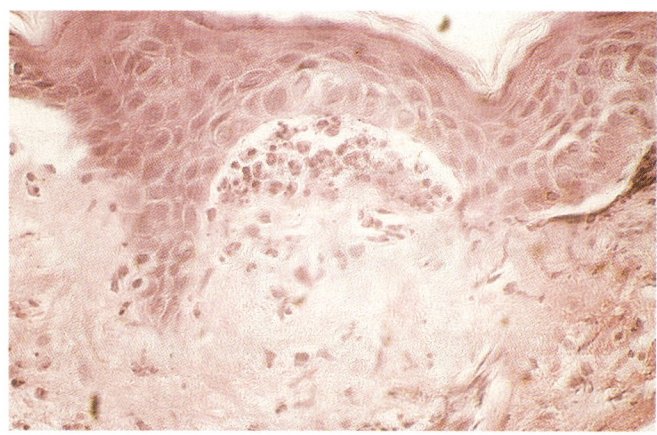

FIGURE 10-10. Biopsy of patient with bullous LE demonstrating collection of polymorphonuclear leukocytes at the tip of dermal papillae and subepidermal cleft formation. (Courtesy Raymond Gammon, MD.)

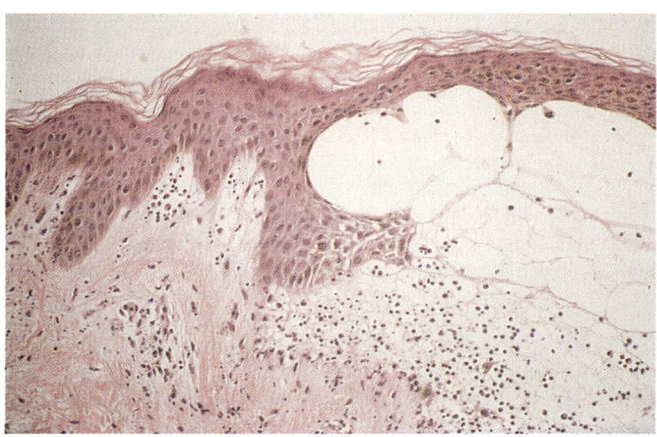

FIGURE 10-9. Biopsy of patient with bullous LE demonstrating a subepidermal bulla. (Courtesy Robert E. Jordon, MD.)

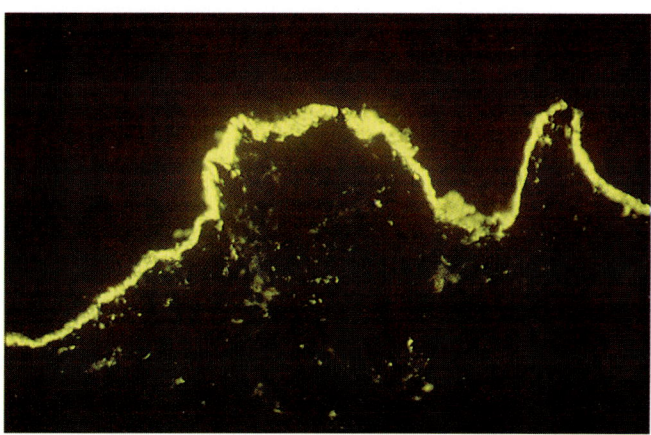

FIGURE 10-11. Direct IF examination of lesion of bullous LE demonstrating thick linear deposition of IgG on dermal side of subepidermal blister. (Courtesy Robert E. Jordon, MD.)

Diagnosis

The diagnosis of bullous LE is based on clinical observation and a history and physical examination evaluating SLE features.

Routine biopsy for H&E staining, with IF studies, especially direct IF examination, are valuable diagnostic tools.

Serologic testing for SLE antibodies (i.e., antinuclear, Sm, U_1RNP, Ro [SS-A] antibodies) using gel double diffusion and ELISA technologies is helpful.

Treatment

In general, the treatment of bullous LE is directed at the systemic features. In the case of the bullous lesions occurring in patients with SLE who are photosensitive and are anti-Ro (SS-A) antibody positive, hospitalization with intense nursing care may be needed to treat the TEN-like disease.

Efforts must be directed to educate and protect the patient from sun exposure. Sunscreens containing titanium dioxide and Parsol 1789 (avobenzone) are recommended. Sun-protective clothing (Solumbra Ultra Sun Protective Clothing and Koala and Frogwear Sun Protective Clothing) is especially effective. Avoidance of intense sun exposure between the hours of 10 AM and 4 PM is also highly recommended.

The putative immune complex and anti-type VII collagen antibody associated bullous LE generally have prominent systemic features, including glomerulonephritis. Oral steroids and immunosuppressive therapy (azathioprine, cyclophosphamide, cyclosporine, mycophenolic acid) are given as needed to control the systemic features. Generally, if the systemic features are controlled, the blistering disease disappears. However, despite therapy to suppress the systemic features, some patients with bullous LE with anti-type VII collagen antibodies may have persistent blister formation.

Differential Diagnosis

As noted, bullous LE is a heterogeneous disease, with respect to pathogenesis. Physician knowledge of the systemic features of SLE is essential. The physician must also be aware that bullous LE is a rare disease, and on rare occasions, patients with SLE may develop bullous lesions of dermatitis herpetiformis, porphyria cutanea tarda, bullous pemphigoid, linear IgA disease, and pemphigus foliaceus.

These diseases can generally be distinguished by direct IF studies of perilesional skin biopsies. Dermatitis herpetiformis demonstrates granular IgA DEJ deposition; linear IgA disease shows linear IgA deposition along the DEJ, and pemphigus foliaceus shows intercellular deposition of IgG.

The direct IF examination of perilesional skin in porphyria cutanea tarda demonstrates characteristic globular dermal deposition of immunoreactants. A 24-hour urine porphyrin quantitation confirms this diagnosis.

Bullous pemphigoid, when occurring with SLE, may be difficult to distinguish from the bullous LE lesions associated with type VII collagen antibodies. Studies of 1 M NaCl-split skin generally demonstrate deposition of the immunoreactants on the epidermal side of the cleft formation. Immunoblot studies will demonstrate reactivity against the 230-kD and 180-kD bullous pemphigoid antigens.

REFERENCES

1. Sontheimer RD, Provost TTP: Lupus erythematosus. In Sontheimer RD, Provost TT, eds: Cutaneous manifestations of rheumatic diseases, Baltimore, 1996, Williams & Wilkins.
2. Kulick KB, Mogavero H, Provost TT, et al: Serologic studies in patients with lupus erythematosus and psoriasis, *J Am Acad Dermatol* 8:631, 1983.
3. Bielsa I, Herrero C, Font J, et al: Lupus erythematosus and toxic epidermal necrolysis, *J Am Acad Dermatol* 16:1265, 1987.
4. Provost TT, Watson R, Simmons-O'Brien E: Anti Ro (SS-A) antibody positive Sjögren's/lupus erythematosus overlap syndrome, *Lupus* 6:105, 1997.
5. Hall PP, Lawley TJ, Smith HR, et al: Bullous eruption of systemic lupus erythematosus, *Ann Int Med* 97:165, 1982.
6. Camisa C, Sharma HM: Vesicobullous systemic lupus erythematosus, *J Am Acad Dermatol* 9:924, 1983.
7. Gammon WR, Woodley DT, Dole KC, et al: Evidence that anti basement membrane zone antibodies in bullous eruption of systemic lupus erythematosus recognize epidermolysis bullosa acquisita autoantigen, *J Invest Dermatol* 84:472, 1985.
8. Gammon WR et al: Evidence supporting a role of immune complex-mediated inflammation in the pathogenesis of bullous lesions of systemic lupus erythematosus, *J Invest Dermatol* 81:320, 1983.
9. Bok E, Roberts LJ, Lieu TS, et al: Epidermolysis bullosa acquisita preceding the development of systemic lupus erythematosus, *J Am Acad Dermatol* 22:587, 1990.
10. O'Lansky AJ, Briggaman RA, Gammon WR: Bullous systemic lupus erythematosus, *J Am Acad Dermatol* 5:511, 1982.
11. Arnett FC: The genetics of human lupus. In Wallace DJ, Hahn BH, eds: Dubois' Lupus Erythematosus, ed 5, Baltimore, 1997, Williams & Wilkins.
12. Yell JA, Wojnarowska F: Bullous skin disease in lupus erythematosus, *Lupus* 6:112, 1997.

Nonimmunologic Acantholytic Diseases

Philip R. Cohen

Hailey-Hailey Disease

Etiology

In the April 1939 *Archives of Dermatology*, Howard and Hugh Hailey described two brothers with a recurrent vesicular eruption that was primarily localized to their intertriginous regions. Five dermatopathologists and a group of dermatologists examined the skin biopsies with various conclusions: three dermatopathologists made a diagnosis of pemphigus, two dermatopathologists thought the sections "looked like" pemphigus, and the dermatologists thought the sections represented Darier's disease. In the same paper, Hailey and Hailey also reported another set of brothers who also presented with an identical clinical picture and whose skin biopsy had been interpreted as Darier's disease. Hailey and Hailey considered all four patients to have a heretofore undescribed familial dermatologic entity, *familial benign chronic pemphigus* or Hailey-Hailey disease.

The pathogenesis of Hailey-Hailey disease has been attributed to a generalized defect in keratinocyte adhesion. The molecular defect for this condition has been localized to a gene mutation on chromosome 3q21-q24.

Several studies suggest that the development of acantholysis in Hailey-Hailey disease is due to disruption of the desmosomes.[1-4] Specifically, immunofluorescence (IF) studies of lesional skin of Hailey-Hailey disease demonstrated abnormalities in the staining patterns for both desmosomal attachment plaque proteins (desmoplakin and plakoglobin) and the desmosome intercellular cement glycoprotein, desmoglein. These proteins diffuse into the cytoplasm of the acantholytic cells. Nondesmosomal attachment proteins (vinculin in the adherent junction and 43-kD connexon in the gap junction) remained intact in Hailey-Hailey disease. The staining pattern for the universal cell surface (transmembrane) glycoprotein (CD44) was partially altered[3,4]; in contrast, in pemphigus vulgaris these proteins are totally or partially (CD44) absent from the cell membrane and cytoplasm of the acantholytic cells, and desmosomal attachment plaque proteins remain present.[1]

Precipitating factors for the development of lesions of Hailey-Hailey disease include hormonal changes (menstruation and pregnancy), minor physical trauma, skin infections (bacterial, candidal, fungal, and viral), increased perspiration (sweating), and ultraviolet (UV) radiation.[4,5]

Clinical Features

Hailey-Hailey disease has an autosomal dominant pattern of inheritance. A positive family history is present in approximately two-thirds of patients. The onset age is typically between 20 to 40 years.

The lesions appear as small, flaccid vesicles that are often on an erythematous base. There is a predilection for lesions to occur on flexures (Figure 11-1) and intertriginous regions such as the side of the neck (Figure 11-2), the axillae (Figure 11-3), beneath the breasts (Figure 11-4), the groin (Figure 11-5), and the perineum. Scalp and mucosal involvement are uncommon. The palms and soles, as well as the dorsal hands and feet, are typically spared as well. Occasionally, longitudinal white bands are present on the nail plates.[4,5]

Pathology

Microscopic examination of Hailey-Hailey disease classically shows well-developed intraepidermal blisters with suprabasilar clefts. There is partial acantholysis of several layers of the epidermis, imparting a "dilapidated brick wall" appearance. The cytoplasm of the acantholytic cells is fairly normal; partial keratinization (dyskeratosis) may be present in an occasional cell (Figure 11-6). Hyperkeratosis overlying the epidermis and eosinophils in the dermis are typically absent.

Direct and indirect IF studies using IgG, IgA, IgM, complement, and fibrin are negative.

Diagnosis

The diagnosis of Hailey-Hailey disease is based on a positive history of other family members with a similar dermatosis, the clinical morphology of the lesions, and their distribution. A Nikolsky's (bullae spread) sign is usually negative. A Tzanck smear preparation should be

NONIMMUNOLOGIC ACANTHOLYTIC DISEASES SUMMARY

ETIOLOGY

Dissolution of the desmosomal attachment is the primary event in acantholysis in Hailey-Hailey disease, Darier's disease, and Grover's disease. Precipitating factors for the development of Hailey-Hailey disease include hormonal changes, minor trauma, skin infections, increased perspiration, and UV radiation. Heat, sweating, sunlight, hormonal changes, lithium carbonate, general anesthesia, and stress can provoke or exacerbate Darier's disease. Grover's disease has been associated with UV radiation, fever and excessive sweating; in oncology patients, occlusive immobility, hospitalization, antineoplastic therapy, radiotherapy, and the diagnosis or recurrence of malignancy may also be related to the development of Grover's disease.

CLINICAL FEATURES

Hailey-Hailey disease appears as small, flaccid, erythematous-based vesicles that have a predilection for occurring on flexures and intertriginous regions; also, longitudinal white bands may be present on the nail plates. Pruritus and malodor are frequent symptoms of Darier's disease; disease-related lesions are typically found in the seborrheic areas (warty, brown papules and plaques), the flexural areas, the hands (nail dystrophies, palmar pits and keratotic papules, acrokeratosis, and hemorrhagic macules), and oral mucosa (white or fleshy cobblestone papules). Grover's disease is characterized by small, pruritic papules and papulovesicles, with or without underlying erythema, on the chest and back.

PATHOLOGY

Acantholysis is a common pathologic feature in all of these diseases. In Hailey-Hailey disease, the acantholysis involves several layers of the epithelium, giving the epidermis a "dilapidated brick wall" appearance; in addition, intraepidermal blisters with suprabasilar clefts are usually present. In Darier's disease, there is dyskeratosis of the acantholytic keratinocytes (corps ronds and corps grains) and cleft formation in which basal cell–lined villi (created by the dermal papilla) project into the suprabasilar lacuna; in addition, hyperkeratosis, papillomatosis, and acanthosis are frequently present. Grover's disease is characterized by acantholysis; in addition, there are at least four distinct histologic patterns that may be present either alone or in combination in a single lesion: (1) the Hailey-Hailey–like pattern, (2) the Darier-like pattern, (3) the pemphigus vulgaris-like pattern, and (4) the spongiotic-acantholytic pattern.

DIAGNOSIS

The diagnosis of Hailey-Hailey disease, Darier's disease, and Grover's disease is based on the symptoms and appearance of the lesions. A positive family history and dermatosis-associated nail changes may be present in individuals with the former two diseases. Correlation of the pathologic findings with the clinical history and lesion morphology may be necessary to establish the diagnosis.

DIFFERENTIAL DIAGNOSIS

The clinical features or the pathologic changes or both of lesion from a patient with Hailey-Hailey disease, Darier's disease, or Grover's disease can mimic those of the other two dermatoses.

TREATMENT

In addition to conservative management and anecdotal therapies, all three dermatoses have been successfully managed with oral retinoids. Surgical treatments have also been efficacious in some individuals with Hailey-Hailey disease and Darier's disease.

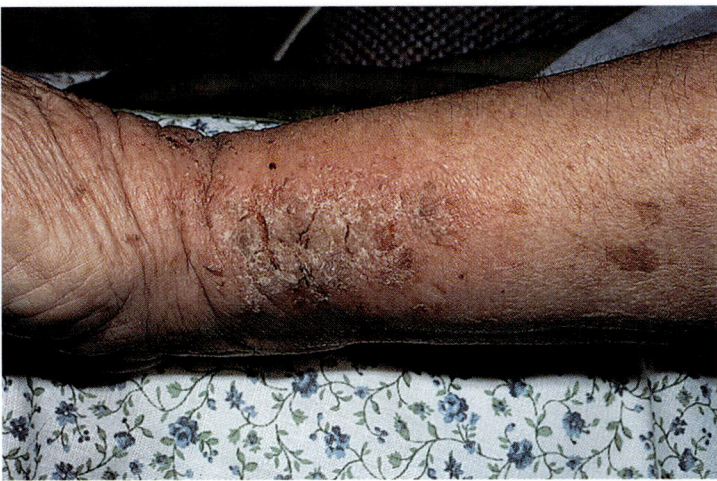

FIGURE 11-1. Weeping, yellow-crusted, erythematous plaques of Hailey-Hailey disease on the right wrist of a 64-year-old woman with a 40-year history of recurrent, weeping pruritic skin lesions with intermittent complete remissions. Her sister and several of her father's relatives had a similar dermatosis.

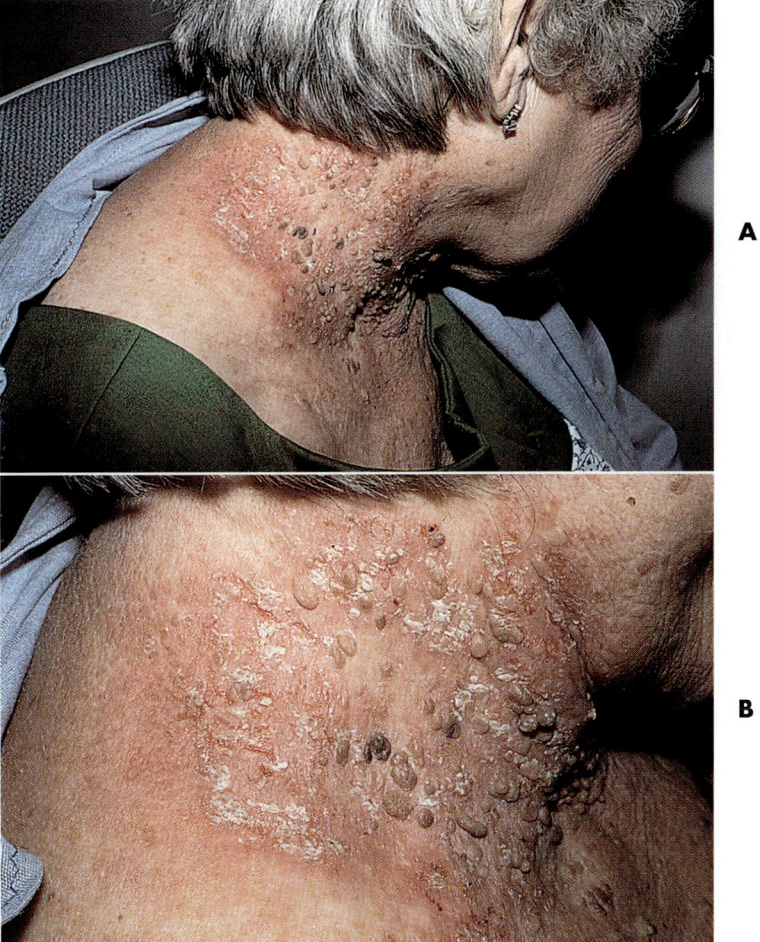

FIGURE 11-2. Distant (**A**) and closer (**B**) views of Hailey-Hailey disease lesions on the right neck of patient in Figure 11-1.

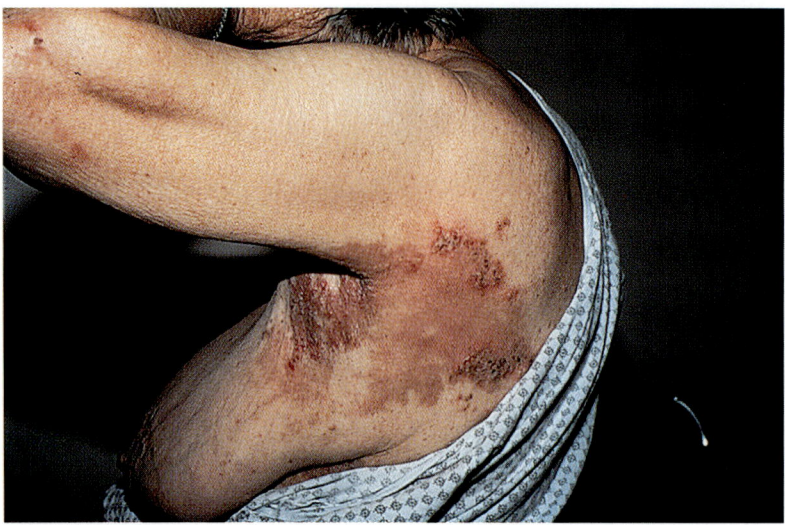

FIGURE 11-3. Intertriginous Hailey-Hailey disease lesions on left axilla of patient in Figure 11-1, with extension to the anterior chest and upper back.

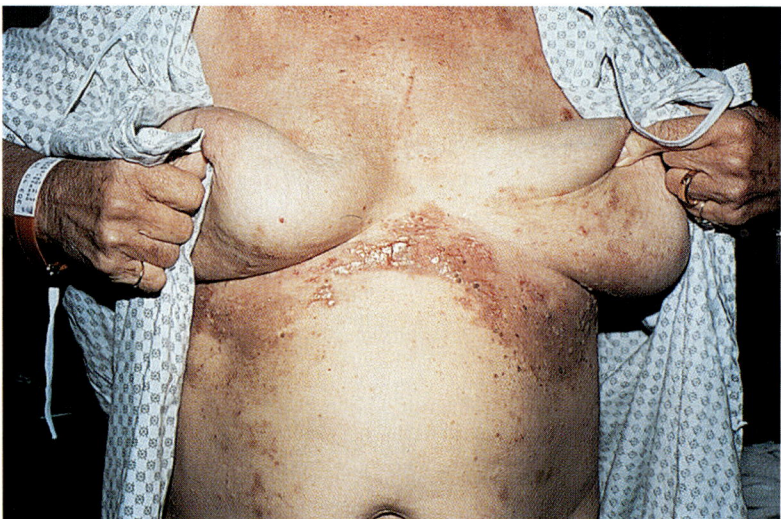

FIGURE 11-4. Inframammary Hailey-Hailey disease lesions beneath the breasts of patient in Figure 11-1.

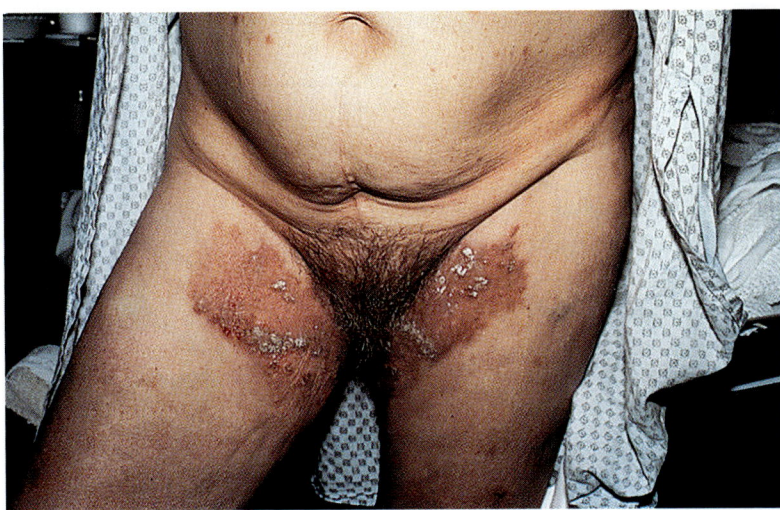

FIGURE 11-5. Bilateral lesions of Hailey-Hailey disease in the groin of patient in Figure 11-1.

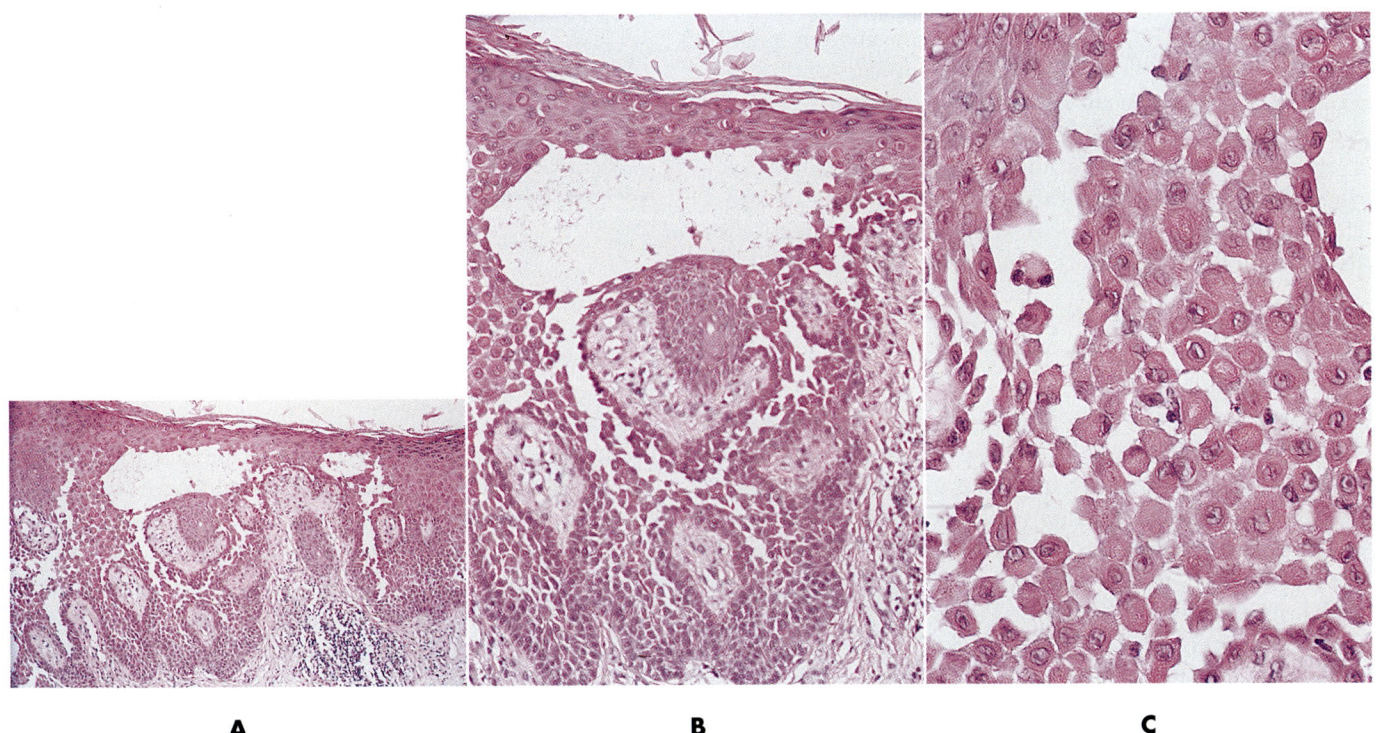

FIGURE 11-6. Low (**A**), medium (**B**), and high (**C**) magnification views of a Hailey-Hailey disease lesion show suprabasilar separation with vesicle formation. There are acantholytic keratinocytes throughout all layers of the epithelium; some have a few intact intercellular bridges, giving the epidermis an appearance of a "dilapidated brick wall." Rare dyskeratotic cells are present. (H&E stain, **A,** ×25; **B,** ×50; **C,** ×100.)

negative—except in individuals whose lesions are secondarily infected with herpes virus. Biopsy of lesional skin for routine microscopic evaluation and for direct IF studies are helpful to confirm the diagnosis and exclude other autoimmune bullous conditions.

Differential Diagnosis

The clinical differential diagnosis of Hailey-Hailey disease includes bullous pemphigoid, Darier's disease, pemphigus vulgaris, and pemphigus vegetans. In contrast to Darier's disease, patients with Hailey-Hailey disease (1) generally have a later onset of their condition, (2) have lesions that are induced by minor trauma, (3) do not have palmar pits or keratotic papules, and (4) do not have both red and white longitudinal nail plate bands and other nail plate dystrophies. The pathologic differential diagnosis includes Darier's disease, Grover's disease, and pemphigus vulgaris.[4,5]

Treatment

Several treatment modalities have been described in patients with Hailey-Hailey disease. Conservative management is often initially attempted with topical (and occasionally oral) corticosteroids. Topical antifungals or antibiotics, oral antibiotics, or both are also commonly used. When there is secondary herpes virus infection, systemic antiviral therapy (acyclovir, valacyclovir, or famciclovir) is initiated. Surgical treatments and anecdotal therapies that have been reported are listed in Box 11-1.

BOX 11-1. TREATMENT MODALITIES FOR HAILEY-HAILEY DISEASE

CONSERVATIVE MANAGEMENT
Corticosteroids: topical (or occasionally oral)
Antibiotics: topical or oral
Antifungals: topical
Antivirals: systemic (if secondary herpes virus infection is present)
SURGICAL TREATMENTS
Carbon dioxide laser abrasion
Cryosurgery with liquid nitrogen
Dermabrasion
Electrosurgery: electrodessication
Excision and split-thickness skin grafts
Oophorectomy
ANECDOTAL THERAPIES
Arsenic
Cyclosporine
Dapsone
Etretinate
Gonadotrophin-releasing hormone analogue (long-acting): Goserelin (Zoladex)
Grenz ray
Methotrexate
PUVA
Thalidomide
Vitamins A, C, E, and K

Darier's Disease

Etiology

In March 1889, Jean Darier—Chef du Laboratoire de la Faculte a l'Hôpitale Saint-Louis—presented a patient at the Societe de Biologie that he hypothesized had a dermatosis caused by a parasite (oval sporospermia or coccidia) that invaded the follicular orifices; he named the condition *psorospermose folliculaire vegetante*. In May 1889, Thibault authored a "These de Paris" on this condition, and in July 1889 Darier published two case reports.[6]

In 1886, Prince Marrow—Clinical Professor of Veneral Disease, University of New York—reported a patient with keratosis follicularis. In June 1889, James C. White, Professor of Dermatology at Harvard University, published a report of a man with an unusual skin disease that had some of the pathologic features of those reported by Marrow; they used the term *keratosis (ichthyosis) follicularis*. Subsequently, later in 1889, White had the opportunity to see Darier's patient at the International Congress of Dermatology in Paris; he realized that his patient and Darier's patient had the same disease. The following year, White saw another patient with the same condition—the daughter of the patient he had reported—and suggested that the condition might be inherited.[6]

The pattern of inheritance of Darier's disease (also referred to as Darier-White disease and keratosis follicularis) is autosomal dominant. The condition is not common. The prevalence ranges from one in 36,000 in northeast England to one in 100,000 in Scandinavia. Recently, molecular genetic studies demonstrated that the gene for Darier's disease maps to chromosome 12q23-q24.1.[6-8]

The pathogenesis of Darier's disease remains to be definitively established. Single studies have demonstrated slightly reduced epidermal zinc concentrations (yet normal serum levels) in patients with Darier's disease and reduced plasma and erythrocyte membrane levels of essential fatty acids (the delta-6-desaturated metabolites of both linoleic acid and alpha-linoleic acid). The relevance and clinical significance of these observations are unclear.

Darier's disease has been described as a disorder of keratinization in which "premature keratinized" cells account for the microscopic features of dyskeratosis and hyperkeratosis of the keratotic papules. Abnormal expression of keratin proteins have been demonstrated by the presence of the following in lesional skin of patients with Darier's disease:

1. The presence of many low molecular weight keratin polypeptide fragments
2. The presence of hyperproliferative keratins
3. The presence of basal cell keratins in some of the acantholytic suprabasal cells

These findings may be secondary to the following:
1. Protein breakdown in degenerating acantholytic cells
2. A nonspecific wound healing response
3. An apparent delay in the expression of suprabasal keratins occurring as a consequence of cell separation

Therefore although changes in keratin expression may reflect the role of an altered structural keratin protein in the etiology of Darier's disease, these changes may merely represent coincidental findings in the lesions of Darier's disease.[6]

Proteases may also have a role in the acantholysis that occurs in Darier's disease. Specifically, plasminogen activation may either be the primary event involved in the etiology of the breakdown of the intercellular adhesions or a secondary event that enhances acantholysis after cell separation has been initiated by other factors. Based on in vitro studies that showed cell dissociation and loss of desmosomes from normal epidermal cells that were cultured in the presence of epidermal cells from Darier's disease, it has been postulated that lesional cells are possibly secreting a protease (an epidermal cell dissociating factor). In addition, immunohistochemical studies have shown that in both skin lesions and cultured keratinocytes from patients with Darier's disease, plasminogen is not only detected in the basal cell layer (as noted in normal skin) but also in the suprabasal acantholytic cells.

More recently, monoclonal antibody studies demonstrated that dissolution of the desmosomal attachment plaque is the primary event in acantholysis of Darier's disease. Several of the keratinocyte junctional proteins are altered in lesions of Darier's disease; there is a loss of the desmosomal attachment proteins (desmoplakin and plakoglobin), desmosomal intercellular cement glycoprotein (desmoglein), and the 43-kD gap-junction protein (connexon). Specifically, the normal peripheral dotted linear pattern of immunostaining on the cell membrane was completely absent and there was diffuse staining in the cytoplasm, demonstrating that the proteins had dissolved from the attachment plaque between the cells and had diffused into the cytoplasm of the acantholytic cells. However, there was preservation of the adherent junction protein, vinculin, and the universal cell surface transmembrane glycoprotein, CD44.[1,2]

Heat and sweating exacerbate or provoke outbreaks of the disease. Sunlight has also been associated with flares of the condition, e.g., erythema that is preceded by an immediate sensation of pruritus, papules that develop 24 to 28 hours after exposure, or papules that appear 1 to 2 weeks after a prior sunburn. Some women have noted perimenstrual or menstrual exacerbation of their disease and varying degrees of improvement with oral contraceptive therapy. In contrast, ingestion of lithium carbonate has been observed to flare the condition. Rare patients have noted severe outbreaks after receiving general anesthesia for surgical procedures. Stress was considered to worsen the condition in more than two-fifths of the patients.[6,7]

Clinical Features

The onset age of Darier's disease may range from the first to the seventh decade of life. Most cases begin between the ages of six and 20 years with a peak incidence around puberty (between 11 to 15 years of age). Although approximately a third of patients notice improvement of their condition as they become older, the disease persists in several individuals. Itching is almost universally present; wool—particularly mohair—caused intolerable pruritus in many patients. Nearly half of affected individuals have significant body malodor. Pain is not a frequent complaint and only present in approximately one-fifth of patients.

Mucocutaneous sites of involvement include (1) the seborrheic areas (specifically, the center of the chest [Figure 11-7], the back, the hair margin—particularly the forehead—the supraclavicular fossae and neck [Figure 11-8], the scalp, and the ears; (2) the flexural areas (axillae, groin, and inframammary in women); (3) the hands (nail dystrophy, palmar pits, acrokeratosis, and hemorrhagic macule); and (4) oral mucosa (fine white papules on either the hard palate or alveolar ridge, fleshy cobblestone papules on the buccal mucosa or tongue, and rarely, fissuring of the tongue). Lesions on the seborrheic and flexural areas typically appear as warty brown papules and plaques. Bullous lesions, painful cutaneous horn, and leukodermic macules (in African-American patients), and linear lesions are less common manifestations.[6,7]

Palmar lesions include either keratotic papules, palmar pits, or both; similar lesions may be noted on the soles. Bilateral acrokeratosis verruciformis lesions have been noted in nearly half of the patients. Less commonly, irregular red or black macules on the palms and soles are present. Darier's disease–associated nail findings include fragile nails, longitudinal bands (red, white, or both) that extend from the proximal nailfold to the free edge of the nail, nails with longitudinal ridging, nails with longitudinal splits (that are also painful), V-shaped notches at the free edge of the nail, and wedge-shaped subungual hyperkeratoses (Figure 11-9). Some or all of the individual's nails may be affected. Finger nails are more commonly and more severely involved than toe nails.[6,7]

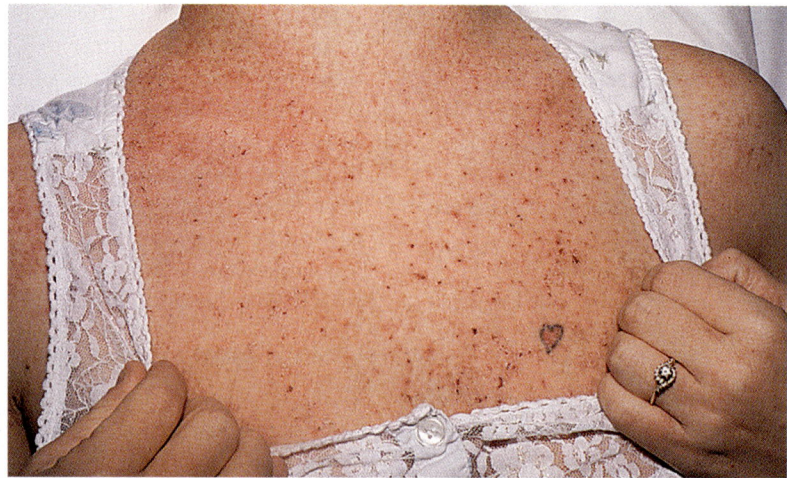

FIGURE 11-7. Erythematous keratotic papules of Darier's disease on the chest of a 28-year-old woman. Her disease initially appeared at 13 years of age and became worse with each of her four pregnancies.

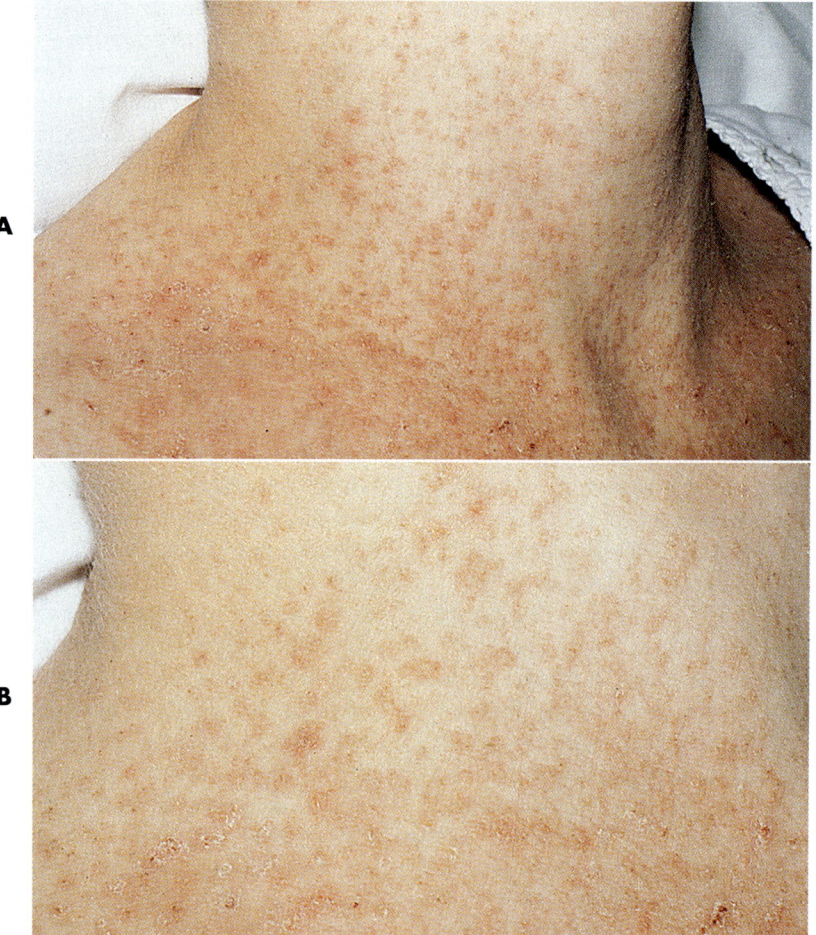

FIGURE 11-8. Distant (A) and closer (B) views of Darier's disease lesions on the right neck of patient in Figure 11-7.

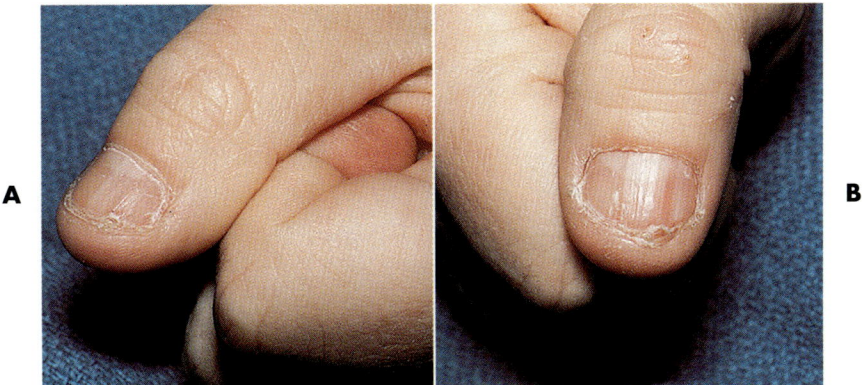

FIGURE 11-9. In same patient in Figure 11-7, Darier's disease–associated longitudinal red bands on the right thumb (A) and longitudinal white band on the left thumb (B) extend from the proximal nailfold, cross the lunula, and reach the free edge of the nail. The V-shaped notch at the distal nail plates is also a dermatosis-related nail dystrophy. *(From Cohen PR: J Am Acad Dermatol 34:943-953, 1996.)*

Patients with Darier's disease may be more susceptible to having superimposed bacterial (most commonly *Staphylococcus aureus*), fungal (refractory *Trichophyton rubrum* or *T. tonsurans*), or viral (herpes simplex) infections. Salivary gland swelling and intermittent parotid gland swelling are uncommon complications that have been observed in patients with Darier's disease. In a series of 163 patients with Darier's disease, a history of epilepsy was present in seven individuals—a prevalence that was six times greater than that of the general population. Depression (secondary to the physical disfigurement and social isolation that are risk factors for suicide and suicide attempts) has also been noted in Darier's patients. Other medical problems, probably occurring only by chance, in patients with Darier's disease include autoimmune thyroiditis, renal and testicular agenesis, and retinitis pigmentosa.[6,7]

Pathology

Microscopic examination of Darier's disease shows hyperkeratosis and often parakeratosis. There is papillomatosis and acanthosis. Acantholytic dyskeratotic keratinocytes are present; they present as corps ronds in the granular and horny layers of the epidermis and corps grains in the stratum corneum and the lacunae. Secondary to the acantholysis, there is cleft or lacunae formation in the suprabasilar layers of the epidermis. Villi are created by the dermal papillae that are lined by basal cells and stick up into the lacunae (Figure 11-10). Hence the term *keratosis (ichthyosis) follicularis* is a misnomer, since (1) the principal pathologic change is dyskeratosis of acantholytic keratinocytes and (2) the hyperkeratosis and dyskeratosis is not primarily follicular and only affects hair follicles as an incidental finding.

Direct IF studies of lesional or perilesional skin and indirect IF studies of serum from patients with Darier's disease are negative for deposits of immunoglobulins or complement within or beneath the epidermis.

Diagnosis

When characteristic papules and plaques are present in a seborrheic distribution, the possibility of Darier's disease is more readily entertained; a biopsy of a representative lesion is helpful to confirm the diagnosis. The presence of typical Darier's disease-associated nail changes (longitudinal red and white bands, nail fragility or longitudinal fissuring, V-shaped notching of the distal nail plate, or wedge-shaped subungual hyperkeratosis) is also helpful in establishing the diagnosis. A history of family members with a similar dermatosis is useful; however, not all patients have a positive family history for the condition.

Differential Diagnosis

The clinical differential diagnosis of Darier's disease includes Hailey-Hailey disease. In patients with Darier's disease with severe flexural involvement and the morphologic appearance, as well as the microscopic features of the lesions, may mimic Hailey-Hailey disease; however, the appearance of keratotic papules on the trunk supports the diagnosis of Darier's disease. The presence of only white longitudinal bands can also be observed in patients with Hailey-Hailey disease; however, patients with Hailey-Hailey disease do not have the other nail dystrophies that are associated with Darier's disease. Because of the distribution and waxy appearance of the lesions, Darier's disease may be confused with seborrheic dermatitis. Epidermal nevi (hamartomas) may mimic the

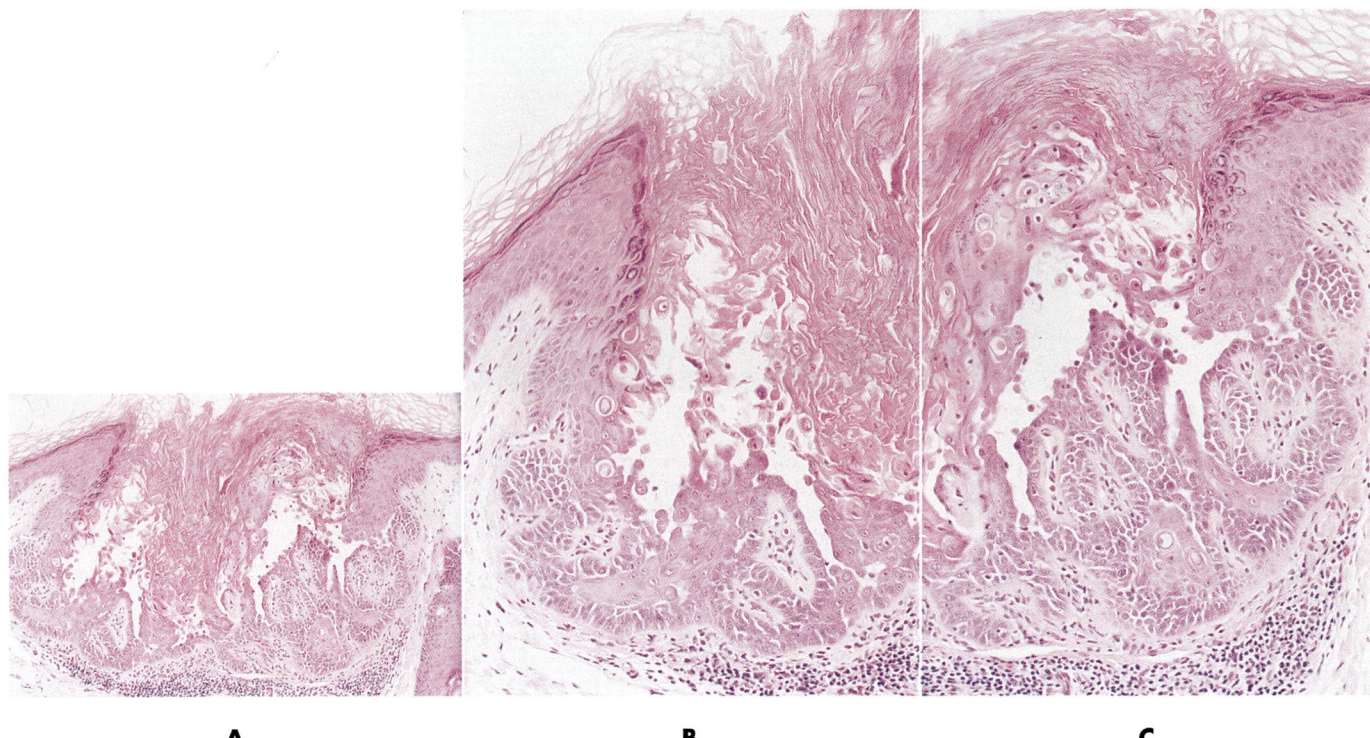

FIGURE 11-10. Low (**A**) and higher (**B** and **C**) magnification views of a Darier's disease lesion show a keratin-plugged crateriform lesion. There are acantholytic dyskeratotic keratinocytes; corps ronds and corps grains are present. There is cleft formation in the suprabasilar layers of the epidermis and basal cell–lined villi (created by the dermal papilla) project into the suprabasilar lacuna. (H&E stain, **A,** ×25; **B,** ×50; **C,** ×50.)

linear forms of Darier's disease. The acral keratoses of acrokeratosis verruciformis of Hopf are clinically similar to those of Darier's disease; however, the microscopic features of the lesions in acrokeratosis verruciformis of Hopf are different from those noted in the dorsal hand lesions of Darier's disease.[6,7]

In addition to Hailey-Hailey disease, the pathologic differential diagnosis of Darier's disease includes Grover's disease, warty dyskeratoma (a solitary, elevated, keratotic papule or nodule with a deep central invagination), focal acantholytic dyskeratoma, and familial dyskeratotic comedones (an autosomal dominant inherited condition characterized by widespread comedonal lesions that are primarily located on the extremities and that have pathologic features similar to those of Darier's disease). Also, similar pathologic changes can be seen in lesions that contain incidental focal acantholytic dyskeratosis[10] (Box 11-2).

Treatment

Conservative management of Darier's disease includes topical corticosteroids and antibiotics. Patients should try to remain cool and wear cotton clothing against their skin. If the patients experience sunlight-associated flares of their disease, they should use a high sun–protection factor sunscreen. For women who experience menstrual or perimenstrual exacerbations of their disease, oral estrogen (contraceptive) therapy may be helpful. False nails may be useful to camouflage the disease-related nail dystrophy and prevent split nails from catching on clothing and other objects. Oral antibiotics may be necessary to treat bacterial colonization or infection of the lesions. Systemic antiviral therapy is necessary when there is superimposed herpes simplex virus infection.

Removal of crusts and scales can be accomplished by using salicylic acid in propylene glycol gel. In some patients, topical vitamin A cream—particularly when used under occlusion—has been helpful; however, therapy has often had to be discontinued secondary to skin irritation. The mainstay of therapy is oral retinoids—isotretinoin, etretinate, and acitretin.[6,7] Yet patients require chronic therapy. In one series of 163 patients, 24% of the individuals were unable to tolerate the retinoid-associated side effects and had to discontinue the drug.[7]

A small number of case reports describe patients with Darier's disease whose lesions have been treated with other modalities: grenz ray or excision and grafting (in patients with hypertrophic lesions), electrosurgery, dermabrasion, and carbon dioxide laser vaporization.

> BOX 11-2. **LESIONS ASSOCIATED WITH INCIDENTAL FOCAL ACANTHOLYTIC DYSKERATOSIS**
>
> **EPITHELIAL LESIONS**
> Benign
>   Condyloma acuminata
>   Seborrheic keratosis
> Malignant
>   Basal cell carcinoma
>   Squamous cell carcinoma
> **FIBROHISTIOCYTIC LESIONS**
> Dermatofibroma
> Fibrous papule
> Scar
> **INFLAMMATORY CONDITIONS**
> Chondrodermatitis nodularis chronica helicis
> Pityriasis rosea
> Pityriasis rubra pilaris
> Psoriasis vulgaris
> **MELANOCYTIC LESIONS**
> Benign nevi
>   Compound nevi with architectural disorder (compound dysplastic nevus)
>   Junctional nevus with architectural disorder (junctional dysplastic nevus)
>   Melanocytic nevus (not otherwise specified)
> Malignant melanoma
>   Acral lentiginous malignant melanoma
>   Malignant melanoma (not otherwise specified)
> **MISCELLANEOUS LESIONS**
> Comedones
> Follicle (ruptured)
> Hemorrhoids

From DiMaio DJM, Cohen PR: *J Am Acad Dermatol* 38:243-247, 1998.

Grover's Disease

Etiology

Ralph Wier Grover reported "... six patients with an apparently unique, self-limited, primary acantholytic skin disease ..." that he observed during the previous 5 years in a paper titled "Transient Acantholytic Dermatosis" in the *Archives of Dermatology* in April 1970. The development of Grover's disease is associated with many factors. These primarily include sunlight (UV radiation), excessive heat (fever), and excessive sweating (perspiration). Although Grover's disease has been described in patients with other dermatologic conditions, a statistically significant association has only been noted with allergic contact dermatitis, asteatotic eczema, and atopic dermatitis.[11]

Grover's disease has also been reported to occur in oncology patients in four settings: idiopathic, disease induced by antineoplastic therapy (recombinant human interleukin-4 and 2-chlorodeoxyadenosine), disease induced by radiotherapy, and paraneoplastic.[12-14] In patients with cancer, Grover's disease was most frequently associated with hematologic malignancies—particularly acute and chronic myelogenous leukemia. A genitourinary organ malignancy was the most common cancer in patients with Grover's disease with solid tumors.[15]

Desmosomal adhesion molecules may have a role in the pathogenesis of acantholysis in Grover's disease. Immunohistochemistry studies have shown the loss of intracellular desmosomal proteins (desmoplakin I, desmoplakin II, and plakoglobin) from the desmosomes and their diffusion into the cytoplasm of acantholytic cells. Desmoglein (an intercellular transmembrane desmosomal glycoprotein) diffused into the acantholytic cell cytoplasm; however, some desmoglein was also demonstrated to still be on the cell membrane. In contrast, a normal staining pattern was observed on the surface of the acantholytic cells for the nondesmosomal transmembrane glycoprotein CD44.[1,2,11]

Clinical Features

Grover's disease most frequently occurs in white men over 40 years of age. Women are less commonly afflicted (female-to-male ratio is 1:3). The lesions appear as small (1 to 3 mm) papules and papulovesicles, with or without underlying erythema, on the chest and back (Figures 11-11 to 11-13). Less frequently, lesions are located on the scalp, neck, and extremities. The lesions tend to be pruritic and excoriations are often present; however, in one review of patients with cancer with Grover's disease, pruritus was absent in 38%. Other associated features include a prolonged febrile episode (excessive heat) and excessive perspiration (sweating); in hospitalized individuals, occlusive immobility (most often secondary to chronic confinement to bed) has also been noted in patients who develop Grover's disease.[11,15]

Grover's disease is classically "transient" in duration and typically resolves within a few weeks to 3 months. However, in some individuals the dermatosis is persistent or recurrent. In 12% of the oncology patients with Grover's disease, the appearance of lesions coincided with either the detection or the recurrence of their malignancy.

Pathology

Although acantholysis is the unifying microscopic feature of Grover's disease, there are at least the following four distinct histologic patterns that may be present either alone or in combination in a single biopsy specimen:
1. Hailey-Hailey–like pattern
2. Darier-like pattern
3. Pemphigus vulgaris-like pattern
4. Spongiotic-acantholytic pattern

The Hailey-Hailey–like pattern has a "dilapidated brick wall" appearance characterized by numerous acan-

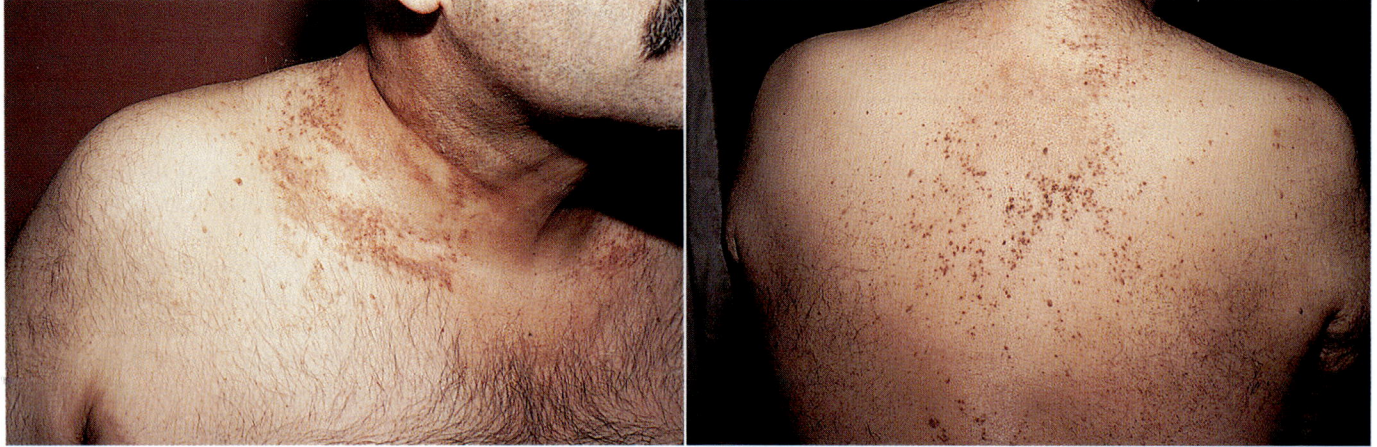

FIGURE 11-11. Patient with paraneoplastic Grover's disease and recurrent transitional cell carcinoma of the renal pelvis whose initial episode of Grover's disease (at age 45 years) preceded the discovery of the associated kidney tumor by 8 months and resolved after nephrectomy and chemotherapy. The dermatosis reappeared 3 years after original onset, coinciding with the detection of bony metastases of recurrent tumor. The cancer continued to progress despite 11 months of antineoplastic chemotherapy and radiotherapy; during these months, the Grover's disease lesions also persisted; pruritic erythematous papules of recurrent Grover's disease are present on the lateral neck and anterior chest (**A**) and central portion of the upper back (**B**). *(From Guana AL, Cohen PR:* J Clin Oncol *12:1703-1709, 1994.)*

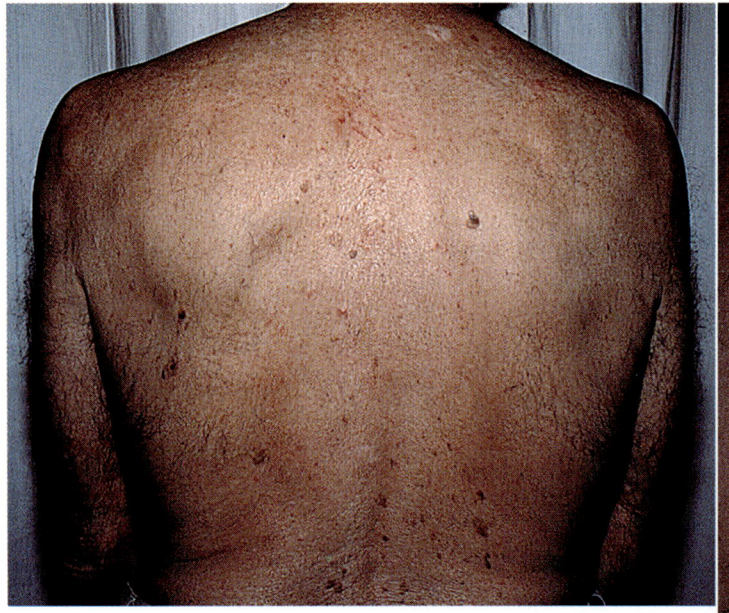
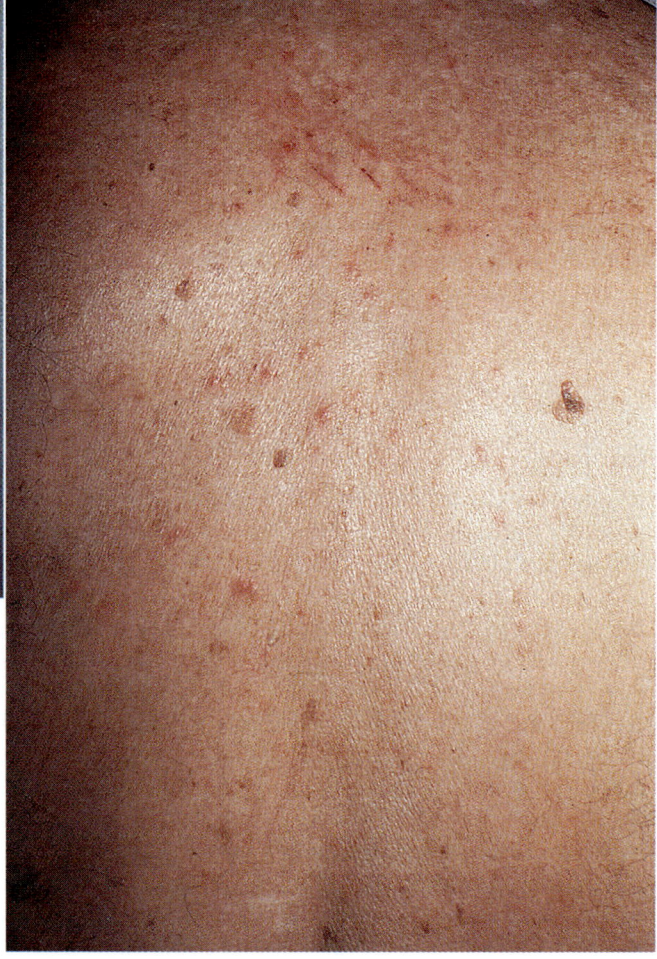

FIGURE 11-12. A distant view (**A**) of the linear excoriations and pruritic erythematous papules of Grover's disease on the back of a 79-year-old man. A transitional cell carcinoma of the bladder had been diagnosed 3 years earlier, and the tumor had been resected followed by postoperative immunotherapy with bacillus Calmette-Guérin. A closer view (**B**) of his central back shows pruritus-induced excoriations (upper area) and Grover's disease lesions (middle and lower areas). The Grover's disease improved during the year after diagnosis; however, 8 months after the diagnosis of the dermatosis, his recurrent cancer was treated with laser resection and thiotepa chemotherapy. Although he subsequently remained free of cancer, he had two additional episodes of the dermatosis. Each episode resolved but the pruritus persisted. *(From Guana AL, Cohen PR:* J Clin Oncol *12:1703-1709, 1994.*

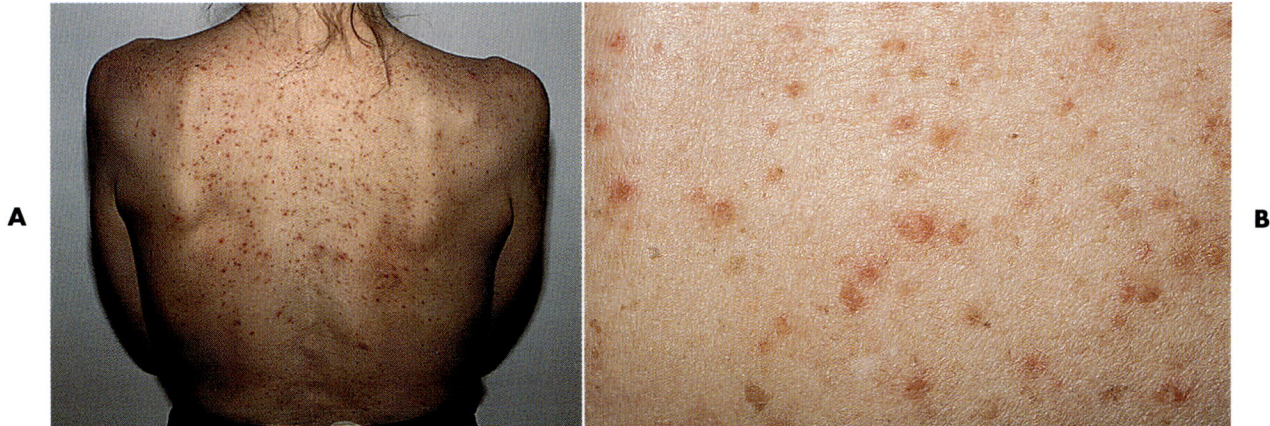

FIGURE 11-13. Distant **(A)** and closer **(B)** views of pruritic, erythematous-based papulovesicles of Grover's disease on the back of an otherwise healthy 49-year-old woman. Her disease initially appeared 1 year earlier and had subsequently been characterized by several recurrences. In addition to pruritus, dermatosis-related features included increased perspiration (night sweats, which had been attributed to her being premenopausal); excessive heat (febrile episodes) were not associated with the development of the initial or subsequent lesions.

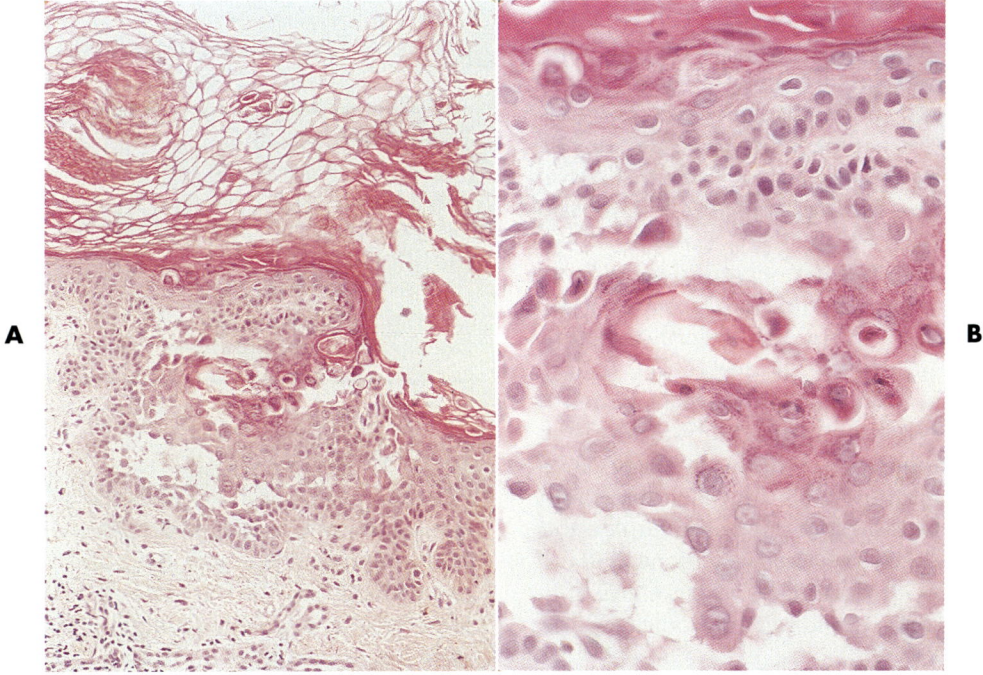

FIGURE 11-14. A low magnification view **(A)** of a Grover's disease lesion from the man in Figure 11-11 shows orthokeratosis, acanthosis, and acantholysis with focal areas of suprabasilar splits; a higher magnification view **(B)** shows additional pathologic features of Grover's disease: necrotic keratinocytes and epidermal cells with pyknotic nuclei. (H&E stain, **A,** ×50; **B,** ×100.) *(From Guana AL, Cohen PR:* J Clin Oncol *12:1703-1709, 1994.)*

tholytic cells that are present within most levels of the epidermis. The Darier-like pattern is the most common and shows a few sharply circumscribed areas of focal acantholysis and dyskeratosis (corp ronds and grains) overlying suprabasilar clefts (Figure 11-14). The pemphigus vulgaris-like pattern shows a few acantholytic cells above discrete suprabasal clefts; the overlying epidermis is mostly intact and few if any eosinophils are present in the dermis. The spongiotic-acantholytic pattern shows tense, well-circumscribed, intraepidermal spongiotic vesicles; a few acantholytic cells are either within or contiguous with the foci of spongiosis. In ad-

BOX 11-3. CLINICAL DIFFERENTIAL DIAGNOSIS OF GROVER'S DISEASE

AUTOIMMUNE BULLOUS DERMATOSES	INFECTIOUS DISEASES—CONT'D	MISCELLANEOUS DISORDERS—CONT'D
Dermatitis herpetiformis	Scabies	Arthropod bite
Dermatosis of pregnancy	Spirochetal	Drug eruption
Pemphigus erythematosus	Syphilis (secondary)	Neutrophilic eccrine hidradenitis
FOLLICULAR DISTRIBUTION	Viral	Papular urticaria
Acne vulgaris	Herpes simplex virus	Seborrheic keratosis
Folliculitis*	(disseminated)	Sepsis
Graft versus host disease	Varicella-zoster virus†	Vasculitis
Milaria rubra	Viral exanthem	**PAPULOSQUAMOUS DERMATOSES**
INFECTIOUS DISEASES	**MALIGNANCY**	Dermatitis
Bacterial	Actinic keratosis	Contact dermatitis (irritant)
Bullous impetigo	Leukemia cutis	Papular eczema
Fungal (disseminated systemic infection)	Metastatic carcinoma	Seborrheic dermatitis
Candidiasis	**MISCELLANEOUS DISORDERS**	Pityriasis lichenoides
Cryptococcosis	Acute febrile neutrophilic der-	Pityriasis rosea
Histoplasmosis	matosis (Sweet's syndrome)	Prurigo simplex

Adapted from Guana AL, Cohen PR: *J Clin Oncol* 12:1703-1709, 1994.
*This includes the following types of folliculitis: bacteria, eosinophilic pustular, perforating, *Pityrosporum species,* and steroid-induced.
†This includes disseminated, nondermatomal herpes zoster and primary varicella.

---

dition, a pemphigus foliaceus-like pattern (in which the clefting and acantholysis are superficial—within the uppermost layers of the stratum malpighii) and a bullous variant (in which the intraepidermal vesicle is either located beneath the stratum corneum or within the stratum granulosum or the stratum spinosum) have also been described.[11,15]

Positive IF results have been observed in some biopsies from patients with Grover's disease. However, a single abnormality was not consistently demonstrated to be associated with the disease. For example, in one study, IF abnormalities were noted in 5 of 11 patients. An abnormal deposit of immunoreactant was found in the lesions of four patients; three of the these individuals had deposits of immunoglobulin or complement present at the DEJ and one person had complement present in the intercellular spaces. Two patients had circulating antibodies to intercellular and basal cell antigens and one person had circulating antibodies to BMZ antigens.

Electron microscopy of Grover's disease has shown variable findings that correlated with the pathologic features observed on routine microscopy. Hence, depending on the lesion's histologic pattern, ultrastructural changes have been consistent with either Darier's disease, Hailey-Hailey disease, or pemphigus vulgaris. Studies done with electron microscopy also demonstrated that the cause of acantholysis in Grover's disease is from dissolution of desmosomal attachment plaques. There is thinning of attachment plaques in early acantholytic cells; later, there is complete disappearance of the plaques and aggregation of the remaining tonofilaments near the cell membrane.[11]

BOX 11-4. HISTOLOGIC DIFFERENTIAL DIAGNOSIS OF GROVER'S DISEASE

Acantholytic acanthoma
Actinic keratosis (acantholytic or Darier-like)
Darier's disease
Hailey-Hailey disease
Incidental focal acantholytic dyskeratosis
Pemphigus foliaceus
Pemphigus vulgaris
Relapsing linear acantholytic dermatosis

Diagnosis

The diagnosis of Grover's disease is based on the symptoms and appearance of the lesions. Correlation of the pathologic findings with the clinical history and lesion morphology may be necessary to establish the diagnosis. Especially in oncology patients, a lesional biopsy for microscopic and culture evaluation can be useful to exclude other conditions that can mimic Grover's disease.[12,15]

Differential Diagnosis

Several conditions can mimic either the clinical morphology or the histologic features of Grover's disease. The clinical differential diagnosis of Grover's disease is listed in Box 11-3. The histologic differential diagnosis of Grover's disease is listed in Box 11-4.[10,11]

Treatment

Although Grover's disease may resolve spontaneously, many patients require treatment either for disease-associated pruritus or for the primary dermatosis. Symptomatic treatments include avoiding exacerbating factors (such as strenuous exercise and sun exposure), taking baths (containing either emollient oils or colloidal oatmeal), using wet compresses (using either calamine lotion, low-potency corticosteroid lotions or creams, or zinc oxide), and applying topical antipruritics (such as mentholated lotions or pramoxine-containing preparations). Oral antihistamines are often used; although they only tend to have limited success in resolving the pruritus and no success in preventing the appearance of new lesions. Topical corticosteroids may also be helpful in alleviating the pruritus; in some patients systemic corticosteroids have been used.

When necessary, systemic retinoids are probably the most effective treatment modality. Isotretinoin, etretinate (25 to 50 mg per day), and acitretin (0.5 mg/kg per day) have been used. A 12-week course of isotretinoin has been described starting at a daily dose of 40 mg; if improvement is noted (after 2 weeks of therapy), the dose can be tapered to 10 mg daily (over the next 4 weeks) and maintained for the remainder of the 12 weeks. Oral vitamin A has also been successfully used in patients with Grover's disease. Appropriate baseline and follow-up laboratory studies are recommended for patients with Grover's disease being treated with systemic retinoids.[11]

Methotrexate, photochemotherapy (PUVA, psoralen, and UVA irradiation), and grenz ray irradiation have been used in patients for refractory or chronic Grover's disease. Systemic antibiotics are often used to treat secondary impetiginization; however, they have not been shown to improve the underlying dermatosis. Therapies that have not been demonstrated to be successful in the management of Grover's disease include 5-fluorouracil cream, liquid nitrogen cryotherapy, and topical antibiotics (clindamycin or erythromycin).[11]

References

1. Hashimoto K, Fujiwara K, Harada M, et al: Junctional proteins of keratinocytes in Grover's disease, Hailey-Hailey disease and Darier's disease, *J Dermatol* 22:159-170, 1995.
2. Hashimoto K, Fujiwara K, Tada J, et al: Desmosomal dissolution in Grover's disease, Hailey-Hailey's disease, and Darier's disease, *J Cutan Pathol* 22:488-501, 1996.
3. Metze D, Hamm H, Schorat A, et al: Involvement of the adherens junction—actin filament system in acantholytic dyskeratosis of Hailey-Hailey disease. A histological, ultrastructural, and histochemical study of lesional and non-lesional skin, *J Cutan Pathol* 23:211-222, 1996.
4. Burge SM: Hailey-Hailey disease: The clinical features, response to treatment and prognosis, *Br J Dermatol* 126:275-282, 1992.
5. Sehgal VN, Jain S: Chronic familial benign pemphigus, *J Dermatol (Tokyo)* 21:382-388, 1994.
6. Burge S: Darier's disease—the clinical features and pathogenesis, *Clin Exp Dermatol* 19:193-205, 1994.
7. Burge SM, Wilkinson JD: Darier-White disease: A review of the clinical features in 163 patients, *J Am Acad Dermatol* 27:40-50, 1992.
8. Berg D, Bassett AS: Darier's disease: Current understanding of pathogenesis and future role of genetic studies, *Int J Dermatol* 32:397-400, 1993.
9. Cohen PR: The lunula, *J Am Acad Dermatol* 34:943-953, 1996.
10. DiMaio DJM, Cohen PR: Incidental focal acantholytic dyskeratosis, *J Am Acad Dermatol* 38:243-247, 1998.
11. Parsons JM: Transient acantholytic dermatosis (Grover's disease): A global perspective, *J Am Acad Dermatol* 35:653-666, 1996.
12. Cohen PR, Kurzrock R: Transient acantholytic dermatosis in cancer patients (abstract), *South Med J* 89(10:1):S30-S31, 1996.
13. Cohen PR, Kurzrock R: Transient acantholytic dermatosis after treatment with 2-chlorodeoxyadenosine (letter), *Acta Derm Venereal (Stockh)* 77:412-413, 1977.
14. Cohen PR, Kurzrock R: 2-Chlorodeoxyadenosine-associated transient acantholytic dermatosis in hairy cell leukemia patients (letter), *Am J Dermatopathol* 21:106-107, 1999.
15. Guana AL, Cohen PR: Transient acantholytic dermatosis in oncology patients, *J Clin Oncol* 12:1703-1709, 1994.

Index

A

Acantholysis
  experimental, 1-5
  in drug-induced pemphigus, 12
  in nonimmunologic acantholytic diseases,
      147-161
    Darier's disease, 152, 155-156
    Grover's disease, 157-160
    Hailey-Hailey disease, 147, 151
  in paraneoplastic pemphigus, 29, 30, 34
  in pemphigus foliaceus, 26
  in pemphigus vulgaris, 1-5, 13
Acanthosis, Darier's disease and, 155
Acitretin for Grover's disease, 161
Acrokeratosis verruciformis of Hopf, in Darier's
      disease, 156
Age
  bullous pemphigoid and, 45
  cicatricial pemphigoid and, 66
  linear IgA bullous dermatosis and, 109
  paraneoplastic pemphigus and, 39
Agranulocytosis, dapsone-induced, 105
Anchoring fibril, 125, 126
Anchoring plaques, 125, 127
Ankyloblepharon, 66
Annular plaque
  in chronic bullous disease of childhood, 113
  in pemphigoid gestationis, 76, 77, 78
Antibiotics
  for bullous pemphigoid, 59, 61
  for Darier's disease, 156
  for Grover's disease, 161
  pemphigus induced by, 12
Antibody
  acantholysis and, 5
  in bullous pemphigoid, 43, 47
  in bullous lupus erythematosus,
      139-140
  in cicatricial pemphigoid, 63, 66-67

Antibody—cont'd
  in epidermolysis bullosa acquisita, 132
  in linear IgA bullous dermatosis, 115
  in paraneoplastic pemphigus, 29
  in pemphigoid gestationis, 75, 88
  in pemphigus foliaceus, 17
Anti-bullous pemphigoid antigen mucosal
      pemphigoid, 63
Anti-desmoglein 3 autoantibody, 5
Anti-epiligrin cicatricial pemphigoid, 56, 63
  bullous pemphigoid *versus*, 56
Antigen
  in bullous pemphigoid, 43
  in epidermolysis bullosa acquisita, 125-126
  in linear IgA bullous dermatosis, 115, 116
  in paraneoplastic pemphigus, 30, 37-38
  in pemphigus vulgaris, 1
Anti-HLA antibody in pemphigoid gestationis, 83
Anti-laminin-5 cicatricial pemphigoid, 67
Anti-p105 pemphigoid, 71
Anti-RO antibody, 139-140
Autoantibody
  in anti-epiligrin cicatricial pemphigoid, 63
  in Brunsting-Perry pemphigoid, 129-130
  in bullous pemphigoid, 43
  in epidermolysis bullosa acquisita, 125-127
  in paraneoplastic pemphigus, 30, 35-36, 37-38
  in pemphigoid gestationis, 85-86
  in pemphigus foliaceus, 17-24
  in pemphigus vulgaris, 1, 2
Autoimmune diseases
  bullous pemphigoid, 43-62,
    associated diseases, 52,54
    clinical variants of, 50
    diagnosis of, 44, 56-59
    differential diagnosis of, 44, 58, 59
    drug-induced, 54
    etiology of, 43-45
    pathology of, 44, 54-56
    treatment of, 44, 59-62

Autoimmune diseases—cont'd
    cicatricial pemphigoid, 63-73
        bullous pemphigoid *versus*, 56, 58, 70
        clinical features of, 64-66
        diagnosis of, 64, 69-70
        differential diagnosis of, 64, 70-71
        etiology of, 63-64
        pathology of, 64, 67-69
        treatment of, 64, 71-72
    dermatitis herpetiformis associated with, 103
    epidermolysis bullosa acquisita, 125-138
    clinical features of, 129-130
    diagnosis of, 126, 131-133
    differential diagnosis of, 126, 136
    etiology of, 125-126
    pathology of, 126, 130-131
    treatment of, 126, 133-136
    linear IgA bullous dermatosis, 109-123
        clinical features of, 109-110
        diagnosis of, 110, 120
        differential diagnosis of, 110, 120
        etiology of, 109, 110
        pathology and immunopathology of, 110, 115-120
        treatment of, 110, 120-122
    paraneoplastic pemphigus, 29-41
        clinical features of, 29-34
        diagnosis of, 30, 36-40
        differential diagnosis of, 30, 40
        etiology of, 29, 30
        pathology of, 34-36
        therapy for, 40-41
    pemphigoid gestationis, 75-97
        clinical features of, 75-81
        diagnosis of, 76, 86-89
        differential diagnosis of, 76, 90-96
        etiology of, 75-76
        pathology of, 76, 81-86
        treatment of, 76, 96-97
    pemphigus foliaceus, 17-27
        clinical features of, 18, 22-23
        diagnosis of, 18, 25-26
        epidemiology and etiology of, 17-20
        histopathology of, 18, 24, 26
        pathogenesis of, 17-24
        therapy for, 18, 27
    pemphigus vulgaris, 1-17
        clinical features of, 2, 6-12
        diagnosis of, 2, 12-14
        etiology of, 1-5
        pathology of, 2, 12, 13
        treatment of, 14-16
Axilla
    Hailey-Hailey disease and, 150
    linear IgA bullous dermatosis and, 112

Axilla—cont'd
    pemphigus vegetans and, 11
    pemphigus vulgaris and, 7
Azathioprine
    for bullous pemphigoid, 60
    for cicatricial pemphigoid, 70
    for epidermolysis bullosa acquisita, 133
    for pemphigus foliaceus, 25
    for pemphigus vulgaris and pemphigus vegetans, 14, 16

B

B cell neoplasm, paraneoplastic pemphigus and, 29
Back
    dermatitis herpetiformis and, 99
    linear IgA bullous dermatosis and, 110, 111
    paraneoplastic pemphigus and, 32
    pemphigus vulgaris and, 7
Basement membrane zone
    anchoring plaques and fibrils in, 125, 126
    bullous pemphigoid and, 47, 52, 54
    cicatricial pemphigoid and, 63
    epidermolysis bullosa acquisita and, 125, 127, 132
    linear IgA bullous dermatosis and, 120
    paraneoplastic pemphigus and, 35, 36
    pemphigoid gestationis and, 75, 81
Benign mucous membrane pemphigoid, 63
β4 integrin, cicatricial pemphigoid and, 63
Betamethasone valerate for bullous pemphigoid, 61
Biopsy
    in bullous pemphigoid, 57
    in bullous lupus erythematosus, 145
    in cicatricial pemphigoid, 67
    in Darier's disease, 155
    in dermatitis herpetiformis, 103-104
    in drug-induced linear IgA bullous dermatosis, 117-118
    in Hailey-Hailey disease, 147
Black fly, 17
Blindness, cicatricial pemphigoid and, 66
Body odor, Darier's disease and, 153
Brunsting-Perry cicatricial pemphigoid-like epidermolysis bullosa acquisita, 129-130
Brunsting-Perry pemphigoid, 66, 129-130
Buccal mucosal biopsy in cicatricial pemphigoid, 67
Bullous pemphigoid, 43-62
    associated diseases, 43
    bullous lupus erythematosus *versus*, 140
    cicatricial pemphigoid *versus*, 56, 58, 70
    clinical variants of, 50
    diagnosis of, 44, 56-59
    differential diagnosis of, 44, 58, 59
    drug-induced, 54
    epidermolysis bullosa acquisita *versus*, 125, 126, 130

Bullous pemphigoid—cont'd
   etiology of, 43-45
   linear IgA bullous dermatosis *versus,* 112, 121
   pathology of, 54-56
   pemphigoid gestationis *versus,* 55, 56, 58, 90, 92-93
   treatment of, 44, 59-62
Bullous pemphigoid antigen I, 43
Bullous pemphigoid-like epidermolysis bullosa acquisita, 126, 130-131
Bullous lupus erythematosus, 139-146
   bullous pemphigoid *versus,* 56, 58, 70
   cicatricial pemphigoid *versus,* 71
   clinical features of, 140, 144
   diagnosis of, 140-145
   differential diagnosis of, 140, 146
   epidermolysis bullosa acquisita and, 125-126
   etiology of, 139-144
   linear IgA bullous dermatosis *versus,* 121
   pathology of, 140, 144-145
   pemphigoid gestationis *versus,* 96-97
   treatment of, 140, 145-146
Buttock
   chronic bullous disease of childhood and, 114
   dermatitis herpetiformis and, 102

C

Cancer
   bullous pemphigoid and, 54/p]
   Grover's disease and, 157, 158
   paraneoplastic pemphigus and, 29-41
      clinical features of, 29-34
      diagnosis of, 30, 36-40
      differential diagnosis of, 30, 40
      etiology of, 29, 30
      pathology of, 34-36
      therapy for, 40-41
   pemphigoid gestationis and, 75, 80
Captopril-related pemphigus, 10
Castleman's disease, 29, 38, 39, 40
Child
   chronic bullous disease of childhood, 109, 113, 114-116
   neonatal lupus erythematosus syndrome, 139
   neonatal pemphigoid gestationis, 80, 81
   neonatal pemphigus vulgaris, 10
   pemphigus vulgaris, 8, 10
Chlorambucil for bullous pemphigoid, 60-61
Choriocarcinoma, pemphigoid gestationis and, 80
Chronic bullous disease of childhood
   clinical features of, 109, 113, 114-116
   treatment of, 122
Chronic lymphocytic leukemia, paraneoplastic pemphigus and, 30, 38
Chrysotherapy for pemphigus vulgaris, 15-16

Cicatricial pemphigoid, 63-73
   bullous pemphigoid *versus,* 56, 58, 70
   clinical features of, 64-66
   diagnosis of, 64, 76, 86-89
   differential diagnosis of, 64, 70-71
   epidermolysis bullosa acquisita *versus,* 110
   etiology of, 63-64
   pathology of, 64, 67-69
   treatment of, 64, 71-72
Cicatricial pemphigoid-like epidermolysis bullosa acquisita, 125
Classic noninflammatory epidermolysis bullosa acquisita, 125, 126
Clinical variants
   of bullous pemphigoid, 50
   of cicatricial pemphigoid, 63
Clobetasol propionate for bullous pemphigoid, 60, 62
Cluster of jewels configuration in chronic bullous disease of childhood, 115
Colchicine for epidermolysis bullosa acquisita, 133-134
Collagen
   bullous lupus erythematosus and, 144
   epidermolysis bullosa acquisita and, 125
Complement
   bullous pemphigoid and, 43, 52, 54
   bullous lupus erythematosus and, 139-143
   cicatricial pemphigoid and, 63
   dermatitis herpetiformis and, 103-104
   linear IgA bullous dermatosis and, 120
   paraneoplastic pemphigus and, 35
   pemphigoid gestationis and, 82, 84, 85
   pemphigus vulgaris and, 1-5
Conjunctivitis
   in cicatricial pemphigoid, 65-66
   pemphigus vulgaris and, 9
Connexon, 153
Contact dermatitis, pemphigoid gestationis *versus,* 90
Cornea, cicatricial pemphigoid and, 66
Corticosteroids
   for bullous pemphigoid, 59, 60
   for cicatricial pemphigoid, 72
   for Darier's disease, 156
   for epidermolysis bullosa acquisita, 133
   for Grover's disease, 161
   for Hailey-Hailey disease, 152
   for paraneoplastic pemphigus, 40-41
   for pemphigoid gestationis, 96-97
   for pemphigus foliaceus, 27
   for pemphigus vulgaris and pemphigus vegetans, 14-16
Crusted lesion
   in dermatitis herpetiformis, 101,102,103
   in paraneoplastic pemphigus, 31
   in pemphigus foliaceus, 24, 25
   in pemphigus vulgaris, 6, 7

Cyclophosphamide
    for bullous pemphigoid, 60-61
    for cicatricial pemphigoid, 70, 72
    for epidermolysis bullosa acquisita, 133
    for paraneoplastic pemphigus, 40, 41
    for pemphigoid gestationis, 96-97
    for pemphigus foliaceus, 27
    for pemphigus vulgaris and pemphigus vegetans, 14-16
Cyclosporine
    for bullous pemphigoid, 60, 61
    for epidermolysis bullosa acquisita, 133
    for paraneoplastic pemphigus, 40, 41
    for pemphigus vulgaris and pemphigus vegetans, 14-15
Cytokines
    bullous pemphigoid and, 45
    Castleman's disease and, 2
Cytoxan; see Cyclophosphamide

D

Dapsone
    adverse effects of, 105-106
    for bullous pemphigoid, 60, 61
    for cicatricial pemphigoid, 71, 72
    for dermatitis herpetiformis, 101, 105-106
    for linear IgA bullous dermatosis, 122
    for pemphigus vegetans, 14, 16
Darier's disease, 148, 152, 155-156
    clinical features of, 148, 153-155
    diagnosis of, 148, 155
    differential diagnosis of, 148, 155-156
    etiology of, 148, 152-153
    pathology of, 148, 155
    treatment of, 148, 156
Dermal-epidermal junction
    bullous pemphigoid and, 43
    bullous lupus erythematosus and, 143
    cicatricial pemphigoid and, 63
    epidermolysis bullosa acquisita and, 125
    linear IgA bullous dermatosis and, 111
Dermatitis herpetiformis, 99-107
    bullous pemphigoid *versus*, 56, 58
    bullous lupus erythematosus *versus*, 146
    clinical features of, 100-103
    diagnosis of, 100, 104
    etiology and pathogenesis of, 99-100
    linear IgA bullous dermatosis *versus*, 109, 111, 115
    pathology of, 100
    pemphigoid gestationis *versus*, 96
    treatment of, 100, 104-106
Desmoglein, 1, 2, 22
    Darier's disease and, 153
    Grover's disease and, 157
    Hailey-Hailey disease and, 147

Desmoplakin
    Darier's disease and, 153
    Grover's disease and, 157
    Hailey-Hailey disease and, 147
    paraneoplastic pemphigus and, 35, 37,
Desmosome
    Hailey-Hailey disease and, 147
    pemphigus foliaceus and, 23
Desquamative gingivitis in cicatricial pemphigoid, 64, 65
Diabetes mellitus, bullous pemphigoid and, 56
Diarrhea, colchicine-related, 56
Dietary therapy in dermatitis herpetiformis, 104-106
Differential diagnosis
    in bullous pemphigoid, 44, 58, 59
    in cicatricial pemphigoid, 70, 71
    in Darier's disease, 148, 155-156
    in epidermolysis bullosa acquisita, 126, 136
    in Grover's disease, 148, 160
    in Hailey-Hailey disease, 148, 152
    in linear IgA bullous dermatosis, 110, 121
    in paraneoplastic pemphigus, 30, 40
    in pemphigoid gestationis, 76, 90-96
    in pemphigus foliaceus, 18
Direct immunofluorescence
    in bullous pemphigoid, 57
    in bullous lupus erythematosus, 139-140, 144-145
    in cicatricial pemphigoid, 67-68
    in dermatitis herpetiformis, 103-104
    in epidermolysis bullosa acquisita, 131
    in linear IgA bullous dermatosis, 115-116
    in paraneoplastic pemphigus, 35
    in pemphigoid gestationis, 81-84
    in pemphigus foliaceus, 17, 21-24
Drug-induced disorders
    bullous pemphigoid, 54
    linear IgA bullous dermatosis, 115, 117-118
Drug-induced pemphigus, 10, 11
Dry eye in cicatricial pemphigoid, 64
Dyskeratosis
    in Darier's disease, 155
    in Grover's disease, 157
Dystrophic epidermolysis bullosa, 126

E

Eczematous lesion in bullous pemphigoid, 52, 54
Edema in pemphigoid gestationis, 81-82
Electron microscopy
    in cicatricial pemphigoid, 69
    in epidermolysis bullosa acquisita, 132
    in Grover's disease, 160
    in linear IgA bullous dermatosis, 115-116
    in pemphigoid gestationis, 84-86
ELISA; *see* Enzyme-linked immunosorbent assay

Enteropathy
    dermatitis herpetiformis and, 99, 102-106
    linear IgA bullous dermatosis and, 121
Entropion, 66
Envoplakin, 37-38
Enzyme-linked immunosorbent assay
    in epidermolysis bullosa acquisita, 131, 133
    in pemphigus foliaceus, 22, 24, 26
Eosinophil
    bullous pemphigoid and, 44-45, 54-55, 56
    cicatricial pemphigoid and, 63
    pemphigoid gestationis and, 67, 68
    pemphigus vulgaris and, 12
Eosinophil cationic protein, 45
Eosinophil-derived neurotoxin, 45
Eosinophilia in bullous pemphigoid, 45
Eosinophilic spongiosis
    in bullous pemphigoid, 55, 57
    in pemphigoid gestationis, 81-82, 89
    in pemphigus foliaceus, 26
    in pemphigus vulgaris, 12
Epidermal antibody in pemphigus foliaceus, 17, 26
Epidermolysis bullosa acquisita, 125-138
    bullous lupus erythematosus and, 125
    bullous pemphigoid *versus*, 56, 58
    bullous lupus erythematosus and, 125-126
    cicatricial pemphigoid *versus*, 70
    clinical features of, 129-130
    diagnosis of, 126, 131-133
    differential diagnosis of, 126, 136
    etiology of, 125-126
    pathology of, 126, 130-131
    treatment of, 126, 133-136
Epidermolysis bullosa acquisita antigen, 125-126
Erosion
    in bullous pemphigoid, 49, 51, 52, 54
    in chronic bullous disease of childhood, 113
    in epidermolysis bullosa acquisita, 126, 129
Erythema
    in paraneoplastic pemphigus, 32,33
    in pemphigoid gestationis, 77
Erythema multiforme
    bullous pemphigoid *versus*, 56
    chronic persistent, 39
    linear IgA bullous dermatosis *versus*, 121
    in paraneoplastic pemphigus, 32,33, 34
    pemphigoid gestationis *versus*, 93
Erythromycin for bullous pemphigoid, 61
Esophageal lesion in cicatricial pemphigoid, 66
Etretinate for Grover's disease, 161
Exfoliative erythroderma
    in bullous pemphigoid, 53, 56
    in pemphigus foliaceus, 24, 25
Experimental acantholysis, 1-5

Eye
    cicatricial pemphigoid and, 63, 64-66
    pemphigus foliaceus and, 26

F

Familial benign chronic pemphigus, 147
Fetus, pemphigoid gestationis and, 80-81
Fibrin
    cicatricial pemphigoid and, 67
    linear IgA bullous dermatosis and, 115
Fibrosis in cicatricial pemphigoid, 66
Fingernail, Darier's disease and, 153
Fogo selvagem, 17-27
    clinical features of, 18, 22-23
    diagnosis of, 16, 26
    epidemiology and etiology of, 17-20
    histopathology of, 24-26
    pathogenesis of, 17-24
    therapy for, 27
Folinic acid before intramuscular methotrexate, 14
Furosemide-related bullous pemphigoid, 54

G

Gastrointestinal disturbance
    dermatitis herpetiformis and, 102-103
    linear IgA bullous dermatosis and, 121
Genetic factors
    in Darier's disease, 153
    in fogo selvagem, 17, 20
    in Hailey-Hailey disease, 147
Gingiva
    bullous pemphigoid and, 49
    cicatricial pemphigoid and, 66
    pemphigus vulgaris and, 8
Glucocorticoids for bullous pemphigoid, 59, 60
Glucose-6-phosphate dehydrogenase deficiency, dapsone and, 60, 105
Gluten-sensitive enteropathy, dermatitis herpetiformis and, 99, 102-106
Gold injection for pemphigus vulgaris and pemphigus vegetans, 14, 15
Goserelin for pemphigoid gestationis, 96
Granulocyte-macrophage colony stimulating factor, bullous pemphigoid and, 45
Graves' disease, pemphigoid gestationis and, 81
Grover's disease, 148, 157-161
    clinical features of, 148, 157
    diagnosis of, 148, 160
    differential diagnosis of, 148, 160
    etiology of, 148, 157
    pathology of, 148, 157-160
    treatment of, 148, 161-162

H

Hailey-Hailey disease, 147-152
    clinical features of, 147, 148
    diagnosis of, 147-148, 152
    differential diagnosis of, 148, 152
    etiology of, 147, 148
    pathology of, 147, 148
    treatment of, 148, 152
Hallopeau type pemphigus vegetans, 11
Hand
    bullous pemphigoid and, 52
    Darier's disease and, 154
    epidermolysis bullosa acquisita and, 126, 128
    paraneoplastic pemphigus and, 32
Hemolysis, dapsone-induced, 105-106
Herpes gestationis, 75-97
    bullous pemphigoid *versus*, 55, 56, 58, 90, 92-93
    clinical features of, 64-66
    diagnosis of, 64, 69-70
    differential diagnosis of, 64, 70-71
    etiology of, 64-66
    pathology of, 64, 67-69
    treatment of, 64, 71-72
Herpes gestationis factor, 82-83
Histopathology
    in bullous pemphigoid, 54-56
    in cicatricial pemphigoid, 66
    in epidermolysis bullosa acquisita, 130-131
    in paraneoplastic pemphigus, 34
    in pemphigoid gestationis, 81-86
    in pemphigus foliaceus, 24, 26
    in pemphigus vulgaris, 12
Human leukocyte antigen
    in bullous lupus erythematosus, 144
    dermatitis herpetiformis and, 99-100
    epidermolysis bullosa acquisita and, 126
    in fogo selvagem, 17
    in pemphigoid gestationis, 73
    in pemphigus vulgaris, 3, 8
Hydatiform mole, pemphigoid gestationis and, 80
Hyperkeratosis in Darier's disease, 155
Hyperpigmentation in pemphigus vulgaris, 8
Hyperplasia, pseudoepithelilomatous, in pemphigus vegetans, 80

I

Immunoblotting
    in bullous lupus erythematosus, 144
    in cicatricial pemphigoid, 69
    in epidermolysis bullosa acquisita, 133
    in paraneoplastic pemphigus, 37-38
Immunochemistry in cicatricial pemphigoid, 69
Immunoelectron microscopy
    in cicatricial pemphigoid, 69
    in epidermolysis bullosa acquisita, 132
    in linear IgA bullous dermatosis, 115-116
    in pemphigoid gestationis, 84-85
Immunofluorescence
    in bullous pemphigoid, 57-59
    in bullous lupus erythematosus, 139-140, 144
    in cicatricial pemphigoid, 67-68
    in dermatitis herpetiformis, 103-104
    in epidermolysis bullosa acquisita, 131
    in Grover's disease, 159-160
    in linear IgA bullous dermatosis, 117
    in paraneoplastic pemphigus, 30, 34-39
    in pemphigoid gestationis, 82-84
    in pemphigus foliaceus, 17-22, 26
    in pemphigus vulgaris, 1-4, 12
Immunoglobulin A
    bullous pemphigoid and, 57-59
    bullous lupus erythematosus and, 139-140
    cicatricial pemphigoid and, 63, 67-69
    dermatitis herpetiformis and, 99, 103
    linear IgA bullous dermatosis and, 109-123
Immunoglobulin E, bullous pemphigoid and, 45
Immunoglobulin G
    anti-epiligrin cicatricial pemphigoid and, 63
    in Brunsting-Perry pemphigoid, 128
    bullous pemphigoid and, 43, 52, 54
    bullous lupus erythematosus and, 139-140, 144
    cicatricial pemphigoid and, 63, 69
    epidermolysis bullosa acquisita and, 125, 131, 132
    paraneoplastic pemphigus and, 30, 35, 36
    pemphigoid gestationis and, 75
    in pemphigus foliaceus, 21, 26
    in pemphigus vulgaris, 1, 2
Immunoglobulin M
    bullous pemphigoid and, 43, 57
    bullous lupus erythematosus and, 139-140
Immunopathology
    in cicatricial pemphigoid, 67-69
    in linear IgA bullous dermatosis, 115-116
    in pemphigoid gestationis, 82-86
    in pemphigus vulgaris, 3, 8, 12
Immunoprecipitation
    in bullous pemphigoid, 43
    in cicatricial pemphigoid, 69
    in paraneoplastic pemphigus, 37-38
    in pemphigoid gestationis, 82
    in pemphigus foliaceus, 22, 23/p]
Immunosuppressive agents
    for bullous pemphigoid, 59-61
    for bullous lupus erythematosus, 145-146
    for cicatricial pemphigoid, 71
    for epidermolysis bullosa acquisita, 133

Immunosuppressive agents—cont'd
  for pemphigus foliaceus, 27
  for pemphigus vulgaris and pemphigus vegetans, 14-15
Imuran; *see* Azathioprine
Incidental focal acantholytic dyskeratosis, 157
Indirect immunofluorescence
  in bullous pemphigoid, 57-59
  in cicatricial pemphigoid, 67, 68, 69
  in epidermolysis bullosa acquisita, 132-133
  in Grover's disease, 160
  in linear IgA bullous dermatosis, 96
  in paraneoplastic pemphigus, 28, 31-32
  in pemphigoid gestationis, 69, 70
  in pemphigus foliaceus, 17-21, 26
  in pemphigus vulgaris, 1-4, 12
Infection, linear IgA bullous dermatosis and, 89
Inflammatory infiltrate
  in bullous pemphigoid, 44
  in dermatitis herpetiformis, 85
  in epidermolysis bullosa acquisita, 130
  in linear IgA bullous dermatosis, 115-116
  in pemphigoid gestationis, 81
Inflammatory mediators
  bullous pemphigoid and, 43
  cicatricial pemphigoid and, 63
Interleukin-3, bullous pemphigoid and, 43, 45
Interleukin-5, bullous pemphigoid and, 43, 45
Intravenous immunoglobulin for epidermolysis bullosa acquisita, 134-135
Isotretinoin for Grover's disease, 161

K

Keratinocyte
  Darier's disease and, 155
  Hailey-Hailey disease and, 147
Keratosis follicularis, 122

L

Lamina lucida antigen, 115, 116
Laminin-5, 63, 69
Laminin-6, 63, 69
Laryngotracheal disease in cicatricial pemphigoid, 66
Leucovorin; *see* Folinic acid
Lichen planus pemphigoides, 52, 55
Lichen planus-like eruption in paraneoplastic pemphigus, 30, 34
Linear IgA bullous dermatosis, 109-123
  bullous pemphigoid *versus*, 56, 58
  bullous lupus erythematosus *versus*, 1468
  cicatricial pemphigoid *versus*, 70-71
  clinical features of, 109-110
  diagnosis of, 110, 120

Linear IgA bullous dermatosis—cont'd
  differential diagnosis of, 110, 120
  etiology of, 109, 110
  paraneoplastic pemphigus *versus*, 29, 30, 33
  pathology and immunopathology of, 110, 115-120
  pemphigoid gestationis *versus*, 93, 96
  treatment of, 110, 120-122
Lip
  paraneoplastic pemphigus and, 29, 30, 31
  pemphigus vulgaris and, 8, 10
  Lupus erythematosus; see Bullous lupus erythematosus
Lymphocyte
  cicatricial pemphigoid and, 63
  pemphigoid gestationis and, 81

M

Macrophage
  bullous pemphigoid and, 44
  cicatricial pemphigoid and, 63
Major basic protein, bullous pemphigoid and, 44
Major histocompatibility complex, pemphigoid gestationis and, 85-86
Malignancy
  bullous pemphigoid and, 43
  dermatitis herpetiformis and, 103
  Grover's disease and, 157
  linear IgA bullous dermatosis and, 109
  paraneoplastic pemphigus and, 29-41
  pemphigoid gestationis and, 75, 80
Mast cell, cicatricial pemphigoid and, 63
Membrane attack complex
  bullous pemphigoid and, 43
  pemphigus vulgaris and, 4, 5
Methemoglobinemia, dapsone-induced, 105
Methotrexate
  for bullous pemphigoid, 61
  for epidermolysis bullosa acquisita, 133
  for Grover's disease, 161
  for pemphigus vulgaris and pemphigus vegetans, 14
Methylprednisolone for bullous pemphigoid, 60
Milia in epidermolysis bullosa acquisita, 128
Minocycline for bullous pemphigoid, 60, 61
Mucosa-associated lymphoid tissue, cicatricial pemphigoid and, 63
Mucous membrane
  bullous pemphigoid and, 46-47
  bullous lupus erythematosus and, 144
  cicatricial pemphigoid and, 63-71
  epidermolysis bullosa acquisita and, 129
  linear IgA bullous dermatosis and, 109
  paraneoplastic pemphigus and, 29, 30
  pemphigus vulgaris and, 6

Myasthenia gravis, 29
  Castleman's disease and, 29
  pemphigus vulgaris and, 10

N

Nail, Darier's disease and, 153
Neonatal lupus erythematosus syndrome, 139
Neonatal pemphigoid gestationis, 80-81
Neonatal pemphigus vulgaris, 10
Neoplasms
  bullous pemphigoid and, 43, 44
  Grover's disease and, 157
  paraneoplastic pemphigus and, 29-41
  pemphigoid gestationis and, 75, 80
Neumann type pemphigus vegetans, 11
Neutrophil
  bullous pemphigoid and, 43, 44
  bullous lupus erythematosus and, 114
  cicatricial pemphigoid and, 63
  dermatitis herpetiformis and, 103
  linear IgA bullous dermatosis and, 115-116
  pemphigoid gestationis and, 81-82
  pemphigus foliaceus and, 26
Niacinamide for bullous pemphigoid, 60, 61
Nikolsky's sign
  in bullous pemphigoid, 46
  in pemphigus foliaceus, 18, 24, 26
  in pemphigus vulgaris, 6
Noncollagenous 1 domain, 125
Nonimmunologic acantholytic diseases, 147-161
  Darier's disease, 152, 152-157
  Grover's disease, 157-161
  Hailey-Hailey disease, 147-152

O

Ocular pemphigoid, 63
Oral involvement
  in bullous pemphigoid, 45, 49, 50
  in bullous lupus erythematosus, 144
  in cicatricial pemphigoid, 64, 65
  in Darier's disease, 152-157
  in epidermolysis bullosa acquisita, 129
  in paraneoplastic pemphigus, 29, 30, 31
  in pemphigus vegetans, 11-12
  in pemphigus vulgaris, 6, 8
Oral mucosal pemphigoid, 63

P

Pain
  in dermatitis herpetiformis, 100, 101-10282
  in pemphigus vulgaris, 8, 10
Papillomatosis in Darier's disease, 155

Papule
  in bullous pemphigoid, 48
  in Darier's disease, 153, 154
  in dermatitis herpetiformis, 100, 101
  in Grover's disease, 157, 158
Parakeratosis, 155
Paraneoplastic erythema multiforme, 40
Paraneoplastic pemphigus, 29-41
  cicatricial pemphigoid *versus*, 71
  clinical features of, 29-34
  diagnosis of, 30, 36-40
  differential diagnosis of, 30, 40
  erythema multiforme-like eruption of, 32, 33
  etiology of, 29, 30
  lichen planus-like eruption of, 34
  linear IgA bullous disease and, 33
  pathology of, 34-36
  therapy for, 40-41
Pemphigoid
  bullous, 43-62
    associated diseases, 52, 54
    bullous lupus erythematosus *versus*, 146
    clinical features of, 44, 45-54
    clinical variants of, 50
    diagnosis of, 44, 56-49
    differential diagnosis of, 44, 58, 59
    drug-induced, 54
    etiology of, 43-45
    pathology of, 54-56
    treatment of, 44, 59-62
  cicatricial, 63-73
    bullous pemphigoid *versus*, 56, 58, 70
    clinical features of, 64-66
    diagnosis of, 64, 69-70
    differential diagnosis of, 64, 70-71
    etiology of, 63-64
    pathology of, 64, 67-69
    treatment of, 64, 71-72
Pemphigoid gestationis, 75-97
  bullous pemphigoid *versus*, 55, 56, 58, 90, 92-93, 96
  clinical features of, 75-81
  diagnosis of, 76, 86-89
  differential diagnosis of, 76, 90-96
  etiology of, 75, 76
  pathology of, 76, 81-86
  treatment of, 76, 96-97
Pemphigoid gestationis factor, 82-83
Pemphigoid nodularis, 55
Pemphigus foliaceus, 17-27
  bullous lupus erythematosus *versus*, 146
  clinical features of, 18, 22-23
  diagnosis of, 18, 25-26
  differential diagnosis of, 18
  epidemiology and etiology of, 17-20
  histopathology of, 18, 24, 26

Pemphigus foliaceus—cont'd
  pathogenesis of, 17-24
  therapy for, 18, 27
Pemphigus herpetiformis, 26
Pemphigus vegetans, 1, 2, 11-16
  clinical features of, 11, 12
  Hallopeau type of, 11
  histopathology of, 12, 13
  immunopathology of, 12, 13
  Neumann type of, 11
  treatment of, 14-16
Pemphigus vulgaris, 1-16
  clinical features of, 2, 6-12
  diagnosis of, 2, 12-14
  etiology of, 1-5
  histopathology of, 12, 13
  immunopathology of, 12, 13
  paraneoplastic pemphigus *versus*, 37, 40
  pathology of, 2, 12, 13
  treatment of, 14-16
D-Penicillamine-related pemphigus, 12
Periplakin, 38
Phenacetin-related bullous pemphigoid, 54
Photophoresis for epidermolysis bullosa acquisita, 134, 135, 136
  in Sezary syndrome, 134
Photosensitivity in bullous lupus erythematosus, 139
Plakoglobin, 1
  Darier's disease and, 153
  Grover's disease and, 157
  Hailey-Hailey disease and, 147
Plaque
  anchoring, 125, 126
  in bullous pemphigoid, 52, 54
  in chronic bullous disease of childhood, 109
  in dermatitis herpetiformis and, 99, 100
  in Hailey-Hailey disease, 149
  in pemphigoid gestationis, 76, 78
  in pemphigus foliaceus, 24
Plaquenil for pemphigus foliaceus, 27
Plasmapheresis
  in bullous pemphigoid, 61
  for pemphigus vulgaris, 14, 16
Plasmin, acantholysis and, 1
Plasminogen, Darier's disease and, 153
Polymorphic eruption of pregnancy, 90-92
Porphyria cutanea tarda, 138
  bullous lupus erythematosus *versus*, 146
  epidermolysis bullosa acquisita *versus*, 126, 131
Prednisolone for pemphigoid gestationis, 96-97
Prednisone
  for bullous pemphigoid, 59, 60
  for cicatricial pemphigoid, 72
  for linear IgA bullous dermatosis, 122

Prednisone—cont'd
  for paraneoplastic pemphigus, 40-41
  for pemphigus vulgaris and pemphigus vegetans, 14-16
Pregnancy, pemphigoid gestationis during, 75-97
Proteases, Darier's disease and, 153
Pruritus
  in Brunsting-Perry pemphigoid, 66
  in bullous pemphigoid, 46
  in Darier's disease, 153
  in dermatitis herpetiformis, 100-10282
  in Grover's disease, 157
  in Hailey-Hailey disease, 149
  in pemphigoid gestationis, 77, 86
Pseudopemphigoid, 71
Psoriasis, bullous pemphigoid and, 52
Psorospermose folliculaire vegetante, 152
Pulse therapy for bullous pemphigoid, 60
Pustule in pemphigus vegetans, 10, 11
Pyrazolone derivative-related pemphigus, 11
Pyridoxine for pemphigoid gestationis, 96

R

Respiratory involvement in paraneoplastic pemphigus, 29, 34
Retinoids
  for Darier's disease, 156
  for Grover's disease, 161

S

Salt-split skin study
  in bullous lupus erythematosus, 146
  in cicatricial pemphigoid, 68, 69-70
  in epidermolysis bullosa acquisita, 132-133
  in pemphigoid gestationis, 84
Scabies, paraneoplastic pemphigus and, 30, 39
Scabies, 59
Scalp
  Brunsting-Perry pemphigoid and, 66
  pemphigus foliaceus and, 24
  pemphigus vulgaris and, 7
Scarring
  in cicatricial pemphigoid, 64, 66
  in dermatitis herpetiformis, 100-102
  in epidermolysis bullosa acquisita, 126, 128
Senear-Usher syndrome, 24
Skin biopsy
  in bullous pemphigoid, 57-58
  in cicatricial pemphigoid, 67
  in Darier's disease, 155
  in dermatitis herpetiformis, 103-104
  in drug-induced linear IgA bullous dermatosis, 115
  in Hailey-Hailey disease, 151

Skin lesion
    in bullous lupus erythematosus, 139-140
    in cicatricial pemphigoid, 63, 65
    in Darier's disease, 153-124
    in dermatitis herpetiformis, 100-102
    in drug-induced linear IgA bullous dermatosis, 115
    in Grover's disease, 157
    in pemphigoid gestationis, 79, 80, 82
    in pemphigus vegetans, 11
    in pemphigus vulgaris, 6
Skip pregnancy, 77
Small bowel biopsy in dermatitis herpetiformis, 104
SS-A antibody, 139-140, 144, 145
Steroid-sparing agents
    for bullous pemphigoid, 59
    for pemphigus vulgaris and pemphigus vegetans, 14-16
Stomatitis in paraneoplastic pemphigus, 29-31, 34, 40
String of pearls configuration in chronic bullous disease of childhood, 115, 116
Subcorneal blister in pemphigus foliaceus, 26
Subepidermal blistering
    in bullous pemphigoid, 43-62
    in bullous lupus erythematosus, 139-140, 144
    in cicatricial pemphigoid, 63-71
    in epidermolysis bullosa acquisita, 125-138
    in linear IgA bullous dermatosis, 109
    in pemphigoid gestationis, 75-97
Sulfapyridine
    for dermatitis herpetiformis, 105-106
    for linear IgA bullous dermatosis, 121-122
Sulfones for bullous pemphigoid, 61
Sunscreen, bullous lupus erythematosus and, 145-146
Supportive therapy for epidermolysis bullosa acquisita, 136
Suprabasilar acantholysis
    Hailey-Hailey disease and, 147
    paraneoplastic pemphigus and, 30, 34
Symblepharon, 65-66
Systemic disease
    Darier's disease and, 155
    epidermolysis bullosa acquisita and, 130
Systemic lupus erythematosus
    bullous lupus erythematosus and, 139, 142-146
    pemphigus vulgaris and, 10

T

Tense bullae
    in bullous pemphigoid, 46, 47, 52, 54
    in pemphigoid gestationis, 79, 87
Tetracycline for bullous pemphigoid, 60, 61
Thiol-related pemphigus, 12
Thymoma, paraneoplastic pemphigus and, 29, 38-39
Thyroid disease
    dermatitis herpetiformis associated with, 103
    pemphigoid gestationis and, 81

Thyrotoxicosis, 81
Tongue
    paraneoplastic pemphigus and, 31
    pemphigus vulgaris and, 9
Topical steroids
    for bullous pemphigoid, 59, 60
    for Grover's disease, 161
    for oral cicatricial pemphigoid, 72
Toxic epidermal necrolysis, 139, 140
Triamcinolone acetonide for bullous pemphigoid, 60, 61
Trichiasis, 66
Trophoblastic tumor, pemphigoid gestationis and, 80
Tumor
    bullous pemphigoid and, 54
    Grover's disease and, 157
    paraneoplastic pemphigus and, 29-41
    pemphigoid gestationis and, 75-81
Tumor necrosis factor-α, bullous pemphigoid and, 45
Type VII collagen
    bullous lupus erythematosus and, 144
    epidermolysis bullosa acquisita and, 125, 126, 133

U

Ultraviolet light
    bullous lupus erythematosus and, 139, 144
    Darier's disease and, 153
Urticarial lesion
    in bullous pemphigoid, 58
    in linear IgA bullous dermatosis, 109, 110, 114
    in pemphigoid gestationis, 76, 77, 86
    in polymorphic eruption of pregnancy, 92

V

Vesicle
    in bullous pemphigoid, 52, 54
    in chronic bullous disease of childhood, 109-110
    in dermatitis herpetiformis, 100-102
    in Hailey-Hailey disease, 147, 150, 152
    in linear IgA bullous dermatosis, 109, 112
    in pemphigoid gestationis, 77, 82
    in pemphigus foliaceus, 24, 26
Vesicular pemphigoid, 43
Vulvar bullous pemphigoid, 51

W

Waldenström macroglobulinemia, 30, 38-39
Well's syndrome, 56
Western immunoblot
    in epidermolysis bullosa acquisita, 133
    in paraneoplastic pemphigus, 37-38